GROUP PSYCHOTHERAPY
WITH PEOPLE WHO
ARE DYING

GROUP PSYCHOTHERAPY WITH PEOPLE WHO ARE DYING

By

STEVEN PHILLIP LINDENBERG, Ph.D.

Certified Clinical Mental Health Counselor
Hershey Psychiatric Associates
Hershey, Pennsylvania

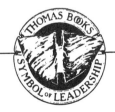

CHARLES C THOMAS • PUBLISHER
Springfield • *Illinois* • *U.S.A.*

Published and Distributed Throughout the World by

CHARLES C THOMAS • PUBLISHER

2600 South First Street

Springfield, Illinois, 62717, U.S.A.

© *1983 by* CHARLES C THOMAS • PUBLISHER

ISBN 0-398-04814-2

Library of Congress Catalog Card Number: 82-19582

With THOMAS BOOKS *careful attention is given to all details of manufacturing and
design. It is the Publisher's desire to present books that are satisfactory as to their physical
qualities and artistic possibilities and appropriate for their particular use.* THOMAS
BOOKS *will be true to those laws of quality that assure a good name and good will.*

Printed in the United States of America
CU-RX-10

Library of Congress Cataloging in Publication Data

Lindenberg, Steven Phillip.
    Group psychotherapy with people who are dying.

    Bibliography: p.
    1. Terminally ill--Psychology.   2. Cancer--
Psychological aspects.   3. Group pscyhotherapy.
I. Title. [DNLM: 1. Psychotherapy, Group.
2. Death. 3. Attitude to death. 4. Terminal care--
Psychology. 5. Neoplasms--Psychology. 6. Neoplasms--
Therapy. QZ 266 L743g]
R726.8.L56   1983   616.89'152'0880814   82-19582
ISBN 0-398-04814-2

To Linda:

> The first thing is to acquire wisdom;
> Gain understanding though it cost you all you have.
> Do not forsake her, and she will keep you safe;
> Love her and she will guard you;
> Cherish her, and she will lift you high;
> If only you embrace her, she will bring you honor.
> She will set a garland of grace on your head
> And bestow on you a crown of glory.

Proverbs 4:6-9

PREFACE

IN August 1975 Cynthia Ann Whitacre was killed in an automobile accident. Cindy was one of those rare people who combined intelligence and sensitivity into a radiant personality. She bubbled with life. She was a guidepost to me in life. She became an inspiration in death.

The fall of 1975 found me at the end of my first year in a doctoral program at The University of Georgia. I was looking for a subject for my dissertation. Cindy's death and the feedback from her family about my caring during those awful days while Cindy lay comatose led me, by the urgency and demands of my own grief, to examine the area of thanatology: death, dying, grief, and bereavement. Never had the questions of life and death burned so furiously at the core of my being.

Carl Jung has described synchronicity as the cosmic order of so-called random events. Approximately six months after Cindy's death in the spring of 1976, I was beginning to develop a prospectus for my dissertation. For obvious reasons, I was interested in working with the bereaved, particularly bereaved parents. In order to understand bereavement better, however, I decided that I must first work with the dying. Since my counseling specialty was group therapy and since no one had clearly established the efficacy and feasibility of group psychotherapy with incurable cancer patients, I decided that this would be a worthwhile research endeavor. It would also be good therapy for me.

At approximately the same time, three women who were dying of incurable breast cancer were seeking the opportunity to explore feelings and issues about cancer treatment. These women are represented fictitiously as Carol, Jane, and Diana in this book. Later Sally, Amanda, Barbara, and Louise joined the group.

All of these beautiful women have since died. Every time I look at a page of this text and think of how my life has been enriched by sharing some of their last days and experiences, they are alive. Their willingness to share their humanness and suffering with me is preserved in my heart. Their story is preserved in this book. May these ordinary people serve to teach you the meaning and greatness of courage and suffering.

INTRODUCTION

I N the fall of 1976, I began my research with seven women who were suffering from incurable cancer. Each one had metastatic breast cancer. My goal was to prove the efficacy of group psychotherapy with the terminally ill. Men were also interviewed as candidates for the group. For one reason or another, none joined.

In all, there were ten consecutive sessions over a period of fourteen weeks. Each of the sessions was tape-recorded. Initial interviews were also recorded as were a presession and a follow-up session. The research was successful. Group counseling and psychotherapy for incurable cancer patients are helpful.

There were two major areas I wished to address. One area had to do with themes addressed by individuals who were dying and the commonality and consistency of those themes between patients. The other had to do with techniques for facilitating group discussions for persons who are incurably ill. With this in mind and with transcriptions of audiotapes in hand, I began to factor out the major themes addressed in this therapy group.

Subsequently, Section I includes chapters corresponding to the major themes: psychological effects, psychosocial dynamics, the family, death and dying, and patients' reactions to treatment. Coupled with knowledge of the literature and personal experience, I was able to outline and integrate topics as they emerged from the transcripts. For instance, the subject of anger was implicitly and explicitly addressed in each of the group sessions. Excerpts from numerous transcribed passages were organized within the text to help the reader gain insight about anger — *through the eyes of the patient.*

Section II speaks to group dynamics and techniques. Exploration, transition, action, and termination are the four phases used as points of reference. Once again, passages from the transcripts are integrated into the text. Group dynamics, technique, sociometry, and personal journals are presented for each session. Sessions are examined in the context of technique and are subgrouped within one of four chapters corresponding to each of the four phases respectively.

Suggested readings are provided at the conclusion of the book and are by no means exhaustive. They are designed to assist the inquisitive reader who desires further information. Readings have been selected and grouped according to major themes for each chapter in Section I. All suggested readings pertaining to technique and group dynamics are listed under the heading of Section II.

The transcriptions were edited in a fashion designed to preserve the spontaneity, vitality, and intensity of the group's interactions. The book is organized in an attempt to develop the character of each member while presenting factual and useful information. In this way the members of the group teach.

Each of the group members was a real living person and is now deceased. Only their names are fictitious. Similarly, those interviewed but not participating in the group as well as staff members, physicians, and others cited were real people whose identities are protected by fictitious names.

I have now been in practice as a counselor for five years. My life has been truly enriched in purpose and meaning through working with the dying and the bereaved. I hope that in some way this work will enrich and enhance your life.

SPL

ACKNOWLEDGMENTS

THERE are several people whose guidance and direction have been instrumental in facilitating research with the women whose stories and interaction in group therapy are the basis of this work. I would like to thank Melvin Moore, M.D., Donald Nixon, M.D., and Sandy Sullivan, R.N., for trusting me and for allowing their patients to be members in the research group.

George M. Gazda, Ed.D., supported my interest while patiently and competently directing my research. He recognized the need for studies that would interface skills from the discipline of counseling with the field of medicine. George's greatest strength lies in his flexibility to cultivate and guide doctoral students. George gave me the green light and showed me how to "get the car into first gear."

I wish to thank Dottie Stoner and Carol Matthews for their typing assistance during the early stages of this book's development. I am especially grateful to Marsha Schmidt for doing the bulk of the typing on the manuscript.

Judy Strickler did much of the research and preparation for the suggested readings in this book. Her help was invaluable.

Posthumously, I wish to cite the courageous women who shared their lives with me. This book is a memorial to the lives of Darlene, Juliette, Kitty, Isabella, Lillie, Betty, and Sara: May God rest their souls.

On August 26, 1967, I married Linda Kathleen Young. Three children and fifteen years later, we find our relationship challenging, interesting, loving, and growing. She has illustrated the figures in this book. Her love and support have provided the base for my freedom to be. Our choice to share free wills continues to be the key to the unlocking of my creative spirit.

CONTENTS

SECTION I: THEMES SHARED BY THE TERMINALLY ILL

SECTION II. THE GROUP:
COLLECTED PERSONS — FALLING LEAVES

GROUP PSYCHOTHERAPY WITH PEOPLE WHO ARE DYING

SECTION I
THEMES SHARED BY THE
TERMINALLY ILL

Chapter 1

THE PSYCHOLOGICAL EFFECTS
OF CANCER

Our whole life is taking a pill or taking this shot. Our whole day is around taking that medicine. You know; I guess I want to live so badly and I want to be normal and I want to do things that other women my age do and I can't because I'm very restricted.

Diana

IF the above quotation is examined carefully, the reader begins to get more than an intimation of the psychological effects of cancer. In a statement similar to other verbalizations, Diana pleads for a semblance of normality in her existence. For a moment, let's analyze the psychodynamics of Diana's plight.

First of all, Diana, speaking in the collective *our*, states that her life is involved with taking medicine. The implied affect includes anger, resentment, and bitterness. Dependency fears are also evident in what is unsaid: "I am dependent on medicine."

One could say that feelings regarding long-term dependence on medication and/or medical procedures are not unique to cancer patients. Cases of chronic heart disease, kidney disease, and diabetes are examples of such conditions. However, cancer patients are unique in that many of the treatment procedures involve chemotherapy: the treatment of cancer with powerful chemical compounds. Chemotherapy often produces traumatic side effects. These side effects in themselves may be temporarily debilitating. In some cases treatment is anticipated with as much anxiety as the disease itself. Some treatments are of such potency as to require short-term hospitalization with constant monitoring during their administration. Such hospitalization interrupts family activities as well as careers and may continue over a period of years. These treatments serve to reinforce feelings of losing control of one's life and cause low self-esteem, further resentment, and depression. More often than not, chemotherapy follows surgery: surgery often of a radical,

5

disfiguring nature.

Also, chemotherapy is often accompanied by the treatment modality of radiation therapy. By itself, radiation therapy often produces uncomfortable and sometimes painful and disfiguring side effects. Thus, when a cancer patient such as Diana complains about taking "medicine," discussion is likely to be encompassing the entire therapeutic milieu with all of the uncomfortable side effects. Personal dignity, self-esteem, and positive body image are constantly barraged with life-saving/life-threatening assaults. Imagine the love-hate paradox: destroying one's self in order to prolong one's life.

Notice that I did not say *save* one's life. Often the possibility of saving one's life does not exist within current medical technology or any other treatment modality. Thus, the principle of delayed gratification (struggling today for a better tomorrow) becomes distorted. The thought often becomes *delayed termination*, a thought that is often suppressed to preserve sanity. Chronic depression, distortion of reality as a coping mechanism, denial, and suicidal ideation become psychological concerns to which the counselor/therapist must be alert.

Analysis of the "I want. . . . " phrases reveals the passion to live, the desire for "normalcy," and the apparent need to experience life consistent with developmental needs and goals. Regardless of which theorist's stages of human development one subscribes to, all hypothesize needs and goals relative to a particular maturational level. With the cancer patient, particularly young cancer patients (Diana was 33.), longevity is often contingent upon the uncertain evolution of the disease. In the case of metastatic disease, the issue is not "if I die. . . . " but, ". . . how soon will I die?" While all of us live with the certainty of death, most can avoid the concreteness of that awareness until death is imminent.

For the cancer patient death is imminent and may be imminent for weeks, months, or years. Hope may spring eternal, but reality is the mainstream of finite awareness in the state of consciousness called life. Hence, the hope of and the desire to live, be normal, and develop becomes the reality of the clause ". . . I'm restricted." Subsequently, "I'm restricted" becomes the anguished cry for help: "*I'm dying!*" In between hope and reality are crowded denial/coping behaviors aimed at the rush to live. After all, one's entire development must be squeezed into an uncertain (yet certain) life expectancy. The life-style of the cancer patient manifests itself as psychological levels within levels, fluctuating between rejection of death versus acceptance of death. Thus, Diana may be saying *"My whole life is dying!"* As the *life* wanes, preservation of the *self* becomes increasingly more taxing. The maintenance of the integral self (ego) becomes the focus of the caring relationship with the cancer patient.

Anger, fear, resentment, bitterness, and depression are fairly obvious affective dimensions of the cancer experience. There are other dynamics that are more subtle.

"THE-DESIRE-TO-SHARE-MY-STORY" SYNDROME

Anyone who has worked with self-help groups knows of the double-bind that the "victim" is faced with. In real life the cancer patient (alcoholic, addict, bereaved parent, etc.) seems constrained by the *perceived* societal expectation: "Thou shalt not show feelings." This commandment has done (and still does) immense psychological and psychosomatic damage in our society. Were the truth to be recognized by the scientific community, suppressed affect would top the list of contributing factors of disease and death among human beings.

In the presence of significant others and the public, the sufferer is expected to carry his or her pain with dignity. The unsaid message is, "I can't handle your pain so please don't stir my fears with your problem." As an aside, society now has its "ears" for hearing such problems in the form of helping persons such as counselors, who have been specially trained to violate the societal norm and encourage the expression of affect.

If, for example, the cancer patient experiences the need to express feelings but the implied consent is not perceived as being given for such emoting, the patient is stressed. Some theorists (*see* Suggested Readings) suggest that the personality of the cancer patient would be the key determinant in not perceiving implied consent since he or she exhibits a repetoire of behaviors characterized by withdrawal from stress producing situations and the suppression of strong affect, specifically anger. Consequently, from this author's vantage point, the problem seems analogous to the "chicken vs. egg" argument: Is it that the cancer patient doesn't *have* implied consent or doesn't *wish to have* the implied consent? It has been this author's

experience that both conditions exist with the latter often more pronounced. The same dynamic seems to exist in the *loneliness* issue
discussed later.

Also, one must consider the existence of the dynamic of the
following: "You can't know my pain unless you've been there!" It
is difficult to argue with this truth/accusation/defense. As the helper,
regardless of one's professional discipline, unless one has or has had
cancer, one is always an outsider. However, even in those situations
observed in which the leader of the group or person interacting in an
authority role has been or is a victim, there exists the inevitable:
"Yes, but . . . ."; "Yes, but doctor, you have a profession that accepts
your long absences from work"; "Yes, but Reverend, God has
chosen you for this work and guides you through this disease"; "Yes,
but my pain is so severe that you could never understand." As the
counselor, no matter how one responds to the allegation, one is
placed in a competitive/combative juxtaposition. If one acquiesces,
the patient's defense/accusation is validated. If one confronts, the
stage is set for a "my-scar-is-bigger-than-yours" interaction.

It also seems clear that there exists a compulsion to share from
the "misery-loves-company" aspect. Often, sharing one's feelings
about cancer with noncancer persons does not seem to be feasible
and does not produce the necessary barometer for assessing one's
level of performance as a cancer victim in comparison to others. It
becomes apparent that only a "self-help" group consisting of other
cancer patients is a viable alternative. The only "living" alternative,
in a psychological sense, becomes a social sharing, and subsequently, a *therapeutic* group consisting of the criteria of cancer as a prere-
quisite for membership.

Consequently, the desire to share one's plight with those in a
similar circumstance involves, for some cancer patients at least, the
question: "Am I normal for a cancer victim?" On a relatively lower
scale of intensity, the syndrome is similar to a group of adolescents
saying, "How are we going to survive old man Lindenberg's class?"
Witness the following excerpt:

Diana: . . . You know, I have to be supermom and
              everybody goes . . . and people do this to all of you
              I'm sure. They look at you and say, Oh wow! I'm glad
              it's you and not me!

Amanda: I find it's embarrassing for me.

Carol: I do too.

Amanda: And nothing is more threatening to other people than your own fears — having to come in touch with your mortality.

Carol: And because of that reason, I don't tell anybody until it come's right down to the point where they need to know.

Steve: It's scary.

Carol: It really is.

Steve: I'm not sure what Diana is saying? On the one hand she was saying, "Yeah. That's not what the real concern is; it's not so much people's discomfort. It's kind of an expectation that I have for myself and an expectation that other people have of me that I'm supposed to be super-together." And, you know, sometimes, I get the feeling from what you're saying, that sometimes they're saying, "You're so courageous." And they don't allow you to be uncourageous; allow you to lean a little bit. And it's their discomfort, that's hurtful to you.

Diana: *And I guess that's why this group session seems to be important to me. It is that I can look you in the eye and I can say I'm afraid: I really am afraid. But, when I leave here and I turn into that super person again who has two children and who look me in the eye [and mama has to feel good]; and a husband who loves me dearly [if I'm OK, he's OK]; I have to keep going. My parents, if I feel fine [if I'm OK], they are OK. And there are days when I don't feel OK but I can't admit that to anybody! I have to keep going! I have to go that extra mile! Not that it's not that important, but sometimes I just want to sit down and cry. But I can't do that.*

ALONENESS (LONELINESS)

Perhaps there is no conscious physical and psychological state that is simultaneously both feared and longed for as aloneness. I say conscious because it would seem that death is the *unconscious* physical and psychological *state* that is simultaneously both feared and longed for by man.

It is interesting how many times one hears the expression, "I am surrounded by people and yet I feel so alone;" on the other hand, paradoxically, "I find peace when I am alone walking in the woods."

Of course, an argument could be made that aloneness is self-imposed whereas loneliness is other-imposed. It would also seem that it is possible to be alone, because of choice, and to be lonely at the same time. This is the point exactly. The cancer patient seems to desire both aloneness and loneliness. He or she wants and fears aloneness.

Cancer patients seem to come from family systems in which stress is dealt with by individual members isolated (withdrawn) from the family group as opposed to the family as a whole dealing with a given stressful situation. Each member is left alone to deal with the problem at hand. Thus, in keeping with this theory, cancer patients come from family systems that encourage suppression of affect, stoicism, suffering with dignity, and retreating to being alone with a problem.

With the possibility that the propensity toward self-imposed loneliness is psychologically ingrained through family dynamics, the cancer patient experiences an other-imposed loneliness because of fear and ignorance regarding cancer. If a person in our society gets a heart attack, he or she is immediately surrounded by caregivers and loved ones. The heart attack can be seen as analogous to being wounded in combat and being sent home from the front. The heart attack victim is the hero in our society. This "wound" achieved in the hazardous pursuit of happiness is rewarded with the "purple heart." A heart attack survived can be a symbol of status much as an ulcer. Lavish attention is given to the patient. Life affords permission to find new directions and to retreat from the rigors of the Protestant work ethic.

On the other hand, consider cancer. There is no status in cancer. To the fearful and ignorant, cancer is leprosy. Cancer is dreaded in that very often the prognosis is incurable. Because of myths and misconceptions, cancer is feared as a contagious disease. Persons who recover are often maimed and disfigured in the process. Sometimes they talk funny, or not at all. Sometimes they go to the bathroom by emptying a plastic bag. Sometimes they lose their hair. Sometimes they are in chronic pain. All of these dynamics violate the cultural concept of health and normality.

Having a heart attack is quick, clean, and neat. If one dies, he or she goes swiftly and efficiently. Funerals are sprite, prim, and proper. Grief is made simpler by the acceptability of the loved ones method of dying. In other words, heart attack people die as they're "supposed to."

Cancer, on the other hand, is neither quick nor simple. Death is often prolonged for years. Death from cancer is an imprecise affair. Prognostications are generally errant. Funeral arrangements are awkward and cosmetics are employed to remind us of the victim's healthier days. Grief, out of practice but not of necessity, is often a prolonged process because of the nature of the dying process with cancer and because of societal injunctions surrounding the experience of cancer. At the time of death, in many cases, emotional and financial resources are significantly depleted. Where, in the case of the heart patient, death is often a surprise; with the cancer patient, death is a release.

The whole dynamic of death heightens the perception of loneliness for the cancer patient. Death seems almost anticlimactic. It is the self-imposed and other-imposed aloneness that seems most tragic. If, as suggested by some, the so-called cancer-prone personality is one that reacts to stress by withdrawal and repression (denial/coping), what could be more isolating than cancer? The following discussion addresses the difficulties surrounding aloneness and loneliness. Jane begins and is at the center of this segment. Diana has called Jane on the phone since the group's previous meeting as a caring gesture.

Jane: I've listened to all your strengths. I must be weak because I stayed in bed very lonely — reached out to my church; to a group in my church — merely to call me, as I said to them — to siphon off some of the loneliness that existed. And out of 100 persons, three called me. And I did feel rejected and I did say to them, "I do need somebody to talk to." And I was not trying to present the picture of great strength and still not of weakness but of having a certain need as a human being.

Diana: And it's your very own need. This is my very own exclusive need. And I don't know. . . . I can't even share it with anybody. I can't even tell my mother, who I'm very close to, because she just doesn't understand it. And it's like you calling me and saying — just saying I'm going to live. I know you don't have anything to base that on. Nothing! But you don't know — you are saying that just to me — that's just for me. And that makes me feel very good. You are not saying it for my children and for my husband. You are saying it just for me. And it makes me feel very good because I have to think about everybody else. And you know, some days the top may blow off my head. I've always thought if you could acknowledge I had a problem, then that's half of it. But I find out that's not half of it even though you know you have a problem.

Steve: I want to make sure of one thing. Did you [Jane] hear what she [Diana] said to you? That your call made her feel very good — your reaching out to her?

Jane: Yes, I did feel good.

Amanda: You may be underestimating yourself.

Steve: On the one hand, you're waiting for people to call you; to say, "I care." On the other hand, you are reaching out to someone else to say I care. I guess the question I want to ask is, who goes first? Is it a thing of waiting and seeing how much love there is in the world for me because I'm alone? Or is it a question of taking a little initiative? I don't know the answer. I think the answer is somewhere in between. But I wanted you to get that feedback. Because after that last week that you had, I want you [Jane] to hear what she [Diana] said to you. She said she felt very good because you gave her something ". . . just for me" from you — for no one else. And that's very important for you to pay attention to that.

Jane: And you see that was the thing that I was looking for in my church. And there wasn't anybody.

Steve: And you were disappointed and hurt.

Jane: That's right. I was very disappointed.

Steve: Crushed.

Jane: Yes and. . . .

Amanda: Jane, let me ask this. Have you made any other overtures other than saying, "I need you, please call me."?

Jane: You know what I did. I stayed in bed and said to myself that I am not going to waste away. I'm going to do something constructive. And I had always liked to work mental health groups. And I made a list of the various facilities and finally did some volunteer work. And I would be continuing to do it only. . . . [Jane's eyes began to water.]

Steve: Where is the feeling of sadness you are experiencing coming from? You just got such a good feedback? I'm wondering where the sadness is coming from in your eyes?

Carol: *I think it's the loneliness, Jane, that you feel that shows in your eyes.*

Jane: And I'm not working at The Mental Health Center now because of this group. And I want to get back. I want to join another group there. This is very intensive work because it. . . .

Carol: I think if you joined other groups like that or worked in a clinic three days a week, if your health permits it, that you would find much joy and happiness.

Jane: There are just special places I like to work.

Carol: Right.

Jane: Mental health groups.

Amanda: Some just feel we don't all have to do something worthwhile.

Jane: For me that's so rewarding that I don't know what other kind of fun I would have.

Amanda: Well, there are some things that you enjoy doing. Maybe you could do them with somebody.

Carol: Jane, why don't you move into a senior citizens home? They have activities [laughter].

Amanda: Oh come on! That's insulting, Carol!

Carol: That's what I'm going to do when I get old.

Jane: You know when I'm 100, I'm not going to be eligible [all talking and laughing]!

Carol: Amanda, you don't like those homes.

Amanda: Well, you see. . . .

Jane: I'm never going to stretch the last mile.

Steve: Jane, did you hear what they did to you? They are rushing to your rescue. They got you involved in the American Association of Retired Persons, senior citizens homes, the clinics again; and they've got all kinds of solutions. So there's a lot of caring for you right here and that's why I couldn't. . . .

Jane: The only thing: I can't accept that kind of caring because I'm too young [laughter].

Steve: Let me see what I want to say. Let me just think for a second. What they are saying to you is kind of an interesting contradiction about where you are. Because a while ago you were feeling sadness and Carol, I think, hit it. *You know, this is the loneliness that comes out. And yet there are four women in here and you've talked to one on the phone, who gave you good feedback. They are all giving you good feedback that, God bless you, you are healthy. You can get out there and do things. They are all saying to you, "There are five of us in here and there are two who aren't here that care about you."* Cindy upstairs! Already we got past our fingers and we are counting on our toes about those people who care about you. And I know it's a little different to have someone call and say, "Hello! Jane! How the hell are you," or something like that, or in Carol's words, "Hello Jane! How are you?" And I hear you getting in touch with the problems you had with your son. But I don't hear you getting in touch with what's happening right here.

Jane: *Maybe it's because I'm unaccustomed to it. I'm unaccustomed to caring or having somebody care for me.*

Steve: *So it's difficult for you to accept.*

Carol: *In other words this is the most family you have had in a long time.*

Jane: *Yes.*

Carol: *We are your family now.*

Steve: I wonder if it's not possible because you don't expect it. I don't know if that's the case. *Could it be that you might be pushing it away?*

Jane: *It could be. It could be the fact that I'm so unaccustomed to it and it's such a strange feeling for me, it's hard for me to grab so that I cannot very closely and intimately respond. I feel it but I feel strange about it.*

Amanda: I gather, Jane, this is not a recent development. This apparently has characterized your entire life.

Jane: Oh, yes.

Amanda: Well, no wonder it's hard for you; you are being asked to change your whole life. That's hard to do. That would be very hard for me to change because I think what I'm doing is all right.

Steve: This is an interesting analogy for me and it just struck me while I was sitting here listening to this. On the one hand we are talking about how hard it is to change our lives, and I think we are talking in a psychological sense after the years of experience and this mistrust in your [Jane's] case [the mistrust, the beating, the not caring, the manipulating]. It probably has as much to do with who you are as it did with those around you. And on the other hand, we are talking about a physical disease called cancer that is intervening in your lives and has forced every one of your bodies to change; the bodies that have been there for as many years as your mind.

Sally: That's changed our whole attitudes, our whole lives.

Steve: I guess the thing that I'm struck with is what Amanda was saying. I don't think she was saying that you can't change. But I think she was saying that it's harder to change when these life-style patterns have been established for so long a period of time. And yet, I don't hear the impossibility of change.

Amanda: No, not impossible.

Steve: Because sometimes your physical situation has forced you to change. And maybe it's important to take a look at the quality of your life, the loneliness, the misinterpretation, the lack of communication of love between you and those you really care about, and the lack of communication because of distance. Maybe there are problems communicating with people who you don't really care about. But you've been forced to put on a facade over the years. Maybe it's time to do something for each of our selves to make the quality of relationships more meaningful and the quality of life more meaningful.

Diana: Yeah, now how do you go about doing that?

Steve: Well, how would you go about doing that?

Diana: I don't know. I can't see my life changing; I can't see. . . .

Steve: *You can't see a way that you could interact any differently with those you care about than you are? Is that their problem or is it your problem? Because we were just talking about Jane pushing people away. It's as much her pushing them away as it is them pushing her away and you all kind of shook your heads at that — up and down. I guess I'm saying, whose problem is it? Is it yours?*

In the next excerpt the affective dynamics of loneliness are explored as more group building takes place.

Steve: Let me just say something. When we were talking about loneliness, feelings, strengths, and stuff your face was long, your eyes were a little glazy, and there was a lot of expression of emotion. You know, a lot of tension.

Diana: Well, I feel like. . . .

Steve: A lot of tension, just like you did right there. That's a little shaky.

Diana: Well, I feel like that Jane is alone and I have a husband who loves me very deeply and children and a family that's close and rallied around. Yet I'm still alone too. I mean. . . .

Steve: So, you can experience the same sort of loneliness.

Diana: So, even though I've got all this, I hope it's not self-

	pity that . . . .
Amanda:	Diana, don't you think everybody . . . .There are some roads you have to walk alone! That's all there is to it!
Steve:	I don't know if I buy into that.
Amanda:	Yes you do, Steve! You just haven't lived long enough!
Steve:	I don't know.
Amanda:	There are some places you have to go by yourself.
Steve:	OK, I'm willing to concede [the point].

Feelings of loneliness and difficulties in building new relationships are themes in the following excerpt. Again, such difficulties are not unique to the cancer patient. However, that such problems existed for each group member seems significant beyond coincidence. Also, note Carol's assertion and Amanda's reinforcement that loneliness is worse than *the disease*. This assertion echoes Jane's complaint heard earlier.

Diana:	Don't you want someone to listen and not come back with advice?
Steve:	That's the thing! That's the thing I guess I react to most. When I share something with someone and they say take two aspirins, drink plenty of water, and walk slowly, I just want to go umm . . . you know . . . I just get angrier than hell, and feel even more lonely. That's what I'm hearing from the group too.
Carol:	After my husband passed away, I was very, very lonely and it's such a horrible feeling. People would invite me to their homes for dinner and yet my world was shut out because I was just so crushed. I guess I was feeling sorry for myself.
Steve:	So, you were doing it as much as they were doing it.
Carol:	Right. And at that time I didn't care to listen to anyone else. *But it was such a deep hurt and I know the loneliness. It's worse than a disease sometimes.*
Amanda:	*It is. You are quite right.* But, is it not possible that in doing the very thing that Steve questions the wisdom of [which is *pretending* no matter how you feel], you

would have gotten over that soon, if you had made yourself go? If you had made yourself enjoy?

Carol: Oh, I made myself do it. I didn't enjoy it, but I knew that I had to get back into social . . . .

Steve: If you [Amanda] are in such control of your feelings, I wonder how it's possible to make yourself enjoy something if you are controlling the feelings that would make it possible for you to enjoy?

Amanda: We are getting a little twisted up here.

Steve: I hope I'm not communicating anger or anything. I find that hard for myself to plug into . . . .

Amanda: Let's see. Let me put it another way. You are invited to go some place, and you are sad and unhappy, and you don't really want to make the effort; but you know you should just for your own mental health's sake. So you say, "I'm going!" Well, if you go with a positive attitude [I'm going to try my best to have a good time], all of a sudden you are having a good time. *That doesn't mean you've forgotten the sadness, because it just overwhelms you at the damndest moments.* But for a time you have been able to push it to the back of your head. And I don't see anything wrong with that! Then the next time it's a little easier. And the next time! And the next time! And finally it's a sad memory. But it's a memory! It's not ever present. It's not an influence on everything you think and do.

Jane: You see, but I didn't have the opportunity in many instances. People were not inviting. Chrismas would come by — Thanksgiving would come by — and I would be alone. And this certainly didn't make me very happy.

Amanda: No, of course not.

Steve: I'm hearing a lot of self-doubt — like you might be asking yourself, "What have I done to turn these people off? What have I done?"

Jane: Yes. *And I would say, "Why am I rejected?" or "What is it about me that is so distasteful?" "There must be something!"*

Amanda:	Were you really rejected or were you just not invited? Did you invite them? And did they say, "No I don't want to come?"
Jane:	No!
Steve:	Did you throw the party?
Jane:	No! They did. You see these were families, and I could not very easily. . . .
Steve:	Your family?
Jane:	No! *I don't have a family. I just have my son!* But I could not easily invite five or six people. If I invite anybody anywhere, I have to take them out to dinner because I don't really have facilities for it. So, actually what was happening, I think, was a combination of many feelings. There's no doubt I was feeling sorry for myself. I was questioning. I wondered, "What was there about me?" Is there something so distasteful? *But there must be something that I'm doing.*

At the end of the previous passage, Jane poses the possibility that perhaps she is doing something, consciously or unconsciously, to keep people away. This verbalization opened the door for confrontation regarding the hypothesis that much of the loneliness encountered by the cancer patient is self-imposed. The following passage deals with that confrontation. Notice the confession of "bribing" people to get their attention in an effort to be involved without being committed to relationship. Such maneuvering ultimately serves to reinforce self-imposed loneliness. Interestingly, Diana identifies with Jane's problem.

Steve:	I'm just wondering, Jane. Is there anything that you might be aware of that could be pushing people away? What you could do to draw people closer to you?
Jane:	Well, I think there are a lot of conditions that would influence this.
Steve:	For instance?
Jane:	I think, I still find there's prejudice [to cancer] even though people are not actually consciously aware of it. I think when I became ill, a lot of people that I had seen before who would invite me gradually rejected me.

Steve: Is it possible that's happening because you expect it to happen?

Jane: Because I expect it to happen?

Steve: What I'm getting at is, is there any way you could be setting that up to happen because you expect it to happen?

Jane: *I think a lot of things I do are not particularly encouraging to people really seeking me out.*

Steve: For instance?

Jane: *Many times I will withdraw and not go to certain functions.*

Steve: Can you be specific when you say withdraw. What other kinds of things do you do that might push people away when they want to get close or when you would like them to get closer?

Jane: I think I have a difficult . . . . I've always had this problem of not letting people get too close because I think my problem has been they expect certain performances of me and it's generally been an exaggerated one. They think I'm supposed to do certain things.

Steve: You know who you sound like?

Jane: Who?

Carol: Diana?

Diana: [to Carol] You've been around me too long!

Jane: *They expect me to be able to do something and I'm afraid. I don't want to disappoint them.*

Steve: *Are you aware of what I'm hearing you say? What you just said was that you are as much responsible for the feelings of loneliness you have for not letting people get close to you as the other people are for making you feel lonely.*

Jane: [tearfully] I am! I am!

Steve: . . . . That you have a responsibility in that.

Jane: *I am! And I'm not exercising that responsibility [in a positive direction] right now.*

Steve: You haven't yet. That's it exactly. I think that's an interesting awareness you have because there's a responsibility in initiating a relationship with people.

One has to take a certain amount of responsibility in doing that. There are risks involved with that. *I think that what you just said is that sometimes you are afraid of the risks.*

Jane: *I am!*

Steve: Because you've been burnt?

Jane: I am, and I have a tendency to do certain things.

Steve: That push people away?

Jane: *No, not that push people away. That I do in order to encourage people to notice me. They are actually almost in the nature of a bribe. I'll do certain things which I don't really have to do and I think that I complicate certain situations.*

Steve: Then I would guess that when people find out that you've done that, they feel like they've been set up.

Jane: I don't know. But maybe I do make people feel that I've done certain things that might impose an obligation on their part which they might not want to execute.

Steve: *Is that kind of a way of using people?*

Jane: *Is that a kind of way of using people? It could be a very subtle way.*

Steve: So, what happens then when you do that?

Jane: What happens? Nothing happens.

Steve: Well, something happens to cause nothing to happen.

Jane: Oh, you mean what happens? I didn't quite understand.

Steve: I guess what I'm saying is that if I were in a relationship with you and I felt that you had in some way manipulated our relationship, our friendship, either through talking about it or through, in some kind of a way, using our relationship just to salve your loneliness, and yet at the same time keeping you at a distance, I'd get pretty angry after a while. I wouldn't want to be around you. I would lose interest in you and I wouldn't call. I wouldn't invite you to a party anymore.

Jane: I don't know if that's exactly true. I can't be objective about it.

Steve: How do you feel about it?

Jane: How do I *feel* about it? Ah, I sometimes *think* that I do certain things which are . . . which I do with the idea that eventually that person will like me. I think I do it for that. I think very subtly I play this game myself.

Steve: Who are you talking to? I see you looking at. . . .

Jane: I was looking at Amanda but I'm talking to the group. *I think that I play this little game. . . .*

Steve: Do you hear what you said?

Jane: Yes.

Steve: Have you known this before? Have you been aware. . . .

Jane: That I can do certain things? That I've been doing certain things?

Steve: Manipulating relationships.

Jane: I am not really manipulating relationships. I am doing certain things occasionally, or not having any contact with the person at all.

Steve: I don't know about the rest of you. I just got lost there a little bit.

Jane: It's actually, either I would be excessive in my desire to be noticed or I would do nothing and if I had no reason to go somewhere, I would not do it.

Steve: Are they ways of getting attention?

Jane: Are they ways?

Steve: Are they ways of doing something to try to talk yourself into a relationship. For example, contacting a lot of people or withdrawing: Are they two ways of getting some kind of attention?

Jane: I think one — they are not exactly two ways of trying to get attention — one, I think. The withdrawing is an evaluation of myself in thinking that I can't score and I can't cope with it so that it's easy for me to pull out.

Steve: So I guess the other question I would have is, Where does trust and love enter into these relationships?

Jane: I can't evaluate that.

Steve: I'm not talking about sexual and marital love you know. I mean the friendship kind of companionship: love, caring, and honesty.

Jane: Yes. I have only my friend I think I'm capable of having this kind of relationship with. And the interesting thing is we totally disagree in our philosophy. But in spite of that there's a certain respect and a certain concern. And she's probably one that I can feel really comfortable with.

Steve: *I guess what I was hearing was that a lot of loneliness and stuff that you experience is worse than cancer. I guess what I was hearing is that you bring a lot of that on yourself by in some way turning some people off when you really don't intend to. But on the other hand there is some intention.*

Jane: *And even many times. . . . Like recently there's a woman at the church, a very intelligent person, who called me on a few occasions. And I could have seen her and gone to church with her. But she was attaching so much significance to me and what she thought I was capable of that I was scared to encourage this relationship. Because I felt that I would be disappointing her; that I was not what she thought I was.*

Steve: I heard that somewhere in this group before. I heard Diana saying the same thing.

Diana: *You're ending up with the same thing I am.*

Interestingly, the group illustrates psychodynamic characteristic of cancer patients that this author has observed: difficulty with the expression of affect and the acceptance of the expression of others' feelings. In the earlier part of the protocol cited above, Carol and Amanda began to offer suggestions for ways that Jane can combat loneliness (such as going to a senior citizens' home). It is more than coincidental that such solutions are offered as soon as Jane's eyes began tearing from the loneliness she was experiencing in the group. The group had difficulty accepting Janes's affect.

THE EFFECTS OF AFFECT

Every once in a while. . . . Like they put me in the hospital this summer because I had literally run out of steam. I was just a complete and total nervous wreck and occasionally that happens. Occasionally, I literally go to pieces. But I don't have anybody in this world other than Cindy [a nurse practitioner] that I can talk to whenever I come in. And then I only open up just a little bit because I've still got to be strong even to them. And I sit here and I listen to all this whether people like me or not. And that, to me, I mean is to Diana — it's so unimportant, you know. . . .

Diana

As stated earlier, the suppression of feelings and the inability and/or unwillingness to share such feelings is said to be one of the most stress-producing dynamics of human behavior. For whatever reason, the suppression (and all of those other sinister things people do with their emotions) of affect has as a "bottom line" the fear of rejection.

On the other hand, the inability to share feelings honestly with significant others may cause rejection of the self. Theoretically, psychological rejection of the self leads to a psychosomatic breakdown of the organism's biological defense mechanisms. With the breakdown of the immunosuppressive defense mechanism comes the susceptibility to disease. Carcinogens, viruses, genetic predisposition, and mutant cells exacerbate the body's vulnerability. The all-consuming depression, anger, and fear of the mind manifests itself biologically consuming the organism. Could it be that cancer is passive suicide? It may be the body's creative mechanism for enforcing the unacceptable outcome associated with active suicide. Perhaps this is one reason that cancer is so dreaded by mankind. The collective unconscious recognizes the disease process for what it is in essence.

Of course, we are examining the effects of affect on at least two levels: (a) *theoretically*, as the psychological basis for organic dysfunction and (b) *situationally*, in the contemporaneous moment of the experience of cancer. While we may not be able to resolve the theoretical question in this text, perhaps the following excerpt can communicate some of the psychodynamics of suppression of affect situationally and the cancer patient's rationale for such suppression with more potency than this observer can write.

Steve: Have you ever sat down and said to someone in your family, "You always look up to me as the Rock of Gibraltar and I would rather you talk to me like a person — like a person that has faults and is scared sometimes and is happy other times, but just talk to me like a person."?

Diana: No! I could not! I cannot because my parents call — "How do you feel?" "Fine! Great! Terrific!" It doesn't matter that I may really feel bad. I don't allow myself to feel bad! But even if I did, I don't!

Amanda: You see, I don't think that controlling feelings is so bad. You are *helping* people you care about. You are helping them to be comfortable and happy because you care about them and that's more important to you than expressing all these feelings.

Diana: But I'm asking you, you know. I see we are alike, but what about those feelings on the inside? The ones you don't, you know, maybe you feel uncomfortable when I say, you know. . . . I am this way to the public but *here* I want to say I need help to adjust because this is something I've got within myself — or with Steve's help or with each of you listening to how you handle it. But whether people like me or not is irrelevant, you know.

Amanda: Of course, I think I have an advantage over you, Diana, in that I live alone. And if there comes a time when I want to let down, okay I can let down and nobody. . . . And I know I have been one of these responsible people all my life. Duty is the blindest word in the English language and sometimes I have to say, "I'm tired of being responsible!" But it was only temporary. . . .

Carol: I *never* get so aggravated that I tell someone to go to hell.

Steve: Do you feel — have you ever felt that type of rational control has taken itself out somewhere else on your person: in your mind or your body?

Amanda: *Maybe. I just know I always thought, "I could slam a plate against that wall!" But, I'd have to clean it up!*

Diana: *You see I've done a pretty good job in covering my feelings. Nobody really knows how I feel.*

Steve: You are covering them up. I think that's a key point right there. But I know how you feel. I mean I don't know how you feel; I know how you are coming across to me. You're angry about having to play this charade and not being able to be yourself.

Diana: But, you see, I don't have any out. I've got to be this way to keep my home like it is — and my children happy and my husband happy and my parents. My mother calls, "How do you feel?" It doesn't matter if I feel like I'm going to drop dead. "I feel good! I feel good!"

Steve: What I'm hearing now is you are keeping up a charade to help others' feelings without taking anything for yourself.

Diana: But, you see, I've said all this before.

Amanda: You know something. It seems to me, Diana, that you are helping other people not to feel uncomfortable and what have you, in a way contributing to your husband. Because if your husband is fearful and anxious and always, "Diana's going to die tomorrow"; if your children think, "Is Mamma going to leave us?" your household would be very unhappy. It would just be gloom, gloom, gloom. So, in a way, you are sort of protecting yourself as you protect other people.

Diana: It's got to be this way.

Steve: But I'm feeling that you are not doing a very good job of protecting yourself. Because if you are so happy how come you sound so angry?

Diana: No, I didn't say I was so happy.

Amanda: She lies a lot.

Steve: But that was what you (Amanda) were either picking up. . . .

Diana: [sarcastically] Well, OK! I feel good! I feel good! Well it's like this little group in here, it's like my husband was here, my father was here, my mother was here and here sits one of my children. Just like you are all looking at me now, they are looking at me. And if Diana feels good, everybody feels good. It's secret. If Diana lays down or feels bad, then the house is quiet.

Amanda: It's an awful burden put on you.

DEPRESSION

Amanda: In your bad moments you say, "Why in the hell did this happen to me?"
Sally: Why did it happen to me?
Amanda: And you have bad moments! And I think anybody who says they don't is just not telling the truth.
Sally: I believe that too. *And sometimes we just get so full of self-pity that we just wallow in it until it's just terrible!*

It has been said that depression is anger turned inward. If loneliness and suppression of affect are the culture medium for nurturing the psychosomatic process of cancer then, certainly, depression fuels the fire (anger/rage) that provides the warmth for incubation.

Depression is the cancer patient's arch rival. Depression envelops these persons; seductive, as this insidious psychological process beckons, "come hither and withdraw." Silently and stealthily, the syndrome of depression manifests itself. The cancer patient finds it extremely difficult to forget depression and succumbs easily. It is a constant struggle. Listen!

Diana: Physically I'm well everyday, mentally it's very bad.
Amanda: You know what, Diana? Do you think maybe what contributes to your depression is the fact that you cannot prevent yourself from thinking about what might have been and all the things you may be missing? The rest of us have kind of had our day. We can't say we were cheated. Maybe that's part of your feelings.
Diana: I think I can talk about it, but it's always there, you know. It's always! It never leaves! You know, I don't cry. Maybe if I did, that would help.
Steve: You do cry in a way, though. *Depression is crying inside isn't it?*
Diana: *Yeah. OK.*
Steve: Can I ask you a question? You sound upset to me. Underneath your voice there's tension — there's, I don't know how to say it. There's a smile on the outside, but there's a tension in here [pointing

	to stomach].
Jane:	*Depression.*
Steve:	*Depression. There's a lot of hurt too.* I was just wondering after we were talking for a while — I wonder if you are feeling a little guilty; a little depressed that you may have said the wrong thing to her?
Jane:	No, I don't at all. As a matter of fact that was very unlikely for me because I like to be told. I think that this group is an intimate group where I think we all ought to let our hair down and to me I would not consider this a personal affront at all. As a matter of fact, I would want the same consideration if there's a need that I have. I can say to the group, "Look I have this need. You are attacking it in a way that is not conducive to my relief." But I would appreciate it.
Steve:	I wonder. . . .
Diana:	That doesn't bother me. *No, I'm depressed. I'm just depressed about a lot of things. And every once in a while it gets more than I can handle.*
Steve:	*And then you get depressed.*
Diana:	*And then I get depressed. And then I've been coming here and apparently I've been letting it out enough, you know. I think I have it under control and then all sorts of things. My legs begin to hurt, my back hurts and it's all nerves. And okay, it's coming out somewhere so it comes out in my body. But then I don't see how this can be any different.*

DENIAL/COPING

Steve:	You give the picture of "everything is rosiness" with the cancer and the disease and the world is "hunky-dory" when we know it's not. And so I guess another feeling that comes along is that you are not being honest.
Jane:	No, I'm *not* being honest.

The question of denial examined philosophically becomes a question of coping. All deny reality at one level or another, particularly if such reality does not include the egocentric mortal self as its chief component.

Hurriedly, through the course of this awareness known as life, one rushes purposefully, albeit ultimately futile, to aggrandize the self. Conceptually, a world without the self is possible. Affectively, imagining one's self as not being is inconceivable. With only faith as the guarantor of immortality, men and women strive to erect or deposit some tangible proof that they "were." Paradoxically, giving up such strivings may allow the individual to have meaning and being that will, in the long run, provide greater assurance that, tangibly, ones life will continue to influence the course of mankind henceforth.

At any rate, the anxiety produced by the stress of the quest for immortal being may have profound consequences. One consequence is anxiety neurosis or existential anxiety. Existential anxiety is literally the fear, at subconscious or unconscious levels, of not being in the world. As the self becomes more and more aware of his or her finiteness and, in a sense, meaninglessness, and as religion, family values, and other psychosocial systems lose their purposefulness or validity, the self perceives, at some level, the absurdity of seventy (plus or minus) years in the face of time, the universe, and eternity.

As a result, this perception becomes translated into physical symptoms through a yet mysterious psychosomatic process. Such symptoms include high blood pressure, fainting, heart palpitations, a feeling of lightheadedness, "weak knees," stomach flutters, hyperventilation, profuse perspiration, and swallowing difficulties. Psychological processes include withdrawal, depression, and phobic conditions, such as agoraphobia.

Another consequence of existential neurosis is a syndrome of behaviors emerging as a coping mechanism. That coping mechanism is denial.

Denial is manifest in all populations, healthy or sick. However, perceived as a coping mechanism, denial — pronounced or sublime — exists in even the most realistic person. During the course of the group sessions, denial was evidenced at many levels. Confronting denial requires a delicate balance to be discussed in more depth later. However, recognizing denial is much easier. Carol presents an interesting series of vignettes.

Carol: [initial interview] I have never considered myself as a terminal patient. I don't know how bad my condition is.

This statement is contrary to fact. All of the group members had been told by the staff that their cancers were incurable.

Carol: [session 2] I started keeping a diary three years ago
                when they didn't give me much hope to live and for
                the first few weeks it was pretty rough. And then
                after that I started getting better and better. And
                everyday was a beautiful day. It's a beautiful world,
                and I just kept getting better so I just quit keeping it.

Here we can recognize the acceptance of death; the attempt to
live immortally through a creative act of permanence in authoring a
journal; new hope; and coping through an ever so subtle denial process. This was a theme in Carol's repertoire of responses throughout
the first five sessions.

Just before session 6, Carol had a painful close encounter with
death.

Carol: . . . and it was so painful. I've never had anything in
                my life. . . . I've had pain, but nothing like this.
Steve: This is the worst you've had in the course of the
                disease.
Carol: That was the worst I've had. Whether it was the final
                stage of the medicine grabbing hold of that tumor
                that's in there. . . . Because yesterday I didn't have
                any pain at all and today it's 1:00 and I haven't had
                any. But . . . if I press in that area, I can feel that it's
                still there and it hurts if I press on it.
Steve: So you know it's there.
Carol: I know it's still there.
Amanda: I expect what you have experienced and what you
                are saying is what all of us. . . . I mean none of us
                have really faced up to our. . . . I remember when
                we first came. *You made some comments that you
                live just one day at a time and, everyday was a
                beautiful day. And I thought to myself, "Everyday is
                not a beautiful day; I don't care what she says."
                So . . . intellectually we go through these things and
                then they really hurt you.*
Sally: *That's kind of a different matter.*
Carol: *That's right. Monday was not a beautiful day.*

ANGER

At the beginning of this chapter, it was stated that emotions are the building blocks of psychodynamics. Later anger, specifically, was examined as a component of depression. While anger is an obvious component of psychological complexes and syndromes, it has been my experience that the obvious often goes unnoticed, complicating otherwise simple solutions. Anger is one obvious psychodynamic of cancer that requires further attention. Once again, *showing* is more revealing than telling.

Steve: When you hear people telling you that you've got youth on your side, that you are young, and that hope is just around the corner, how does that make you feel?

Diana: *Like I could throw my coffee up all over the floor.*

Amanda: See, Diana, I feel the same way.

Barbara: What did you want?

Diana: . . . To throw my coffee up!

Steve: But she's not saying that to hurt anybody.

Diana: No!

Steve: Let's talk about that a little.

Amanda: I think what you are saying is maybe what I feel. I'm not discounting a miracle. That would suit me fine. But I'm not putting all my eggs in a miracle basket because I just think. . . .

Diana: Well it's just, you know, I get humored from Cindy and from the doctor. I get humored from my husband and my parents. I get humored from my friends and all. And they pat me on the shoulder and tell me what a good girl I am and how strong I am. And I know — I told my uncle when I was home — I was tired, you know. I'm tired of being told how gallant I am. Or I'm always told what an inspiration I am. But I think what I'm saying is you're not going to hear too much how I feel because I'm, you know, I've lived on top of it for seven years. I experienced a breaking down in the group and here I preached I want to get down to basics. I want us to get down to the problem instead of talking about how to make instant coffee. Now I'm sitting here and I'm saying I experienced it with Jane and maybe what happened with Jane just kind of brought my mind to it. But I'm saying I feel like I've been on a charade. I've been on it continually because there's so much you don't know about me. You couldn't possibly know about me but you wouldn't want to know and I put on my smile and I'll be set. So it's easier to just make you all happy. I feel better, don't you? If you know I feel good, you feel better. And I feel better by you feeling better and it really doesn't matter what's inside.

Steve: If it's so easy, how come you sound so angry?

Diana: Well, sometimes. . . .

Amanda: It's not easy!

Diana: *Sometimes you want to. I saw Rhoda get mad one day on a TV show and she just screamed. OK! That's what I want to do.*

Steve: *That's what you are doing here? I mean that's what I'm hearing. You are screaming.*

Diana: *Yeah, OK, I'm screaming!*

Steve: *Your hands are shaking, your body's. . . .*

Diana: *OK! But then you go back in and it's OK!*

Steve: *You put on your charade again, so that anger just eats at you more and your sense of self. . . .*

Diana: *And every once in a while it gets more than I can handle.*

FEAR

Fear is a survival mechanism. The cancer patient as much as anyone wants to survive and fears the consequences of death. More significantly, he fears the process of dying. Dependency, pain, loss of self, and loss of control are dreaded more than the damned disease itself.

The fear of rejection that may have altered the body's natural immunosuppressive defense system psychosomatically now becomes the fear of rejection by significant others because of the stigma of cancer.

Of course, there is fear of God. In the biblical sense this fear is translated into reverence, respect, love, and awe. To the dying, fear is the more literal fear of judgment.

Fear can be most debilitating and draining, both emotionally and physically. While "ye that fear the Lord shall be saved," those who fear dying and struggle to survive are often emotionally and physically spent as a result.

In the following passage, notice how fear and denial interact ever so subtly.

Diana: Do you get scared before you go in to see the doctor? Do you have any. . . .

Barbara: Oh, I don't, I don't.

Amanda: I can't honestly say I do.

Barbara: In fact, I look forward to it, because I feel like every time I come for a treatment, I'm getting better. And I really do. And even when I was coming once a week, I couldn't wait until Friday. And when I was off of any kind of medication or treatment for two weeks, then I was scared to death. I thought, "What's going on? What's going on?" Then when I started back every Friday, I really looked forward to it and now I do every three weeks. I look forward to it.

Amanda: Diana, I can't honestly say that I feel like Barbara, that I'm getting better and better. I think someway, someway, I've a reprieve. I don't really think I'm getting better. I think I'm on plateau, and that's OK with me.

In the next passage fear and anger seem to combine producing resentment and frustration.

Diana: Oh, goodness. The fact that I feel like I'm on a collision course a little bit, and that I can't seem to think about anything else; it's been worse this time since April than it was the other time. I don't know. I can't deal with it. I just can't seem to get it all together. I want to be strong on the outside to everyone around but I'm not strong on the inside.

Amanda: I think you underestimate yourself.

Carol: I do too, Diana. If you are not sick everyday and you don't have to fight nausea and stuff, I would say you are getting better or, like Amanda, you may be on a plateau and everything is just holding it's own.

Amanda: *To say, anybody in this room never was scared, I* *think is not true.*

Barbara: *I just went into a state of shock.*

Amanda: *Because the first time I felt that lump, you know how when your stomach kind of turns over. And I made up all sorts of reasons why. I mean, I had been playing with my little granddaughter and all that kind of thing. But I did have sense enough to go to the doctor which didn't do me any good for a year and a half. And then when the lump showed up again after I really thought it was clear sailing, I was that naive. Now, a combination of not being naive and believing what you want to believe, that once the surgery was over, that was it. And then when these lumps reappeared, my stomach flip-flopped again. So it would be a plain untruth to say that I was never scared, when maybe it's just be basic nature to be optimistic, to be realistic, I think. I just don't think that, if I pray hard enough, I'm going to get well because the Lord wouldn't do me any other way. I just think somehow I'm going to find the strength to manage whatever comes and I'm going on that basis. I'm not going to say, "Golly, how can I face this? Will I have enough money? Will I have enough this?" I'm just going to do the best I can and let the Lord take care of it.*

Carol had a close encounter with death that she shared during our sixth session. While this encounter will be discussed in more detail later, this is an appropriate place to examine her fear of death.

Steve: As you thought about not coming out of it, as you thought about dying, what kinds of feelings were you experiencing?

Carol: *Well, I was afraid.* I didn't — well, I don't know what to expect when people are dying. I don't know whether you just close your eyes and God takes you away. I really don't know. *I was frightened and I didn't know what to do.* And I know that my face was just racked with pain and my Kathy said, "Let me call the doctor." And I said, "No need calling him.

He's just going to tell me to take pain pills and I've already done that."

Steve: You were at home when this was happening on Monday? It was so severe?

Carol: Monday night, 7:30. And it lasted until 9:15.

Steve: So, you were having about two hours where you thought, "This was it," and so you really were scared.

Carol: And when it finally stopped, I was so exhausted I just fell asleep. *I really was frightened.*

Steve: Besides fear you were wondering, is this how it ends? Does God just take you? I was just wondering if you can share some of how you hoped it would be or how you experienced the room and the presence of your daughter and things like this.

Carol: Well, I was in her bedroom. We were watching TV. I don't have one in my room, so I was in her room. But the pain was so severe that I would leave her room so that I wouldn't have to have her watch me double over with pain and moaning and groaning. I don't know. *I really was frightened Monday.*

Steve: But fear seems to be the only emotion you seem to be in touch with at this point as you are sharing it with us. I wonder, as you look back on that, what other kinds of things were going through you.

Carol: Well, I thought that if death could come quickly and take me away from this pain I felt that I could find relief.

Steve: *So it was kind of a mixed feeling of fear and yet almost desiring the pain to go away and if it took death to take that pain then you were willing.*

Carol: *Aha!* And it was so painful. I've never had anything in my life, I've had pain, but nothing like this.

There are other fears that the cancer patient encounters. One is an unconscious fear of not having lived a meaningful life, which will be discussed in the next chapter. Another is the fear of the dreaded disease itself.

Sally: No, the doctor just said, "Well you know I'm going to do it, and if I get in there. . . . You know what they tell you. "If I find it," they take it out. But I don't know. *I went in there, well just like Carol said, with terrific fear.* I remember looking at that clock as they rolled me into that operating room and I just thought, well, . . .

Steve: It must be strange. I'm hearing Carol's fear and I heard some other things from Amanda, and from you, Sally, as if it's almost a repeat thing. "What happened to my mother is now happening to me today." I get the feeling that this compounds the scariness and the fear of the whole situation.

Amanda: Well, it has to!

Carol: Sure, it does!

Sally: And then you go in there and you don't know which way the ball's going to bounce. You are hoping against hope that it's just going to be a biopsy, you know, and I took the whole "tattle of rags" to come home the next day. And you go in today and have this operation and they find you a free bleeder and you stay in there and they pump blood! Blood! Blood! They scour around to get the blood! And you nearly die on the operating table. And then you don't get awake until way in the next afternoon and you are right in there by yourself. *And, by gosh! You find out what is happening!*

GUILT

Guilt is a balancing mechanism of the psyche. It is the fulcrum between impulse and responsibility. It is a *post facto* psychological mechanism of caution. However, unfortunately, it is not a mechanism of *control*. As Alfred Adler once wrote, "People who feel guilty have no intention of changing." Guilt is the salve of the soul. When one behaves wrongly or inappropriately, whether in the eyes of the observer or the actor, guilt is the submissive posture the mind assumes in the face of one in power or authority.

For example if I deprive my child of a $200 toy, whether by choice or necessity, I may choose to feel guilty as a submissive *gesture*. Whether or not I share this with my child (who is in power), I have no intention of changing my behavior.

Guilt can also evoke submissive *behavior*; for example, "Son, your Aunt Margaret would love to hear from you. It would be nice if you called." *Guilt* sets in! How could I be so terrible? I may call Aunt Margaret submissively, and I may say that we must keep in closer communication. Contemporaneously, I am very genuine. In reality, I probably would not have contacted Aunt Margaret without Mom prompting me and "tripping" my guilt.

Guilt is second only to anger as a causative psychodynamic in so-called neurotic and otherwise unproductive behavior. It is also a dynamic that brings us full circle in this discussion of the psychological dynamics of cancer.

Certainly, guilt and remorse are at times genuine affective expressions in wrongdoing even if, as such, these expressions do not herald behavioral change. However, perceived guilt is often a method that persons with a poor self-concept use to perpetuate unproductive behaviors.

In cancer patients, and maybe in some other populations, guilt is utilized to reinforce the suppression of affect, particularly anger. As such, guilt has both psychological and psychosocial implications in the course of the disease.

In the following passage, Sally is discussing her daughter, who had a history of severe psychiatric problems. Sally had just finished sharing her fear of cancer. She wanted to tell her daughter, but. . . .

Sally: I couldn't tell my child. I just told her I was going to have a biopsy. I wasn't going to tell her what I was going through for anything in the world. But fortunately, my very best friend in the world was here from Birmingham and she found out I was going in the hosptial. [She teaches school.] And she says, "I don't have to go home." She says, "I'll stay with Sally for a while. And she stayed ten days. And my doctor said that was one good thing that happened to my child. Of course, I'd never been sick. She's never been sick. She's never seen anybody sick.

Amanda: Sally, I don't believe that.

Sally: What?

Amanda: *I just don't think that burden of guilt should be placed on you. You couldn't help it 'cause you had cancer and to say that was the thing that contributed to your child's illness. . . .*

Guilt is a subject to which we will return in the next chapter.

Chapter 2

PSYCHOSOCIAL DYNAMICS

There are different kinds of pain. There are pains that can be alleviated by drugs. You can take a person with cancer and give him all kinds of drugs. They can be terminal and they are not even going to feel it. But what are you going to do with somebody who has emotional pain? That's much harder to deal with. I feel that cancer isn't the ultimate in pain. I don't feel badly about it. I really don't worry about the fact that I have extensive metastasis. I never even think about it. But I do know how my son treats me presents a pain that I feel every day.

Jane

EXISTENCE constitutes systems and matrices. Jane, who had accepted metastic cancer and its ultimate prognosis, shared a complaint that is much more painful. It is a complaint shared by others who do not have cancer. Such problems point out that psychosocially speaking, cancer populations do not appear to differ significantly from other populations. In other words, cancer patients seem to have the same kinds of concerns that you and I do. Cancer exacerbates existence. Systems and matrices become strained. Problems press for resolution quickly. Solutions seem unattainable within uncertain time constraints. Follow-up becomes impossible. The psychosocial situations and dilemmas about which most persons procrastinate become truly existential for the cancer patient. The situation needs immediate resolution, for tomorrow may never come. The psychodynamic manifested most often in terms of psychosocial concerns might be thought of as anxiety neurosis.

Psychosocial effects and dynamics are those behaviors that have a primary etiology in the self. The self chooses how it will react in response to a given stimulus from the system and/or matrix in which it exists. In the case of psychosocial effects and dynamics, the self is much more "other-directed" than "inner-directed." The matrix and/or system in which the self exists conditions responses that the self chooses, often preempting alternatives. More often than not, these matrices and systems include other people. Sometimes these persons are *significant* others. In other cases these persons may be

39

agents of social systems or designated representatives of institutions.

Conceptually, there is a gray area between psychological and psychosocial. (For instance, there is some overlap as in the case of aloneness.) While some might argue that there is no difference, diversity yields to controversy and from controversy emerges change. For the purposes of this book, there is a distinction.

Clearly, psychological effects include anger, fear, rage, depression, and anxiety as examples, while psychosocial effects include family dynamics, cultural variables, others' attitude, vocational problems, social stigma, and medical bills. Less clearly, other psychosocial concerns include self-esteem, body image, and sexuality.

FAMILY DYNAMICS

But even with my family, you know, sometimes it seems to help to just lay it on the line; just tell them I feel like hell.

Diana

So begins our discussion on family dynamics. Diana's impassioned plea to just be able to scream expresses a wish that is sadly often contrary to fact. Chances are that, if theory is correct and cancer-prone persons suppress affect, Diana's wish is analogous to this author's attempts to lose weight: complaint and protest, but rarely behavioral change.

If the unstated condition of the family system is little or no communication of affect, complicity enforces the contract. Thus, braggadocio and verbalization regarding intent or desire to express feelings in the family only camouflages intent. The disease is discussed only as an observer and only when such discussion is unavoidable. Hollywood aside, in most cases it is not discussed. Feelings are just not expressed.

GUILT

In the preceding chapter, guilt was briefly discussed as a psychological effect of cancer. Guilt is also a psychosocial phenomenon of cancer. It manifests itself on at least two levels: (a) from the perspective of the patient (victim), and, less obviously, (b) from the perspective of the family members. Let us examine the latter first.

It has been my observation that the family members of the cancer patient's family system often exhibit and feel guilt, consciously and unconsciously. This dynamic is best ascertained from observing the behavior demonstrated by these persons as opposed to actual verbalization. The chief way in which this guilt is manifested is in the way family members comply with the unspoken contract of not communicating regarding the affective component of cancer, thus encouraging the suppression of affect and its psychological consequences.

Of course, such supposition is theoretical. However, carrying this theory one step further one begins to observe some other dynamics. Cognitively, the family and the patient cooperate in acknowledging cancer. Dutifully, someone in the family makes sure that the patient gets to the clinic for chemotherapy and the like. (Incidentally, such "making sure" does not always mean that the family member transports the patient to the clinic. Often such "making sure" consists of emotional, guilt-laden telephone calls to the victim from concerned sons, daughters, parents, aunts, uncles, cousins, lovers, and so on who are not able for one reason or another to be with the patient.) Here we see *applied guilt* and conditional love and acceptance. It's as if to say, "If you don't go to the doctor, you will make me very upset and distressed. I won't be able to sleep, eat, or work. Mom, you must continue to go or you might get worse." That the patient may die is seldom voiced. Denial/coping is at work. The other type of guilt, conscious or unconscious, manifested in the phone call is *implied guilt.* To the genuinely (or otherwise) concerned party, calling and using applied guilt is a way of alleviating self-imposed guilt for not being there in this time of crisis. After all, he or she would be there if the caller needed help.

Interestingly, this guilt syndrome may be escalated. For instance, if Mom will not go to the oncology/hematology outpatient clinic, the guilt-bearing person may call the oncology unit describing to any or all who will listen each heart-wrenching detail involved in Mom's lack of interest and commitment to treatment. In several cases that I have observed, receptionists, secretaries, nurses, physicians, chaplains, and department heads have been besieged by the statement, "Please! Can't you make her come?" The implication is that the oncology unit is not doing its job. The guilt-laden party can project guilt, convert it to anger, and blame the "damn system" for not treating the patient comprehensively. In this case the unconscious motive of expression of anger is the attempt at absolution of guilt.

Few concepts are without positive dimensions. Guilt is no exception. In the case of the patient who has a family system prodding him or her to keep appointments, treatment can be accomplished to whatever end. Ideally, a cure is effected. In less fortunate circumstances, the quality of life, such as it is, is maintained and often prolonged. In socioeconomic systems in which support systems are minimal, diffuse, or nonexistent, compliance with treatment plans is erratic at best and the prognosis is poor. Thus, the guilt-laden support system has positive dynamics. How much more positive this system would be were the family to work through the guilt.

An aside that is raised by this discussion of guilt is the conceptualization of the cancer patient as a victim. It would seem that such a characterization is a way in which society anthropomorphizes cancer in order to focus all of its armies against the enemy. The fact that it is improbable that cancer has a mind that selectively attacks innocent bystanders, thereby victimizing them is inconsequential. Cancer is much easier to visualize by people as an enemy that victimizes. It is much easier to win financial support to defeat the "crab" that overwhelms and consumes. Such conceptualization also obviates any responsibility the victim may have felt for allowing the body to be susceptible to cancer through a breakdown in the immunosuppressive response by the way of psychomatic vulnerability.

At worst, the concept of the patient as victim perpetuates the whole denial process arising out of suppression of affect. It is easier for the physician to see the patient as the victim rather than as an unwitting coconspirator. And what about this poor victim? For the victim, "poor me" can become a crutch that debilitates rather than supports. For the observer, empathy is difficult, sympathy is profuse, and pity salves anxiety. Bringing us full circle, conceptualizing the patient as victim compensates for *survivor guilt*. Survivor guilt is the unconscious process of tragedy that results in a "better-him-than-me" rationalization. The reflex caused by survivor guilt presses into preconscious as, "Oh God! How can I even think that about my wife (child, mother, father)?" The concept of victim allows guilt to become anger directed at the menace that attacks helpless loved ones.

Guilt will be examined from the patient's point of view as this chapter unfolds. In the meantime, let us examine the psychosocial dynamic of self-concept as it applies to cancer patients:

Self-concept + Self-esteem = Self-worth

Self-concept consists of an image one perceives as "me." It consists of many stimuli both internal and external. Internally, self-concept arises from idiosyncratic behaviors as well as conscious and unconscious strivings. One's self-concept may arise from an inner-directed interaction with reality toward self-determinism versus other-directed interaction with reality toward predetermination. At a scientific level, one's self-concept may be predetermined by nature (i.e. genes). At the sociological level it may be other-determined by nurture (i.e. socioeconomic background). What is perceived as truth in this matter may be a constant and persistent matter of inquiry or it may be a matter of faith. The truth probably consists of a balance.

Self-concept is shaped by cultural and religious backgrounds. It is shaped by body image, others' opinions, sexuality, response to sexuality, career goals, fulfillment of career goals, and roles in life.

Self-esteem consists of the affective or *feeling* component of self-concept. It is essentially conceptualized as how a person feels about himself. Simplified, if I conceive of my self as being competent, motivated, and organized and as having meaning in the world, I may feel self-love. On the other hand, if I see myself as inadequate, scared, and disease-ridden and as losing control, I may feel anger and bitterness in myself culminating in a conglomerate of feelings called depression.

The sum total of one's self-concept and one's self-esteem is one's self-worth. Self-worth is the combination of affect and intellect that helps one to exist in the world with meaning. It determines the way one attacks or withdraws from life's situations. It determines which compensating behavior one takes to counter inferiority or superiority strivings. Self-worth may motivate toward perceiving the world as good or evil. The inner sense of self-worth determines the life-style of individuals and the death style of individuals. In short, maintaining a system of self-worth and perceived reality produces so-called "normal" or "abnormal" behavior in response to environments that are either organically or psychosocially created.

While a sense of self-worth may be genetically predisposed,

because of man's adaptability it is not necessarily fixed throughout one's life. As cancer flourishes at the expense of healthy tissue, similarly, it destroys the sense of self-worth. Although there are many factors influencing the self, there are some that seem to especially stand out with cancer patients: body image, stigma of cancer, sexual activity and sexuality, self-sufficiency through the opportunity for gainful employment, and others' attitudes.

Body Image

In a discussion of self-worth, body image is a major component. When a cancer patient sees himself in the mirror, that person can see the visible ravages of the disease. In women, one or both breasts are gone. In men, testicles may have been removed. Without elaboration, such a loss, especially considering society's emphasis on the breast in one example, is devastating to both body image and sexuality. Missing limbs, testicles, ovaries, a uterus, a vagina, a lung, one or both kidneys, a larynx, one or both eyes and/or hair all contribute singularly or plurally to the weakening of a positive body image. Should the cancer patient already possess a poor body image, such insults complicate ego deficits to the point of absurdity. Ostomies, scars, radiation burns, and physiological responses to chemotherapy further add to the sense of losing control of oneself and a weakening sense of self-worth.

In the following passage, Diana and Barbara discussed body image and how it relates to self-esteem.

Diana: But yet it's like when we talk about my weight; it doesn't matter to me that you all can't see that I'm fat. I know that I've gained 20 to 30 pounds and it's very important. This is what I've told Steve. All I have left is my appearance. That's all that I have and you know the fact that my complexion has gone to pot . . . well you all didn't know me before. You don't know what I looked like, which wasn't too great, but. . . .

Amanda: You are making the comparison.

Diana: You know, I know and it did something to my self-esteem. And I lost that. So besides dealing with cancer coming back, I'm having to learn to deal with

	the weight gain.
Steve:	And you get this from your husband; you get this from your children; you get this from your family and friends; and they mean well. She is not sure that this happens with the rest of you all.
Barbara:	Oh, it does!
Amanda:	[to Diana] I think you are wrong about that. Excuse me, Barbara, go ahead.
Barbara:	I feel the same way. I can look in the mirror, I know what I look like, and I'm not used to being this fat. I've got a fat face, no hair hardly, and I'm ugly. I know that. But then when I get around this group, you look so good, you just look so well.
Steve:	I did the same same damn thing, didn't I. Because when I came in you were saying about your wig and I said. . . .
Carol:	Is that a wig?
Barbara:	It's natural. . . .
Jane:	That's not a wig!
Barbara:	Oh, yes, it certainly is too. You want me to take it off?
Jane:	I didn't know. When you said you didn't have any hair, I thought, gosh, she's got more than I've got.

Of course, this counselor did not exactly finesse Barbara's disclosure of her wig. Chronic human imperfection is a terminal condition even for counselors.

During the course of the group, there were many references to scars and disfigurement. One would expect such discusions. Diana, in particular, had difficulty with disfigurement, weight gain (as a side effect of hormone therapy), and body image in general. Presumably, this factor was in part due to her relatively youthful age and the fact that of all the group members, she was the only one that intimated ongoing sexual activity. Because of her ability to confide in one of the nurse-practitioners on staff, Diana began to build her sense of self. Her trials and tribulations in search of gainful employment coupled with having been in the geographical area for only one year combined to undermine this sense of self-worth.

Diana:	I know I'm being picky and choosy about where I go and so I'm hitting up against a brick wall.

Amanda: You're not being that picky and choosy to really hope that you don't get one.

Diana: Maybe I just want someone to say, "Yes, we want you." Then the decision is left on me whether I want it or not.

Amanda: You make the decision.

Jane: You know these are very difficult times and I found myself. . . . Of course I'm considerably older than you are. . . . But I had a rather imposing background in merchandising and when I realized I couldn't get a job. . . . First of all, I didn't even think in terms of cancer, I thought in terms of age. What I did in order to save me; save my sanity . . . I took a volunteer job and found it a very rewarding. . . .

Diana: But you know I've been doing that for eleven years. Having children, you know; I've been volunteering in some way or another. I guess the confidence has gotten built up in me and it's been, I've been coming ten months . . . and I started out in a hole, literally, with so much gushing over me. OK! *And just these last few months all of a sudden my self-worth has gotten built up.* I've begun to think, "Well, maybe there's something in me left." OK! But how else can I prove I'm worth something?

Steve: I think you are touching on something that's really . . . *the sense of self-worth.* If we can get in on that a little bit, we can get more to the core of what this job hunting experience is about. It's just one part of something that's very important to you. I noticed a while ago that when we talked, you know when I talked about it I guess, the underpinnings coming out with your sense of worth especially with the move from where you used to live to here and only being here a year, there was a change in your facial expression. Like even now, I see it. And you went from a yelling angry [making facial expression] this kind of a thing, to a very introspective thing.

Diana: So what are you saying I do?

Amanda: Pin him down!

Diana: If I was home, it would be so different. But I would be in my little cocoon. And I could say I wanted a job, and I would have one just like that!

Steve: Somebody would provide it for you.

Diana: Yea, somebody would provide it for me!

Steve: That would meet the need but what would that do for your *self-worth*?

Diana: Probably wouldn't do much for it.

Steve: The *self-worth*: Part of the investment in self-worth is being able to do it yourself.

Diana: Yeah, because, you know, when you get to thinking about it you see what's on the outside. *I see what I look like everyday when I get dressed and it's very ugly. And I've had to deal with that, maybe being my age and not being able to have any more children, not ever. . . .*

Steve: *So the feelings of lack of self-worth are tied in part to a sense of rejection.*

Diana: *. . . And I think the medication I was on, the male hormone, that nearly, I really can see that, nearly destroyed me because I would work hard at being feminine, hard at it. I would be overmade-up and maybe overdressed, I don't know, to try to make up for that. And now since I'm off that, it's like, you know, my whole attitude is changed.*

Steve: But you still sound angry.

Diana: *But there's nothing we can do about it. It's not going to change the fact that. . . .*

Steve: I think your reactions to your feelings of rejection. . . .

Diana: But Steve I've been this way seven years!

Steve: Seven years of anger. Is that what you are saying?

Diana: Yeah, but it's a whole lot better now than it was. We can't change this. *We can't change the way I look!* We can't change the fact that I have cancer and that I feel terrific today but maybe tomorrow I may be just like I was ten months ago.

The Stigma of Cancer

The stigma of cancer in our society has already been discussed.

More need not be said except by way of illustration. Again we hear from Diana. She has just returned from a traumatic experience at a job interview; a process that will be examined in more detail later in this chapter.

Diana: But I'm not willing to lie about it [cancer]. If I can't get the job . . . and it's like the bank that had an opening. . . . And he [the manager] said, "Aha! Terrific I'm not going to have to go through all this. I hate to interview people." You know, "Fine! They are willing to train me," and all this good stuff. . . . And I sat there waiting for him to see my health history, 'cause he goes through it, "good, good, good". . . . And he looks and he just. . . . His mouth just drops open. And you know it all took a complete change. And I said, "I wondered when you were going to see that." He said, "Oh! Now I don't have to go into any more details about it," he said. Then he talked a little bit further. And he was through. *There was this stigma that goes along with cancer* and so. . . .

Amanda: It's not cancer so much as it is a debilitating illness.

Diana: But this is what he said when it was obvious the interview was over. And it was obvious I was hired until he saw the health history. And then he said, "By the way. I am chapter president of The American Cancer Society."

Amanda: You say, "Good! That gives us a lot in common!"

Diana: Yeah. So I thought, "Well, boy! This ought to show your stripes," you know. I ought to get the job just because of that. But I didn't.

Steve: You sound pretty angry right now.

Diana: Because we come here and we try to deal with cancer and we go out into the world and it's thrown right back in our face. You know, gosh you get so built up, you know it seems like I really feel terrific. I've profited from my group. Maybe my confidence has gotten built up. I charge out and I get slapped right back in my face!

Amanda: I'll tell you what. A visit from, what are their initials? . .

Sally: Economic opportunists. . . .

Amanda: Economic opportunists. . . .

Diana: Well, since it's against the law for them to discriminate against cancer, well, he could say anything other than that.

Sally: It's the same thing with age. Same thing with race and color. But it seems to me that in those kinds of circumstances as far as the insurance is concerned, couldn't they have a waiver?

Amanda: I'm not sure, Sally. I think with the larger an organization is the less leeway there is.

Diana: You see, I wouldn't want their insurance. I couldn't get it. But on top of that I wouldn't want it if I could get it.

Sally: Well, it's mandatory.

Amanda: That's it!

Sally: I was thinking about the waiver part of it.

Diana: You know the fact still remains. . . .

Sally: The county, when they would hire somebody with a disability like a veteran for instance or an amputee or something like that. . . .

Diana: They hire people who have diabetes.

Sally: Yea, and I also think they waive that part in the insurance. Well go to the handicapped place.

Steve: The advice and suggestions are helpful in getting you information. . . .

Diana: But what kind of job am I going to get. Working at a table putting? . . .

Amanda: At Goodwill industry?

Sally: I don't know but they have a marvelous. . . .

Steve: Well, it's a rejection because you know you are otherwise able to do stuff. And it's the anger at the man for being such a hypocrite. I mean, I'm feeling that. He was all smiley and then he tells you something; he gives you a little bit of sugarcoated pill and says, "Well, I'm with the local chapter of The American Cancer Society," as if, you know, he's setting you up to pull the rug out from under you. You say, "Well I understand your problem but you have to understand mine."

Amanda: But in his defense now, Steve, 'cause I had just encountered some of the same thing. . . . I was just
horrified, I don't see how anybody stays in business.
If he had said too much to you about why he turned
you down you could have really filed some sort of
complaint or suit against him and there they'd be.

Steve: That may be. That's probably so but nevertheless it
doesn't help, I don't think it helps Diana with her
feelings right now.

Amanda: No, I don't believe it helps Diana, but maybe it could
help somebody else.

Diana: The only thing left for me to do is to volunteer my
services. You know there's plenty of places that
would take me for free without blinking an eye.

Steve: But it's almost gotten to a point where you would
like to be doing something even if it doesn't pay.

Diana: No, I really would like to get paid for it.

Sexual Activity (Sexuality)

Since sexuality is part of one's self-concept, cancer has a
devastating effect. Cancer may make sexual activity impossible.
However, only the broadest generalizations are possible. While
many intimate issues were discussed during our experience together,
curiously, sex was not one of those subjects.

It would seem that there are several reasons that this subject was
deleted. At a fairly concrete level, of those members in regular attendance (Jane, Amanda, Carol, Diana, and Sally) all were widows except Diana. Furthermore, Jane, Amanda, and Sally were older than
age sixty and not sexually active. Carol had had one date since being
widowed and indicated no sexual activity since her husband's death.
Many authors have cited the difficulties regarding the availability of
sexual partners for older men and women. This seems especially
acute in the case of women since their survival rate is significantly
greater than a man's. Cancer could only exacerbate this dynamic.

Because the group was so open regarding a variety of intimate
concerns having to do with bodily functions and social encounters
and because of a collective system of morals and values that might be

considered traditional and conservative, it is doubtful that anyone in the group except Diana was engaged in sexual activity. (Whether they fantasized such activity and/or masturbated was undetermined. Such fantasy activity was never verbalized.)

In Diana's case, one would presume that she had the opportunity for sexual activity with her husband. Interestingly, she never reported such activity as being the case. It is very possible that there was no sexual activity for a number of reasons. One was that Diana's body image was badly scarred from surgery to remove both breasts (radical mastectomy in both cases), both ovaries and interventions to remove excess fluid in the lungs and around the heart. Hollywood aside, it would take a special loving relationship in order for Diana to feel sufficiently sexually confident in her femininity and the expression of femininity to overcome her negative body image. Another condition for sexual activity would be that her husband would have had to overcome perceptual conditioning (bias) and cognitive dissonance in order to free himself sufficiently to become sexually aroused. From other indicators, it is questionable whether or not Diana's husband would have been so inclined.

In the case of couples who are both healthy and who have been married as long as Diana and her husband (approximately 11 years), there seem to be a natural relaxation of the passions of earlier times with regard to sexual expression. Such relaxation seems to result in exploration of creative approaches to sexual fulfillment. Sex becomes more comfortable and less hurried, thus becoming more of an experiment in intimate communication between husband and wife. Ideally, satiation of passion yields to deeper levels of sexual communication for more meaningful loving experiences. In a sense, sex for procreation becomes sex for *re-creation*, a re-creation of the spiritual and philosophical essence of an intimate relationship between a man and a woman. Such activity results in an amalgam of wills, emotions, and soul vital to successfully maintaining courage in an often frightening world.

Of course, the above analysis of sexual experience assumes fairly healthy and "mature" modes of communication between a man and a woman. It further presumes an open, accepting relationship; one which, for the most part, welcomes the challenge of difficult circumstances in the world, frightening as they might be. Sadly, such a relationship did not appear to exist in the case of Diana and her husband. In the case of male-female relationships where passion is at a low level and love making has not grown toward *re-creation*, sex becomes perfunctory and/or non-existent. The personal, marriage, and family problems that arise from such an evolution of sexual activity are voluminous and need not be discussed further. Suffice it to say that it was my perception that the nature of Diana's sexual relationship with her husband was such that sexual activity was virtually nonexistent. Her body image and energy level were so weak as to all but preclude any extramarital activity.

Whether or not the lack of verbalization of sexuality and sexual activity is "normal" for cancer patients is doubtful. It seems that such lacking would be peculiar to the study group. Perhaps one of the group's hidden agendas was that sex would not be discussed. Such lacking may be further attributed to the fact that the members of this group were metastatic, incurable cancer patients.

If Maslow is correct, it would seem, at least for persons whose developmental stage still includes the possibility for reproduction (for instance, in women, prior to menopause), that the more intense the threat to basic survival, the higher the probability of regression from so-called higher levels of being. Since reproduction is a basic survival need for the species, it would seem to follow that the drive for sexual activity would increase proportional to the threat. On the other hand, one supposes that an argument could be made that, for those persons who are transcending toward meeting more "being" needs, the need for sexual activity would diminish inversely to the level of being: The higher the level of being, the lower the need for sexual activity. Such sexual activity that might exist at this level would be solely for *re-creation*. Certainly, more research is needed in this area.

Perhaps more enlightening is the experience of a twenty-two-year-old male Caucasian cancer patient whom I will call Carl. I worked with Carl in individual counseling for several months. Carl was a "free spirit" who dated frequently with many of the dating experiences culminating in sexual intercourse. Carl had testicular carcinoma. He discovered his cancer while performing self-examination of his testicles. Since his type of cancer was particularly dangerous and virulent, the affected testicle was removed. He also has a resection of the retroperitoneal (in the abdomen) lymphatic system in an attempt to prevent metastasis. This resection resulted in an unfortunate, but not unusual, complication. In the course of surgery the nerve regulating ejaculation was severed rendering Carl unable to ejaculate. One of Carl's biggest frustrations was not being able to . . . "shoot my wad." Carl was capable of erection, intercourse, and orgasm. He was not able to ejaculate. Any ejacula secreted collected in the urethra and was passed during urination. This was a definite blow to Carl's body image and, subsequently, his sexuality. His situation demonstrates another dimension of the difficulties surrounding sexual activity and sexuality encountered as a psychosocial dynamic of cancer.

Self-Sufficiency

The psychosocial manifestation of the psychodynamics of loss of control is the ability to be self-sufficient both vocationally and economically. The loss of control in the ability to provide for one's self is second only to fear of being alone. In many of the cases being discussed, self-sufficiency was the most important aspect of existence. With the exception of Diana, all of the women in the group were over the age of fifty. On the other end of the scale, with the exception of Jane, all the women in the group were beneath the traditional retirement age. Furthermore, all of the women in the group except Diana were widowed or divorced. The need to be productive and self-sufficient was a major theme of the group.

Exactly what one considers to be self-sufficiency may be a matter of conjecture. For some persons self-sufficiency includes the ability to find one's way to the unemployment office and collect either social security disability or social security for retirement. Self-sufficiency may be a subsistence level in such cases. However, for middle-class Americans, the utilization of disability benefits, food stamps, and other such "welfare" programs is tantamount to the loss of self-control; the loss of self-sufficiency. For the women in the group such dependence on the welfare system would compromise self-esteem and independence. It would have been humiliating.

Self-sufficiency at a vocational level consists of the ability to seek gainful employment, acquire gainful employment, maintain such employment with the opportunities for maintenance or advancement and the ability to change jobs at will. In an economic sense, self-sufficiency consists of the ability to use funds gained vocationally to maintain a standard of living and be able to meet expenses. The ability to be economically independent directly affects one's sense of self-worth, self-concept, and self-esteem.

Even in the case of Diana, where the husband's income was sufficient to maintain both she and her children at a comfortable standard of living, there seemed to be a need to find gainful employment. Such an ability would allow the cancer patient, in this case Diana, to maintain a sense of dignity: "I could survive if I had to!"

An argument could be made for the fact that many cancer patients might be able to get a sense of self-satisfaction from volunteer work. Jane was a volunteer until three weeks prior to her death. However, while being a volunteer produces some sense of altruism, it does not provide the same sense of satisfaction for most persons that is afforded by having a paycheck as tangible evidence of productivity. The tangible evidence of a job well done is often necessary to provide a base to reinforce altruistic giving.

There is a genuine need for business and industry to make concentrated efforts to afford sufficient flexibility within their scheduling concerns to allow cancer patients to continue as productive members of society through vocational employment and possibly vocational rehabilitation. The sense of independence and dignity could be maintained by negotiating with employers for flex-time and flexible schedules to accommodate the course of the disease and its treatment rather than being dismissed from a job.

The course of cancer is an erratic one. So is the course of treatment. Often chemotherapy and radiation therapy require the cancer patient to be able to have several hours weekly, bimonthly or monthly for the administration of those treatments. Occasionally, treatment causes side effects that may result in hospitalization. Some of the treatments require hospitalization in order for them to be administered and properly monitored. For instance, during the course of counseling it was necessary for Carol to be hospitalized on several occasions in order to monitor drug administration. On at least one occasion during the course of the group, Carol entered a crisis stage that also required hospitalization. In response to her long service and competency, Carol's company allowed her to use all of her sick leave and vacation time, and when that was exhausted, time off without pay. Toward the end stage of Carol's cancer it was necessary for her to be absent from work more frequently. Her company responded in a very flexible and yet accountable manner. Her ability to continue on the payroll even though her work schedule was often erratic and interrupted, allowed her to maintain her health insurance policy, a policy vital to meeting the horrendous cost of chronic end-stage cancer.

Carol was most fortunate. In some cases it is necessary for cancer patients to take jobs that they would otherwise be overqualified for in an effort to maintain survival income or supplement a spouse's income. For instance, one interviewee reported that on crossing state lines, she inadvertently terminated her health insurance policy. When she tried to have the policy reinstated, she was advised that she was not considered a good risk for health insurance coverage. Similarly, her husband's policy would not allow for her coverage for the continuation of a disease already acquired and previously covered elsewhere by another health insurance policy. As a result this woman was extremely distraught over payment of medical bills incurred in the treatment of her cancer. The psychological stress produced by the loss of insurance coverage was sufficient enough to require further medication for situational anxiety. She was unable to participate in our group because she could not afford (financially) to take time for her mental health.

Some of the difficulties just discussed become more evident when reading excerpts from the group sessions. Being as young as she was, Diana felt very much the need to be productive vocationally. The story of her trials and tribulations in finding gainful employment follows. It should be noted that Diana's case is not atypical.

Diana: I started to say, you know, I went in for a job and, you know, I'm not employable and I had filled out applications and filled out applications. You know, I'm getting so I can walk right in and say, you know, are you accepting any applications. And I think this has dealt a blow to my pride. I was telling Steve at lunch I thought I could go and get a job. I really thought I could. I thought my children are in school, I didn't have to work. Maybe that's not a plus in my favor but I really thought I could go out and get a job. And I'm beating myself against a brick wall! If I'm honest and forthright with them, there's just no way.

Amanda: Well I wouldn't tell them anything about my health situation.

Sally:	I wouldn't either!
Diana:	Well, you know, it's on the applications and this is the encouragement I'm getting . . . that eventually they are going to find out about it and. . . . But no one is a big enough person to accept me like I am — it scares them. I want to work in a bank. Hours would work out with school — a day off in the middle of the week would work out with my coming to the doctors.
Amanda:	Big organizations have a very impersonal personnel policy.
Diana:	So, you know, I haven't worked in eleven years either.
Sally:	But you have some working experience?
Diana:	Heavens, yes! I'd do anything!
Sally:	Does unemployment have something to do with it?
Diana:	. . . I guess it does.
Sally:	I think it must have something to do with it.
Steve:	I can't help feeling that to fill out applications like that must give you some feelings of inferiority. It just must kind of be a gut-wrenching thing to have to lie to be worth something to get a job.
Amanda:	I'll tell you, Diana, if you have always gotten jobs fairly easily, well I had that happen to me once, oh a thousand years ago. And . . . I got that application stuck through the window and I was very furious. You need to know what it's like to really hunt for a job. That was the only time I ever had to hunt for one. But it is. It's sort of an upsetting experience.
Jane:	But you know I lied I felt this way about it. I didn't feel guilty. I thought to myself, "They are forcing me to lie." I would prefer not to lie.
Amanda:	Now Jane. . . .
Jane:	But they are forcing me to lie!

Very often, cancer patients are forced to lie about their cancer in order to acquire even part-time employment. Such lying further compounds psychosocial dynamics relating to self-concept in that such behavior further adds to the burden of guilt for having cancer and constitutes a further suppression of affect. Having to lie is humiliating. It encourages the patient to cope by living in a world where the reality forces denial. In Diana's case, even when she told a prospective employer that she wished no hospitalization coverage, the employer informed her that the company required such coverage for all employees whether they wanted it or not. Due to the fact that Diana was "uninsurable," the company would not be able to take the risk of employing her.

In the following segment, Diana began to explore her feelings about being rejected while trying to find employment.

Sally: Diana, is this the first time you have been turned down?

Diana: This is the first time I've seriously looked for a job in eleven years.

Sally: Well, why don't you. . . . I don't know what department, whether its unemployment, but it's with the state labor department down there, across from city hall. If I were faced with this, I think I would go up there just for my own information to the labor department and state my case and ask, "Now what can I do?"

Diana: Yeah, but they are going to say how much money does your husband make and then they'll tell me to go home and enjoy it.

Sally: No they won't!

Steve: Sally, I think what you are trying to do is help her look at alternatives for the job thing and I guess what I'm feeling is that the job situation is just one part of what is going on. It's one part of the anger. I wonder if it wouldn't be more helpful to Diana to try to look at. . . .

Diana: But I wonder how you are going to be able to do that?

Steve: Well, let's just talk about it a little bit. I think Amanda said it and I think you've all said it. "We have to accept that there are certain limitations we are going to encounter in the way people interact with us." The job's just one of the interactions. But you haven't accepted that. You are still angry and bitter about it. I don't know if we can work that through in here. But I think as you talk about it a little bit, maybe we can get a handle on it and help at least get it out to a point where we can look at it.

Diana: But I don't know if I can say any more [pause]. OK, let's look at it this way. I don't have to work. I've never had to work. The first jobs I've ever had the guy said, "I want that girl over there!" *He hired me not on my ability but on my looks. So all of a sudden my looks are catching up with my age.* OK, so I'm being very picky and choosy about where I'm going and always, if they slap it in my face, I can go home and, you know, watch TV.

Steve: Doesn't the work represent part of your *self-worth?*

Diana: Right . . . right!

Steve: *Your self-concept?* "I would like to know that I could support myself if I had to. I would like to know that I have worth in that part of my personhood." And when you are having things like that pulled out from under you anyhow because of the way the doctors treat you, and the way interviewers treat you, and because of the ways some significant people in your family are treating you, it's just one little *dig, so to speak, at your sense of worth and integrity.*

Amanda: And it doesn't help you a bit to tell you that there are people who really have to support a child or children who are going from place to place looking for a job. I mean, that's not your problem. That doesn't help you a bit! It's as if somebody told me, "I never have found any comfort in somebody else's misfortune."

Sally: The employment market, the labor market right now. . . .

Diana: So I wouldn't spend my time to go downtown to the unemployment office. You know, it's not that important. And maybe all I'm really doing is just complaining. You know, maybe. . . .

Amanda: Oh, I don't think you are just complaining.

Steve: I think the word is *venting.* You are just letting all of this out.

Sally: Gosh! She can't just let one instance of somebody looking at your record and saying. . . .

Diana: [shouting] But he's representing all of them!

Steve: He represents lots of people. It's specific to this situation I guess, Sally, that's what I'm feeling. It's specific to this individual case but that man represents a lot of men — a lot of women and men in their interactions.

Continuing with Diana's difficulties in finding gainful employment, a brief passage illustrates the feeling of self-worth that is attached to gainful employment versus the sense of fulfillment that Jane shared regarding altruistic fulfillment through volunteer efforts.

Diana: I know I'm being picky and choosy about where I go and so I'm hitting up against a brick wall.

Amanda: You're not being that picky and choosy to really hope that you don't get one.

Diana: Maybe I just want someone to say, "Yes! We want you!" Then the decision is left on me whether I want it or not.

Amanda: You make the decision.

Jane: You know these are very difficult times and I found myself . . . of course I'm considerably older than you are.

Diana: [scarcastically] Are you subtracting twenty years from your age?

Jane: But I had a rather imposing background in merchandising and when I realized I couldn't get a job. . . . First of all, I didn't even think in terms of cancer — I thought in terms of age. What I did in order to save me; save my sanity. I took a volunteer job and worked at the mental health center and found it a very rewarding. . . .

Diana: But, you know, I've been doing that for eleven years. Having children, you know, I've been volunteering in some way or another. I guess the confidence has gotten built up in me and it's been, I've been coming ten months and I started out in a hole literally with so much gushing over me. OK, and just *these last few months all of a sudden my self-worth has gotten built*

up. *I've begun to think, well, maybe there's
something in me left. OK, but how else can I prove
I'm worth something?*

In the excerpt that follows, Diana shared some reflections on her
feelings about finding a job voiced one week earlier.

Amanda: Diana, I had a thought about you the other day.
  Diana: [sarcastically] Terrific!
Amanda: I really think you should go back to that bank
        manager and say. . . .
  Diana: You know, I don't think I wanted a job that bad. I
        feel like I'm going through a period of time. My feel-
        ings towards this. . . . I think about this. I feel terrific.
        My medication has been changed. But I thought
        about this this morning. As great as I feel and as
        much on top of the problem I can see that if I came
        in today and saw Dr. Norris and he said
        uh-oh . . . and he said it's gotten worse, I feel like I
        would hit rock bottom again. I feel like this is a
        period I'm going through. I'm on top of it, but I've
        been on top of it before.

Resolution is achieved through rationalization. Such resolution
compromises self-esteem and self-worth. Suppression of affect is
reinforced. Denial as coping obviates responsibility. The quality of
existence deteriorates through a harsh reality imposed by society's
ignorance. Hope is strained, tears fall, and muffled cries fuel anger
and resentment. Another nail is driven in the coffin as cancer overwhelms organ systems and sensibility.

OTHER'S ATTITUDES

Since none of us live in a vacuum, much of our sense of self-
worth and self-esteem is determined by the way others perceive us.
It is also determined in both the way we choose to perceive others'
perceptions as well as how we choose to behave in order to either
fulfill or reject others. For the cancer patient, others' attitudes, and
perceptions of others' attitudes are a significant variable in ones
determination, consciously or otherwise, to belong. As we will see in
the next chapter, the attitude of "significant" others, for example
other family members, is an extremely important variable in

psychological and psychosocial adjustment to the cancer process. Since the cancer patient seems to be one who typically suppresses feelings and seems to have difficulties in establishing warm and loving relationships, it is no surprise that as a general rule, cancer patients are extremely sensitive to how others feel about them but seem to be impotent regarding taking action to build closer relationships.

Earlier, we heard Jane accept the possibility that she had responsibility in maintaining her loneliness. Similar types of insights seemed to come into awareness for other group members as well. The patients' perceptions of others feelings and their anticipation of rejection by others seems to fuel the anger process. The slow-burn type of anger also entwines with a self-fulfilling, ominous type of guilt that slowly but gradually serves to reinforce the cancer patient's withdrawal from life. This type of paranoia serves to continue a self-concept of worthlessness and inadequacy. Once again *cancer*, in the psychosocial matrix, reinforces dependency and loss of control.

In the following excerpt the group discussed the difficulties in sharing feelings and thoughts about cancer with other people. It is particularly interesting to note the perception that one must be strong in the face of adversity for the sake of others. It seems consistent, again, with a denial/coping process that "no one can understand my pain, therefore, why should I share it with them?" Also, notice that the subtle animosity and anger towards other people exhibited at the end of the passage seems to be an indirect way of saying, "Why me?"

Diana: I feel like I'm coming across as a very weak person.

Jane: No, I think there is something very warm and very compassionate about Diana. That's why it was very easy for me to talk to her. And the strange part is that even though I revealed the fact that I did have this need when I was ill for somebody to talk to me, nevertheless, the impression that I give is one of self-sufficiency. People will say, "Oh, she doesn't need any help! She's so self-sufficient."

Steve: But isn't that responding to their expectations? Isn't that what people expect you to be and so you respond to it?

Jane: Yeah. And I could be dying! I don't know how to cope with that situation.

Steve: So who are you being fair to? I guess the question I'm asking all of you is, "Who am I being fair to when I get into that kind of a strong world?" Because the expectation in our society is to be strong — to be strong in the face of adversity. I'm not advocating coming apart and coming unglued and just falling apart, but. . . .

Sally: Sometimes I wish I could have that opportunity.

Steve: The opportunity?

Amanda: For five minutes. I don't want to be that way all the time.

Carol: I came unglued when my husband died.

Sally: That's what I'm saying. Sometimes I think, "Well, it looks like the whole world is closing in on me!"

Steve: And you'd just like to have some place or somebody that you could say, "Hey! I have needs for ten minutes of your attention to allow me to lean."

Carol: Well, Diana, I feel that you think that you are sorry for yourself; that nobody has problems as big as yours are. And this is not true.

Diana: You think I feel that way?

Carol: Right. I feel that you feel that you are sorry for yourself.

Diana: I don't know, I've had this for so long that it's just a natural part. Maybe I go on the defensive, and I say I don't because I feel like I can handle this where other people that I know and am close to couldn't handle this. You know, they'd just go all to pieces. Maybe so. I'm open to whatever. If it's self-pity, then I want to acknowledge the self-pity and have it go away.

Carol: I don't want anybody feeling sorry for me because I have cancer. I had no control over it. It was something that just came and I don't want anybody feeling sorry for me. I don't want anybody saying, "Oh, poor Carol! She's had so many problems these past weeks.."

Amanda: But you know I'm not sure that that's sympathy in an unpleasant sense. I think it's that they really care

about you and they are so sorry that this had to happen to you.

Diana: But most of the time people are saying, "Oh, I feel so
terrible about your problem." And in the back of
their mind, they are saying, "Oh, I'm glad it's not me!"

Steve: Better you than me!

Carol: Right!

Many persons do not know how to react appropriately when encountering a cancer patient. One of the reasons that people do not
have this knowledge is due to their own fear and ignorance about
cancer. Many people are subconsciously revulsed by the thought
that the person across from them or who they may have to shake
hands with has a disease that is the "most horrible" of experiences in
life. Another reason seems to be ignorance. Many people feel that
cancer is contagious. There is no scientific evidence to substantiate
this fact at all. But ignorance and bigotry, as we have seen in many
instances in our society, seem to flourish even in the face of a reality
that the "offending" person or process poses no hazard. In other
situations, people mean well but just seem to react inappropriately
because of their own difficulties in sharing feelings at a deep level. In
part this can be attributed to a societal norm that encourages
withholding strong affect. Much of it, however, can be attributed to
the fact that most of us have not taken enough time to feel comfortable with ourselves to really give of ourselves in human interactions.
The cancer patient needs warmth and caring beyond the ability and
levels that most people are able to exhibit. Therefore, in ambiguous
situations where another person encounters one who is known to be
a cancer victim, the awkwardness of the situations often triggers
anger, bitterness, and an increasing sense of isolation in the patient.

In the following excerpt, some of the group members discuss this
problem.

Amanda: Well, Diana has made it very plain. And I can
understand how she feels. You just get sick and tired
of hearing. . . . Like I don't get a gallon of this inspiration business, but I do get a lot of very warm
handshakes. Like I didn't really expect it. But it
doesn't bother me as much as it seems to bother you.
I know what you are talking about. And I also know

Diana: that you are probably a properly well-brought-up young lady who simply cannot bring herself to say, "Oh, shut up!" when they say how great you are.

Diana: No, no.

Amanda: And I'm afraid that's just the penalty you'll have to pay!

Diana: And yet I really feel bad, you know, to even say, "Please don't pat me on the back because I love you and I don't want it." Now I'm going to put you all on the defensive, you know, you're not going to stop. . . .

Carol: You know what I get tired of hearing in the office is, "Oh, Carol, you look tired! Why don't you go home." You know it's two more hours that I can put out. I can't afford to go home all the time. I'm running out of sick leave. If I go home, I get docked. And they say, "Oh, you look so tired." Why don't they just leave me alone? I can make it the next two hours, then I can go home and rest. This is what I have to fight.

Jane: Well, I think I'm the only one here who doesn't have that kind of problem. Nobody seems to pay too much attention to me.

Steve: I appreciate that sharing, but I think we are getting to the core of something here. I'm hearing that you would like to find ways to communicate to people that you don't want that kind of warmth without hurting them.

Amanda: If you can find the ideal solution to that little problem, you've got us bodily!

Steve: Well, I don't know. There's been some people who are a lot more expert than I am who have come up with ways of expressing your feelings without hurting somebody and being just a little assertive.

Amanda: *That's* what you need, Diana!

Diana: Well, to me it would be like hurting somebody and you know. . . .

Steve: I agree, there's going to be people you are going to bump into like you are saying; like at church or at the office. They are going to give you that warm, gooey handshake.

Amanda: That's not fair, Steve! They really mean well by it. It's just not fair.

Steve: But I had a funny thought. I might say something like, "Didn't you expect to see me here?" or something like that, just to be humorous.

Amanda: But that would be unkind. That would put them in a very difficult position.

After all has been said, notice once again the prevailing theme of suppression to preserve the feelings of others. The cancer patient has decided that it is better to suffer and allow the anger to fester inward and fuel the psychological exacerbation of cancer rather than to take the risk of offending another person. Unfortunately, they also seem to fail to take the risk of getting to know other people at deep levels.

One of the difficulties in maintaining relationships with others is that once a person discovers that another person has cancer, fear and ignorance manifest themselves as withdrawal from the patient by the other. While this dynamic has been spoken to earlier, from the cancer patient's point of view, there is an "investment" in maintaining privacy regarding the course of the acquisition of cancer, the course of treatment and the final prognosis. While in some cases this penchant for privacy may seem like denial, in most cases it is strictly a matter of coping with rejection by other people. Employers may exploit the frequency of necessary treatment as a reason for dismissing the patient from employment due to "absenteeism." The real reason may not be the absenteeism, but the effect on the morale of other employees having to work with someone who has cancer (contagion, disfigurement, and so on).

The cancer patient also has an investment in keeping the fact that he or she has cancer from other people. In being accepted by others (peers and superiors), the cancer patient maintains a sense of self-worth and identity. He is able to maintain the concept of being productive and of having control over life. This produces a feeling of well-being through self-sufficiency. By feeling that one is a useful member of society the rejection experienced upon the discovery by other people that one has cancer and all of the inappropriate attending behaviors that accompany this discovery make the cancer patient feel singled-out and isolated from the group. While some isolation may be desired at the unconscious level, the conscious suffers great emotional pain.

The following passage speaks to the point of discovery.

Diana: Well, I think one of the things, yesterday, in signing up at this employment agency was the fact that she didn't ask me about my health and I didn't tell her.

Carol: I don't ever tell if they don't ask.

Diana: It seems like if someone's around very much, well, eventually they know about it. But it seemed so appealing to move here because I would be meeting a whole new bunch of people and nobody would know my health. But, of course, eventually everybody does.

Carol: It comes out.

Diana: Yeah. When you go trotting to the doctor every week.

Amanda: But you know, Diana, you just have to accept that some people are simply not very receptive and they mean so well and they think they understand, but they just don't!

Carol: They don't!

Amanda: That's all there is to it! And you can't make them! So, you sort of have to make allowances.

Steve: Are you saying that that's a skill you acquired over your years of experience and you've been sensitive enough to people to know when certain types of people just aren't receptive?

Amanda: They just really are not. You could knock them over the head with a brick and they still wouldn't.

Steve: Some of you women are more mature and have had more experience in life than she [Diana] has. Was there a time in your lives where you couldn't understand the insensitivity of people to your own situation even before the cancer?

Carol: I have to say no.

Steve: You would say in your own life there wasn't a time when you felt that people . . . when you felt angry with people who couldn't perceive the hurt that you were having?

Amanda: I felt anger, but I didn't feel hurt. Like, "How could you be so stupid?" rather than, "Oh, these people don't understand."

Steve: And you are somewhere in between at this point.

Diana: Because, you know, I don't cry. Maybe if I did that would help.

Steve: You do cry in a way though. Depression is crying inside, isn't it?

Diana: Yeah, OK.

All of the excerpts so far demonstrate the cancer patient's frustration in social situations. In the following brief citation, Diana, Amanda, and Carol share their anger and method of coping with anger in response to others' attitudes.

Diana: But don't you think a lot of people who come up to you and give you the warm handshake and the pat on the back, in the same sense as if they say how are you. They don't want you to tell them how you are. They don't anymore want to know how you are than the man in the moon.

Amanda: I think it's a salvation, because I sometimes need that distance, particularly from the women in the church. And believe me, if you make the fatal mistake of saying how are you, believe me, they'll tell you for about thirty minutes.

Carol: Well, when my friends come up and say how are you, it doesn't matter whether I'm hurting inside or not. I say, "Oh, I feel great today!" And they don't ask me anymore.

SUICIDE

In closing this chapter on the psychosocial effects of cancer, the subject of suicide needs to be addressed. While some may not consider the necessity to list suicide as a psychosocial process, it is this author's opinion that such is the case. The primary justification for grouping suicide as a psychosocial dynamic is the observation that while suicide may be a selfish act of destruction, it is devastating to the survivors. Also, it is often precipitated by mitigating circumstances in the victim's social milieu.

It is often through the use of suicide that one exacts a final revenge upon those seen as either persecuting or insensitive to the pleas for help by the "victim." The use of the word victim is curious because, generally, the society thinks of the actor as victim. However, family and significant others are very often more victimized, for suicide ends any future role of victimization on the part of the actor.

At this point it might be appropriate to make a theoretical statement. On occasion one reads about a cancer patient committing suicide (at times described as euthansia) in an effort to avoid the final anguish and pain of the dying process. These dramatic gestures are often played up in the media. However, during the course of the group, suicide was only mentioned on one occasion and that was by Diana. Suicide is an active commission of expressed affect. If one can consider the possibility that cancer is a "passive suicide" in itself, psychosomatically speaking, theoretically, acting out suicidal feelings or thoughts would seem to be infrequent. It would certainly be interesting to determine the frequency of active suicide and suicidal gestures by cancer patients as opposed to those who never verbalize or act on such feelings.

It was during her initial interview that Diana first shared her feelings about suicide. During this interview she expressed that at times she felt like pressing the accelerator of her car to the floor while she was driving and aiming her car at a concrete pillar and ending all of this. Again, Diana raised the subject during our seventh session as a group. The following excerpt finds Diana sharing her feelings of suicide and Amanda reinforcing that she had similar thoughts from time to time. At the end of the passage the therapist confronted Diana with the possibility that she might be committing *psychological* suicide; stopping her long enough to at least consider the possibility that she might be doing that to herself.

Diana: But I can sympathize with Carl [a young man who was unable to join the group]. Is that his name? I can really sympathize with him.

Steve: With just wanting to end it all and be gone because the pressure gets to be too much?

Diana: Then you made me think about other people and so I began to think about it. But there again you told me to do the very thing that I am doing in talking about suicide. You said you've got to think about the people that are left with the burden of a suicide. OK, but you are telling me I've got to think about these people who I'm thinking about anyway.

Steve: Even so though, sometimes the pressure gets so much that you do think about suicide, that you think about doing away with yourself. And I guess I was just kind of bouncing it off of you when we talked about that individually. I was just trying to look at suicide as one of the alternatives.

Amanda: I think we've all thought about it. I mean I don't think you should take this as all directed at you Diana. It's just kind of a general topic. Anybody who hadn't thought about it. . . . I have not. Maybe because I'm a coward. I just don't want. . . .

Diana: Well you haven't done anything, so you know. . . .

Sally: I have.

Jane: I have.

Steve: What I'm hearing, Diana, is you are putting so much into doing things for other people to make sure that they are comfortable at the expense of your own comfort. And I wonder if that isn't a type of psychological suicide.

Diana: I never really thought of it this way. That's like saying something to do about your [Steve's off-color] language. Though it was very offensive to me. It took Amanda to come out and say something and me saying no, no, no. Because I wouldn't hurt you [Steve] for the world.

Steve: The feeling I get from you is that you underestimate me. You are not allowing me the responsibility for my feelings. You are saying that you are so strong that your strength can support not having to hurt me. That you'd rather suffer — hurt yourself than have to hurt me. And what that does to me is makes me feel that you are not being honest with me.

Diana: And I guess I never would have been.

Chapter 3

THE FAMILY

NOW that psychological effects and psychosocial dynamics of cancer have been discussed, it is important to direct attention to the primary unit in which the cancer patient (and indeed all of us) finds himself. This unit, of course, is the family.

In all of our lives, the family is the most influential environmental factor governing behavior. The cancer patient is a member of the family at several different levels. First of all, the cancer patient is a child. Whether parents are alive or dead, that aspect of the cancer patient's existence is carried throughout life.

For the cancer patient, the role of a child is the chief role that he plays in the family once the disease has been contracted. If, for instance, the cancer patient choses not to be married, such as in the case of Carl, then he moves into an adult-child role without having any spouse or parenting role in the so-called traditional family. In nontraditional settings, such as cohabitation with another person without contractual obligations of a marriage, the person may find himself in the role of spouse.

For the cancer patient who is married, the role of spouse or parent is another level at which one experiences the family. For those persons who are in the role of spouse, in the presence of their own children, they are also in the third role: that of parent. The parent role is one of authority and leadership. Whereas, in the role of the child, one can be very dependent; and in the role of spouse one can be interdependent; from the child's point of view at least, the parent is supremely independent and fully functioning. As such, one is able to make decisions and impose on children some of those decisions. As a parent one has the responsibility of being consistent with loving discipline.

Having outlined three primary roles as a family member (child, parent, and spouse), it is also important to note ancillary roles. In these roles one may be an aunt, uncle, cousin, godparent, and so on. These are roles within a family system that may differ with intensity, depending on certain variables. For instance, in some cultures being an aunt or uncle carries with it tremendous responsibilities for nurturance and guidance of the younger generation. In other ethnic groups, aunts and uncles may not even be blood relatives. For instance, in the case of a friendship, one might be introduced as an aunt or uncle to the friends' children. The role of aunt, uncle, or cousin is more important in the concept of the extended family than in the immediate family. At the extended level, one is expected to perform in a loving, autonomous, and approachable fashion. It is a question of responsibility to love without being "responsible."

The role of sibling is a fourth role and an important one. Sibling relationships often determine modes of interaction in society as one becomes an adult. After a person has left the biological family unit, the role of brother or sister shifts significantly. It may become a role of distance or it may become a role of close, loving friendship. Often the expression "you can choose your friends but not your relatives" is heard. Many times these are normal feelings that persons have toward siblings and "inherited" siblings, such as brothers-in-law or sisters-in-law. As a result the old nemesis of guilt is often subliminally present in that if one does not care to affiliate with a sibling, one may have feelings of guilt due to parental injunctions stating that the primary relationship is paramount throughout life. It's as though the expression "blood is thicker than water" is used for manipulation toward forcing a relationship that otherwise might not exist. For the cancer patient, sibling difficulties become more pronounced and more complex from the onset of cancer. Oftentimes well-meaning brothers or sisters will offer cancer patients who are widowed (widowers) a place to live. Such was the case with Carol. A sister of hers in Minnesota had invited her to come and live with her during the last weeks of her life. Such invitations offer difficult choices for the patient: to go or to not go, to be gracious and accept, or hurt feelings and reject.

Often brothers and sisters volunteer such care out of guilt and anxiety. Afterall, what kind of a brother or sister would allow a blood relative to die without trying to somehow intervene? The guilt becomes compounded because the cancer patient is often aware that the offer is made out of responsibility more than out of a genuine, loving concern for the dilemma of the patient. The cancer patient (and this is sometimes the case of parents who take their children in as well) begins to feel even more burdensome because of the guilt-

offered care. For the patient this dynamic perpetuates a sense of loss of control, frustration, and hostility towards life in general and the disease process in particular. Often these dynamics seem to be manifested indirectly in asides since, as was earlier explored, the cancer patient has such difficulties expressing feelings to those he or she cares about.

Cancer patients belong to family systems that are "centripetal" in terms of communication patterns. The centripetal family typically reacts to stress with stoicism and the isolation of family members, forcing family members to deal with the crisis with a "stiff upper lip" and to depend upon their own emotional resources. When cancer strikes such a family, there seems to be a tendency for family members to continue reacting in a communication pattern to which they had become accustomed. Therefore, the stress of a family member having cancer and the possibility of dying may produce a "stoic isolation." While the children of a cancer patient may react in frustration and even some panic, their actions often seem to be more indirect than direct. For instance, when Amanda refused to cooperate with chemotherapy alleging that she would rather die with dignity, her daughter became very panicky and proceeded to call the oncology unit. Rather than intervening directly with mother and trying to communicate concern, the daughter avoided painful confrontation in the family unit indirectly by attempting to manipulate the oncology department. In the case of other group members, it seemed that the primary family reacted more typically in withdrawal from the patient. The patient complied willingly, suppressing anger at being isolated and rejected.

In examining the cancer patient as a family member (as a child, a parent, an uncle/aunt, a cousin, a brother/sister), it is fitting to address the issue of the cancer patient as a grandparent. As grandparents, persons are free to attempt to correct self-perceived errors of parenthood made at the expense of their own children. It is a situation in which love and affection withheld from children can be projected onto the grandchildren in an apparent effort to make amends and to demonstrate that reconciliation is possible. It is also an effort to express love unconditionally, for as a grandparent there is very little responsibility (generally) for the outcomes of childhood management.

The role of grandparent is also a milestone. People often offer

silent prayer and consider their lives fulfilled if granted the attain-
ment of a mature age. This ideal age is determined by the criterion
of living ". . . long enough to see ones grandchildren." The ability to
see one's grandchildren is seen as the end of the primary responsibility for siblings. It is though the seed has been planted and the tree has
grown and borne fruit. It is now time for the "harvest." The harvest
may be seen as grandchildren. Success is the enjoyment of the fruits
of one's labor in raising children through the practice of uncondi-
tional love for childrens' offspring. Often this is the time for reconciliation between parent and child over strife that has occurred
throughout the family's history. This is particularly true if the relationship between the parent and child has been a stormy one.
Grandchildren are often significant factors in deepening loving relationships between parent and child. They can also be a devisive element in the relationship between parent and child in that parents as
grandparents often interject their modes of child management in the
form of advice with regard to the management of grandchildren.

An in depth analysis of family dynamics is not the purpose here.
Essentially, it is important to be aware of the many different roles
regarding family dynamics in order to appreciate the immense struggle that the cancer patient has in coping with the onset, progress,
and ultimate course of cancer.

To illustrate these dynamics, it is best to examine, case by case,
the relationship between group members and their respective
families. Jane, Sally, Carol, and Diana all verbalized the difficulties
they were having in helping their families cope with the process of
cancer and regarding the management of family dynamics. Only
Amanda did not share significant difficulties regarding her daughter.
However, Amanda did share some thought and feelings concerning
"little Amanda" from which difficulties with her family might be
discerned.

AMANDA

The most interesting aspect about Amanda and her relationship
with her only child, a daughter, was that her daughter's name was
also Amanda. As stated previously, "little Amanda" was the one who
attempted to manipulate Amanda into chemotherapy in an indirect
fashion by contacting the oncology unit. In general, the closer a rela-

tionship, the more direct the communication. The relationship between Amanda and her daughter may have been one of some
distance and difficulty.

It was also Amanda who discovered the lump in her breast while
playing with her granddaugher. On the surface such an event may
seem to have been happenstance, and quite possibly it was.
However, at a deeper level, imagine the connection between
discovering a life-threatening disease while also discovering intimacy
with a grandchild. The course of discovery of cancer while playing
with a grandchild was even more significant in lieu of the fact that
Amanda saw her grandchild at infrequent intervals.

At the very time that Amanda had an opportunity to function as
a grandparent and rectify some of the distance between she and her
daughter, her life began to end more imminently. Perhaps several
factors combined to produce the psychological environment that
allowed the breakdown of Amanda's immunosuppressive system
permitting the cancerous aberration of her tissues. While just a supposition, it would appear that widowhood was not as significant a
trauma to Amanda as having her only daughter and namesake leave
her home ("breast") to move almost 1,000 miles away. The loss of
that relationship may have been the catalytic factor in the body's unconscious relaxation of defenses. The birth of a granddaughter sym-
bolizing the end of a significant role for Amanda as mother and the
beginning of a new role of lesser significance (grandmother) may
have further contributed to this hypothesized breakdown.

The loss of the "significant something" in Amanda's life may have
included the loss of her role as primary figure for her only daughter,
a significant love object for most of Amanda's productive years. It
may have been the primary psychological factor in the onset of her
disease. The loss of Amanda's vitality and ability to continue in her
job as a top-level administrator could also have been an object of
loss. However, Amanda voluntarily left her full-time position when
the course of her disease was pronounced as metastatic and incurable.
Therefore, since leaving her job was after the fact, the suggestion was
that the significant loss was of a love object (in her daughter, Amanda).

DIANA

Many instances have been illustrated regarding Diana's verbalizations. It comes as no surprise that, therefore, many of the family problems caused by the intervention of cancer are exemplified in Diana's case.

Diana was a person who acted out because of her overt anger and denial of that anger. In the following excerpt, Amanda was confronting Diana and the group as to whether or not Diana had considered confronting her husband and children with the fact that at particular times she just did not feel well. As the dialogue continued, Diana began to verbalize many of the frustrations that she had experienced with cancer. She acknowledged that she was engaged in a charade with her family.

Amanda: Diana, I wonder what would happen if sometime when you really don't feel good, if you would say, "Now look. I don't feel so good today. Now just let me feel bad. Don't bother me. I'm going to feel better tomorrow. I know I will. But just kind of let me be sick today!"

Diana: OK. Then they would. And the house would be very quiet. And everybody would get in a very somber mood.

Steve: Well, why would it be quiet?

Diana: Because, "Mother" doesn't feel good.

Steve: Well, who communicates that the house should be quiet because mother doesn't feel good?

Diana: That's just the way it is. Not that my husband is telling the girls to be quiet or this type of thing, but you know. . . .

Amanda: But you need to "feel" once in a while. And they need to just let you feel bad. You're not planning to do this on a permanent basis. You are going to bounce back. "But I just kind of have to have a day off today."

Jane: You know, I don't think it's rather unusual for people to respect a person who doesn't feel well. I think if a person doesn't feel well, that generally there isn't a lot of noise and people do consider. . . .

Steve: You [Diana] sound like you are taking that personally. That it's personally your fault that everybody should be feeling cheerful all the time and they shouldn't be made to suffer because you have cancer. They should have a normal kind of life. And what you are saying is that a "normal" life means happiness and that we all pretend and play charades and I guess I'm wondering about that.

Amanda: Because, you see, if your illness was a stomachache or a headache, nobody would think anything about it. But the fact that you do have cancer; whenever you say you don't feel well, it's an enormously threatening statement because the next thing that pops into their heads [or immediately thereafter] is, "She's going to die." And it just is hard for them to handle. But I think maybe Steve's right. You ought to give them the privilege of sharing some of this.

Steve: Like what would happen, for instance, if you would say something to the effect with your family, "I'm not feeling too well today and it's important for me to rest. I'm down. I'm feeling a little depressed. And it's not your fault."?

Diana: And they are not going to say anything! They never do say anything!

Steve: I'm not sure that's important. Just let me finish. And then say to them that "I know that you are afraid when I get sick because I have cancer that I'm going to die; that this may be the final time that I'll get sick. But that's not how I'm feeling right now. I'm just a little depressed. I don't feel that kind of sickness so I don't want you all, you know, worrying too much about that." I wonder what would happen if you were more honest about it?

Amanda: This may be a process of education, Diana. The first time they are going to tippy-toe around with faces *that* [indicated with hands] long and then the next time it won't be quite so bad because you will have bounced back in the meantime. And pretty soon they might treat you very casually when you don't feel well.

Diana: I don't know. It's always been this way. I have an eight-year-old who's not known anything. On Sundays I rest or read a book during the week and my children know I have cancer. But I don't think it's something I could sit down and say.

Steve: Right. Is it possible that the charade that you play is communicated to them and they play their own charade because they don't know how else to act around you?

Diana: OK, that could very well be.

Steve: And maybe the reason they don't talk to you about it is because you've never given them, and I put this in quotes, "permission" to talk to you about it because you want to suffer in silence.

Diana: OK!

Steve: But what I'm feeling you are doing is you are eating your heart out. But then when we see you, because it's free in here, you just let it all go. You are loud. You are angry. You are frustrated. And that's OK for in here. But the fact is that maybe you are unwittingly setting this thing up to happen because you are not giving your family permission. You are not saying, "It's OK to talk about my cancer and the fact that I'm depressed and the fact that I might be dying." That, "It's OK for you to have those feelings. Don't feel guilty about those things, they are going on in me too." Open the doors so that some other people can talk to you about it. And sure, there might be tears and there may be pulling of hair and jumping up and down, but it's out there where you can deal with it. And to me, that might make more support, I don't know how you feel about it.

Diana: I don't know.

Amanda: I would disagree with Steve a little bit about the depression. That too has connotations that people frequently are not able to handle. Physical illness they can sort of understand, but anything that borders on mental illness they get awful uptight about. And they might have thoughts about it. "Oh, she'll do something to herself!"

Diana: Well, I don't know. It's been like this, Steve, for so

	long, that if the way I am has caused them to be the way they are, it works to make everybody happy. You know the children. . . .
Steve:	Everybody except you.
Amanda:	Except you!
Steve:	And I'm not sure. . . .
Diana:	But actually, *you don't know!!*
Steve:	You don't know if they are happy because you are all playing a charade with each other. Do you see what I'm saying? I mean, my guess is that if you are playing a charade, maybe they are doing the same thing because they think that's what makes you happy.
Diana:	OK! That could very well be.
Steve:	So there's no communication.

Interestingly, Amanda, in her counseling role, offered Diana suggestions. Significantly, in Amanda's own life, she had difficulty in following her own advice.

In the next excerpt, Diana continued her dialogue with Amanda and the therapist. Here she discussed the difficulty in verbalizing her problems with cancer with her children. Again, the possibility of a charade is approached from the standpoint that perhaps the reason that Diana's children responded to her in what she described as a "normal" way instead of more involved way was because they did not know what Diana wanted them to do in terms of responding.

Diana:	But I don't see how we can sit around a table and talk about . . . you know with the kids there.
Amanda:	Well, I would think that would be very hard on you.
Diana:	You know, I try to make their lives as normal as possible and I think about. . . . I probably talk with my mother and dad more about the way I feel than I have. . . .
Steve:	Can I ask you this? If it were another problem besides cancer and it were causing this much of a breakdown in communications in the family, would you not discuss it?
Amanda:	What if you had migraine headaches? I mean real ones where you had to go to bed and pull the shades down and you were sick and everything like that. You would not only expect them to let you be sick.

	You would . . . they would have to! Because you would be incapacitated.
Diana:	But the thing about it is, I'm not sick! I mean not really sick. I may have a terminal illness, but I'm not sick!
Steve:	But have you told them that? Have you sat down and said, "Look, I know you love me and I know you think what you are doing is making me feel good, but I'm not sick right now. The disease is a long-term, progressive one and right at this moment I'm not particularly ill."?
Diana:	Yeah! But they are not treating me any way. Everything appears to be normal on the home front.
Steve:	Maybe they don't know what you want.
Diana:	I want it to be like it is because I think what we've got going is really something good. And I think when the day comes and their mother dies, that they are not going to remember a sick, mully, grubby, complaining mother. They are going to remember someone who was good.

Immediately following the above exchange, the therapist confronted Diana with the fact that what she seemed to be saying was that were she happy with the status quo (i.e. if she was happy with the way in which she was relating to her children), she would not sound so angry (both verbally and nonverbally). Interestingly, Diana reinforced what had been suspected all along. It came as no surprise that she was grieving over those parts of her life that she would not be able to share with her husband and children. Symbolically, most of the things she seemed to grieve were those material milestones that mark most upwardly mobile, young couple's lifetimes.

Steve:	If you were happy with the way it is you wouldn't be angry.
Diana:	OK! It has created a problem in me because I can't tell you what I'm fighting. It's the fact that I'm living with death and I'm thirty-two years old! And I would like, you know, I want my husband to go up in his company. But I want him to do it so that I can enjoy the things that it's going to bring. OK! Therefore, it makes me unhappy to think that most probably I

won't enjoy those things. But what can be done? What can be done about that? OK, I would like to play tennis, and I do play rarely. But it's just that I'm very limited in what I can do. But that's still . . . that's me! And it's something that even though I can't deal with it, I'm going to have to live with it. You know . . . say my husband's not going up in the company any faster than he's going up. I can't buy everything I want because there's not enough money to buy it. I've always tried to, you know. They say live every day and all this. The hell with it! Someone who's limited. . . .

Amanda: I think that sums it up!

Diana: The person who wrote that [live every day. . . .] didn't have a terminal illness and it's just that we can't plan for the future, Steve! We can't! We can say, well we'd like to go to Washington, D. C., next summer. . . .

Amanda: Yes, you can! Yes, you can!

Diana: But I think inside, "Who knows?"

Steve: But you are eating your heart out today. I'm not saying live each day as it comes, but I'm saying, in not planning for the future and being afraid for the future, in a sense, and being angry about the future and feeling all those pressures, you are missing today.

Diana: Yeah! But as we talk about going to Washington, D. C., I'm thinking inside, "Am I going to be able to?" I don't say to my husband, "Am I going to be able to?" He thinks I'm going to live to be seventy.

Steve: You said it to us! You said it to us!

Diana: He's never thought I was going to die! I've always thought I was going to die! He really thinks and it's craziness! He really thinks I'm going to live to be a little old lady and it doesn't help by me saying I probably won't live to see thirty-five.

Steve: I think what I'm hearing now is that you want . . . you wish you could communicate with him the reality without hurting him.

Diana: Yeah! But by me saying. . . .

Steve: . . . So that you could feel better about what's going on.

Diana: OK! But what's on the inside of me would only pull him down. If I said the things that I say to you, it would only make him unhappy. He would worry about me. He has an awesome responsibility in his job, plus the responsibility of having a wife who has cancer. So if I vent all of my feelings on his. . . .

Steve: So you just eat your heart out.

Diana: So I just eat my heart out! It's OK!!

Steve: It's not OK! If it were OK, you wouldn't be angry. I'm going to keep hitting you with that.

Amanda: Well, Steve, let me tell you something! Let me tell Diana something! [to Diana] If this is a deliberate choice and it's a price you are willing to pay for keeping everything on a normal keel, then pay it and shut up about it!

Diana: Right!

Notice that in Diana's verbalizations of her frustration about not being able to plan for the future and to be able to be a part of her family's milestones as the family matures, Amanda emphasized that missing those milestones, for Diana, must be the most tragic aspect of her condition. Suddenly, feeling as though Diana was confessing an innermost fear, Amanda supported her by suggesting that Diana plan for the future and attempt to make plans to make a trip to Washington, D. C., the following year. The therapist began to confront Diana with her apparent need to try to make the most of each day and let the future be what it will be. However, immediately after doing so, the the therapist also succumbs to supporting Diana in what surely must be gut-level, anticipatory grief by encouraging her to plan for the future. In a sense, it is encouraging her denial/coping. Finally, near the end of the previous excerpt, Amanda rallied to Diana's support confronting the therapist and retreating from her assertion that perhaps it might be better to discuss feelings generated by cancer with loved ones. Of course, Diana "parachutes," picking up Amanda's "conspiracy of silence" by saying, "Right!" This interaction gives one a look into the innermost, intimate thoughts of the cancer patient (Diana) and how infrequently and intermittently such intimacies are shared. This is one of the real tragedies of cancer: the *conspiracy of silence.*

The tragedy of the conspiracy of silence is verbalized further in the following excerpt. The word *trapped* triggered further self-disclosure by Diana regarding the dilemma she found herself in through being more open with her loved ones. Notice that Diana was confronted regarding her rationale for perpetuating the conspiracy of silence and vehemently defended her intent to continue her charade. She was supported adamantly by Amanda. After some intense confrontation, Sally confronted Diana with the fact that if Diana were at peace with her decision she might not have the inner turmoil exhibited during this session. Jane confronted the possibility that Diana had tremendous guilt feelings about her illness and that the only way that she might absolve her guilt was by suffering in silence. This seemed to be a tremendously accurate insight, for Diana continued to talk, stating that she was putting her family through hell.

Diana verbalized her need to protect her husband. She then related how much grief he had gone through when their eleven-year-old daughter was born and almost died. Diana was then confronted by the therapist to the effect that her verbalization of her inner turmoil might be a sign of weakness. She acknowledged that such was the case and that somehow everything would work out for the best. Diana continued to rationalize and resist the challenge being put to her: to share her "self" with her family. She asserted that the problem was essentially hers and not theirs. Other group members particularly Sally, reiterated the importance that Diana reach some solution that would bring peace to her self. Emotionally, Diana began to vent the extreme difficulties that she had gone through since the onset of her cancer through a cycle of onslaughts by the disease and remission. While Diana verbalized that her disease might never go away, with the group's cooperation, the therapist continued to confront the need for her to improve the relationship with her husband to bring her more peace of mind. The therapist confronted her more vigorously and repeatedly with occasional support and insights from the group. It became obvious that Diana's resistance toward sharing feelings of anger with her family was firmly entrenched.

Eventually, Diana shared the pain that she has suffered on a least two occasions where she had been given predictions of ". . . six months to live." She related as to how aggravating such predictions were to her mental health. Diana verbalized the fact that perhaps her mental outlook would be different if she were in her fifties, like most of the other members of the group, as opposed to being thirty-two. From the vantage point of thirty-two, there was more of life to be grieved for than for someone closer to the societal norm for dying.

Toward the end of the session, Diana acknowledged that she was not satisfied with her conspiracy of silence. She verbalized that she must be rebelling against her decision to maintain the silence and that this perhaps was causing the inner turmoil. Diana verbalized her admiration for Amanda's apparent strength, for it appeared that Amanda was at peace of mind and not as angry. Of course *appeared* is the key word. Finally, Diana left what might be interpreted as an opening for behavioral change at the end of the excerpt — that perhaps Amanda's sense of peace would "rub off" on her.

Amanda: Don't you think it's a feeling that you are kind of trapped?

Diana: Yeah, but I know I'm going to have to live with this.

Sally: She doesn't see another way out.

Diana: Right. And I know sometimes that it nearly blows the top of my head off. I realize that and I think the times I've come in here and blown and gone back out.

Steve: Don't you think you communicate that out in the outside world?

Diana: Steve, I really don't! I promise you, I really don't!

Steve: My guess is that your nonverbal behavior communicates your charade. That it is an act. But I can't be sure because I've never seen you outside of here.

Diana: You know I really don't think it does because it's like a button is switched off when I leave here and I go home.

Steve: But that's not how you are reporting about how your children and your husband react to you whenever you go off — that they don't act honestly with you. They don't react honestly the way you would think they would react. What you are saying is you can't really tell how they feel because when you are down they are down. When you are up, they are up. So my feeling is they are mimicking the way you are coming across. Your charade. . . .

Sally: They *are* down when she's down. That's right!

Steve: It's the way you are coming across nonverbally.

Diana: But most probably, Steve, if I had nothing worse than a migraine headache, if mother doesn't feel good, your family has to be the same way. Your little girls sense when your wife feels good or feels bad and so when she feels bad and they know mother feels bad, well, then normally as they get older. . . .

Steve: Aren't you doing with your family what you accused some of the doctors of doing with you? Not telling them the whole truth?

Diana: But I don't see what good it would do.

Amanda: I think you are right about the children's reaction.

Diana: And I want to be able to handle it and not blow up all of the time.

Steve: Now, I think we can help you with that because I think there is a way to handle it without having to devastate your family.

Diana: I'm rejecting everything you are saying because it works outside! My children are very happy, you know, they do well in school. They get along well with other people, you know. There are signs if there is a problem. My husband and I have a beautiful relationship. We really do. And I feel like things are going to have to keep going the way they are going, even though I know sometimes I. . . .

Amanda: It's a high price, but you are willing to pay it.

Diana: Right!

Steve: I guess what I'm feeling is . . . the frustration that I'm feeling. . . . I guess you pick up on my frustration.

Diana: Right! And if anything is worked out with my anger, it's something that I'm going to have to do without involving my family.

Steve: Well, let me bounce off part of where my frustration is coming from, OK? You've got a limited life expectancy. I mean that's something you've shared with me and you are aware of, and what I'm frustrated about is that I'm hearing that in the real world you are holding back anger. I'm not advocating going out and blasting everybody in your family with your anger. If that's the way I'm coming across, that's not what I'm trying to say. But with a limited life expectancy and playing a charade at the expense of yourself because of the risk of destroying what seems to be, from what you tell us, an idyllic relationship for a woman with cancer and her family, a lot of love and caring there. . . . What I'm feeling is how much more enriched the relationship could become; how much deeper it could become; how much more meaningful and closer you all could become in the challenge of the limited life expectancy.

Diana: OK! Let me tell you. . . .

Steve: How long do you put that off, I guess?

Diana: OK! If I go home and I unload on my husband the way I feel, do you know what he's going to do? He's going to put his arm around me and he's going to pat me on the shoulder and he's going to tell me what a good sailor I am. Right now I've had that from other people. But I don't have that from my children and my husband. And if I go home and I unload what's on the inside . . . because you know it came to a boiling point this summer and they put me in upper gate [mental exhaustion and depression] and Cindy talked to my husband and you know she said, "It's nerves. There's nothing wrong with her." But still at that time it came to a boiling point and it will again.

Steve: Because when he would tell you, you know, that you are a good sailor and a good soldier, that would be condescending.

Diana: Because that would be just what everybody else is doing. It's telling me, "Boy, you are really handling this!"

Steve: I wonder what would happen with him if he did that and you said, "You know, that's what everyone else does to me. And that makes me madder than anything because you are not treating me as a person. You are treating me as a make-believe fairy princess and I don't like that!" I mean, it seems to me that the interaction stops prematurely; that you never got to finish; that you weren't just venting; but you never got to express. . . .

Diana: But you see, he's been through this with me! He is just as involved in it as if he had had cancer himself because he's been told all the bad things first and then it's come to me. So he is just as emotionally involved in this as I am. In fact he probably has his own problems facing the fact that he's not . . . maybe . . . not going to have a wife someday.

Amanda: He might want to blow up too!

Diana: Yeah!

Amanda: Each one of them is trying to protect the other and I don't know that that's bad!

Steve: I don't know that that's good.

Diana: But what I'm saying is, you know, it would kill me to probably know the way he really feels.

Steve: I don't think so. I think you are stronger than that.

Diana: Maybe so. But I'd still have to carry that around. And maybe the four of us are playing a charade and I go right back to what I said before. I just don't see any. . . .

Steve: I wonder if it could be any worse than what you are carrying around right now: the anger, the frustration, the bitterness of not knowing, the lack of feeling of worth. I guess what I was hearing Jane saying a while ago — not knowing and fantasizing what could be going on could be worse than what's actually going on. I mean, there's a risk on both sides. I think you are right.

Amanda: I do know as far as your children are concerned. . . . I remember this from my childhood. . . . And I think my own child felt the same way. . . . Mothers aren't supposed to get sick. Mammas aren't ever supposed to be tired and feel bad or anything. And when you get old enough to realize that they do, it's an awful jolt. I remember my daughter saying, you know the first time I found out you couldn't do everything, anything. . . . It was an awful jolt to me because they really feel that way. And yours are that young. They think you can do anything. Mamma can fix it. And you just hate to undermine that image.

Steve: How are you [Diana] feeling right now?

Diana: I'm feeling just like I felt when we started this. There really isn't . . . it's going to have to be this way.

Steve: Of course, that's your decision.

Diana: Well, I feel like it's the best one! I feel like it's worked up until now. Steve, if we are living in a fantasy world, it's brought us all pretty close together and we've got something very special at our house and we probably wouldn't have had it if I had been a very well person. And I can't see it changing; I can't see me changing.

Steve: I think there are three ways it could go. It could continue the same way; it could go in a negative direction . . . your worst fears, you know . . . just maintaining the way you are now. . . . It could get worse or it could get better. And I guess I'm trying to look at how it could get better. And I guess that's what we are all trying to share with you. At least that's what I was trying to share.

Diana: OK! You've heard it all. It's like we all heard Jane. OK! You've all heard the same thing! Do I take a stick and hit it?

Amanda: No! I'll tell you if you want to know how I feel about it. I think you have grown; and I think you are intelligent; and I think you have a lot more strength than you give yourself credit for. And I think you are making a deliberate choice and you have the right to make that choice. *And if you are willing to pay whatever psychic price is involved, OK! Pay it and just don't feel that somehow you should be doing something else! Your house is running smoothly. Everybody is happy. And if you've got to be something of a sacrificial lamb, OK! It's worth it to you!* And I think you've made that deliberate deci-

	sion. And I personally think you have a perfect right to.

Diana: *But if I made it, and I think I have, somehow I'm not satisfied with it or I wouldn't blow up.*

Steve: I don't think you are satisfied. Well, how does the rest of the group feel? I noticed I didn't see a lot of agreement over here with what was just said. You feel differently [to Sally]?

Sally: Well, I just. . . . Each one of us are individuals. We have our own way to work out our own problems. But I know one thing. If I have a decision to make, I've got to be at peace with myself when that decision is made. And I'm just thinking about. . . . She's not at peace.

Steve: You are talking to Diana now?

Sally: Yeah!

Steve: Well, try to look at her.

Sally: [looking at Diana] Well, if you are not at peace with your decision, naturally, you are going to continue to have that inner turmoil. But some way or other, somehow there's got to be an answer so you can get your peace and I think if you get your peace internally, then you are going to feel fine.

Diana: But I'm going to have to get that peace within myself and not by unloading on those who are closest to me.

Sally: I never have gotten peace from anybody else.

Steve: I guess the word *unloading* is starting to bother me too because that's how I must be coming across, but that's not what I'm saying.

Sally: I think and pray about my situations and I usually get my answer. And I'm not saying that I've always done right. If I make a mistake, I accept it and try to profit and go on. You can't go back.

Steve: There's a difference for me between *sharing* versus *unloading*, and I'm going to make a distinction. Sharing is a way of expressing your feelings: "This is how I feel. I'm not accusing anyone in here and I'm not trying to make you all feel bad, because I know you love me and you care about me and this is just how I feel." Now "unloading" is saying, "Not only is this how I feel, but it's all your fault! And I've been carrying this around for eight years." Now that's a little different.

Jane: [to Diana] My feeling has been that you have a tremendous guilt feeling about the fact that you are sick and that you feel that the only way to make it up to your family is for you to condone this: to suffer through it; not to disturb the status quo in any way. And I think personally that there are certain considerations that you deserve, and that. . . .

Diana: You know, but I've put my family through hell!! *Literally through hell!*

Steve: But you see, this thing is taking its toll on you anyhow. Even if you think you've got it under control, the fact that you've shared with us; the fact that you laid it on the line; that it came to the boiling point last summer; that you were in the hospital and it was nerves. . . .

Amanda: May I ask how it came to a boiling point? I'm not familiar with that.

Diana: I don't know. It just . . . it comes out of my body. I know what's wrong with me! And I start having . . . my legs hurt; my back hurts. . . . I start having symptoms of all various kinds and I know what it is. But I can't do anything about it!

Steve: And if I were your husband, let's say for instance, I wonder how I would feel seeing this happen to you? I wonder if I might feel that I had a part. . . . If I might not be feeling some guilt that "Gee! This is my fault Diana is this way. What could I have done to have prevented this? Because this has something to do with her illness." But it's honestly psychological. I mean, it's primarily in your head instead of a result of the cancer if I'm reading you right. And I wonder what kinds of feelings would be going on in me as your husband: "If I really love and care about you. And by sharing your feelings with me and letting me

	carry part of this, that I could have prevented that kind of devastation, that kind of hospitalization."
Diana:	OK! Maybe we don't have that kind of relationship because Diana tries to be strong. You know . . . immediately. . . . I can remember last summer, when they called him and he came up here and they said, "This is our plan of action and this is why we are doing it." And, you know, immediately I said, "Why has this happened . . .?"
Steve:	What you may be saying to your husband is that "Diana is strong" and that you are not!
Diana:	Yeah!
Steve:	I mean, you may be saying that without saying it.
Diana:	That's like when our eleven-year-old was born. She nearly died and he cried and I didn't. Because I didn't cry! Because one of us had to be strong!
Amanda:	Men are bad about that, *I'll tell you!*
Steve:	I beg you pardon?
Amanda:	Listen! Actually, the one time my late husband went with me to the pediatrician just because he wanted to see what was going on. And Amanda had to have a measles shot, or a DPT, or something like that. Do you know that grown man asked the office nurse to hold that baby and I said, "What'll you do if she ever really gets sick?" He said, "I'll do anything to keep her from getting sick!" Men are weaklings in that sense.
Diana:	OK! Maybe eleven years ago started out this way and maybe I began. . . .
Steve:	Let me say this . . . another thing I'm hearing. I'm not sure you are saying this. Maybe it needs to be cleared up. It is that sharing feelings, anger, and turmoil that's inside yourself is a sign of weakness.
Diana:	Yes! We've said these same things before, have we not girls? I mean, you know. . . . You're not bringing in anything that hasn't been said before.
Steve:	I'm just asking. I'm just wondering out loud. . . . Is that the case?
Diana:	Yeah! I guess it is! But apparently for my self-confidence, it's very important for me to be on top

	of this.
Steve:	Well, is what you are going through psychologically now a sense of strength?
Diana:	Somehow. . . . Somehow it'll be OK.
Amanda:	Well, I believe Sally may have helped a lot when she said if you make the decision, it's a deliberate one. It's yours and it's one you feel you must make. But if you find no peace having made it, then you've missed something somewhere.
Diana:	OK, then somewhere I missed something because I need. . . .
Steve:	That's what your group seems to be telling you.
Diana:	I need . . . but I'm going to have to find it by myself. It's nothing that Sally or my parents or my children. . . .
Steve:	Why?
Diana:	Because it's something. . . . The problem is mine! It's not theirs!
Sally:	Well, let me say this for whatever it's worth. What seemed to me the problems with other people . . . and I had listened to their ideas that they had put forth . . . I had to think about the spirit in which those ideas were given to me. So I take them as ideas and mull them over. They are not mine. I've always felt like if those ideas were expressed, they were avenues to help me make and enrich my own decision. And so then I just always try to get off as quietly as I can and get this head of mine sort of calmed down. Because when you always feel and see turmoil in the middle of a storm, you can't see anything. And then sit down. And then think. And most of the time I would get an answer. It might have been something somebody just had given me. It might be a combination of several ideas. It might be something entirely different. Well, anyway, I would know whether it was right or wrong. I say this because inwardly I'm at peace about it and all hell couldn't break me loose from the decision of the way I'm going to look.

Steve: But inwardly Diana's not at peace with herself.

Diana: No, she's not! And that's where the whole problem's coming from. She's in just such a state. And she just rattles off all the time! All the time! And she's just living in a rabbit stew. And unless she's busy doing something to distract her mind, that's right there every minute with her! Isn't it? And I tell you . . . and I mean sometimes right now. . . .

Jane: You know, isn't it an obsession? Because there's this fear of sharing this fear with these people and letting them know that you are a human being.

Diana: Like I say, they've been put through hell by me! You know, this is the way I am today. *X* number of years ago I'd look you straight in the eye and tell you I was going to die. And I lived my life as if I was going to die. And I had two babies. And it was hell! That's all I can say!

Sally: Well, change it around and say you are going to live!

Diana: OK! Then I spent three years believing I had overcome the illness. Went straight out and tell you I was well! No way was I ever going to have cancer again. And then it happened again! So the first three years, I was in chaos. The next three years I thought, "Boy! I got on the ball! I know where I'm going, and what I'm going to do!" And now? Here I am and *nothing! I have faith in nothing! Nothing makes sense!* I know what it is to pray and to believe and all this good stuff. And I put that into practice and it didn't work for me! So, right now, these two months, I have no foundation. You can't tell me anything I haven't tried. So for right now. . . .

Steve: Yeah, we can!

Diana: You can tell me. . . ?

Steve: You haven't tried sharing.

Diana: Oh, I don't know, Steve, I guess I did share that one time! My family . . . it's been up and down like this, OK? For right now this is my problem! For right now everybody else is fine and dandy! Whether they are fine and dandy or not, we are all putting on a pretty good charade! It's working, and occasionally I reach the boiling point. . . .

Steve: It's not working or you wouldn't be that angry. You are just rejecting that. If it were working so well, how come you are not so happy?

Diana: I don't know! I'm not! I think it's only something I can work out!

Steve: Well, I agree with that. And what I'm saying is that we are all trying to help you look at it so that you can make. . . .

Diana: No! And I feel like we talked about this before. And I don't want to talk about it every week! You know, I know that what it is to keep telling the same problem over and over again. It gets boring and you say, "What the heck!"

Steve: Well, I don't think, if you are picking that up from me, I. . . .

Diana: No! No! No! I'm just saying. . . .

Steve: It's not boring. There you go trying to take . . . trying to interpret what we are doing and take that on to make more frustrations. You are doing it with us too.

Diana: But still, the consensus is it is my problem and it's something that I'm going to have. . . .

Amanda: But it doesn't go away.

Diana: It doesn't go away! It hasn't gone away in seven years and it'll never go away, Steve! It'll always be with me and that's why. . . .

Steve: Well, I think the problem's going to be with you because you have cancer. I think that's the core of the problem. I agree with you. It's going to be there. But that you can do nothing about it. That you are so impotent that you can't feel better about the relationships with people. I just don't buy that. I think you're saying that. But I don't buy that.

Diana: But no one's really given me. . . .

Steve: But I see evidence in the rest of the group here, where people are trying to build relationships; and are trying to take care of some unfinished business; and are trying to be a little more open. . . . And they are making strides in that way. And it's producing better mental health, frankly; better interactions in the real world.

Diana: You know, I'm not willing to sacrifice the security in our home just to get out what I feel.

Steve: I'm not sure it's an all-or-nothing proposition. You make it sound like it's either-or.

Diana: Well, it is!

Steve: Why can't it be some of each?

Diana: How?

Steve: I'm feeling that you have to make a decision about the way you are going to approach it and the risks involved.

Diana: You know, I can go home tonight and I can share with my husband, but all I'm going to get is sympathy. All . . . that's all I'm going to get! I'll tell you now! And that's all I will get!

Amanda: Could you be as mistaken about that as Jane was about her son's possible reaction?

Diana: No!

Steve: Well, when you felt that coming, what would happen if you said, "I'm not saying this to get sympathy. I'm saying it to get it out so. . . ."

Diana: He would sit and listen quietly.

Steve: He would sit and listen quietly and then what would happen if you said, "It's important for me to know how you feel about this, honestly, without hurting your feelings." Maybe just start with him: "This is one time I just want to know your honest feelings and if you can't express them, I can appreciate that. But don't give me any sympathy."

Diana: I *can* it, you know [sarcastically]!

Steve: "No! No! No!" You sound like my kid taking her medicine, because daddy. . . . "OK, I'll try it, but it's not going to work." Because you are going to set it up for failure.

Jane: You know, I was so certain of what my son's behavior was going to be. It wasn't anything like that. It wasn't anything I anticipated. And you can say you haven't tried it and you can imagine, "This is the way

	he's going to react." It may not necessarily be so.
Diana:	I don't know.
Amanda:	Diana, are you really so afraid your house of cards will come tumbling down?
Diana:	Yeah.
Amanda:	I don't mean to say that to put it in a confusing tone. I just think if you pull the wrong block out, the whole wall will fall in.
Steve:	You [Amanda] are being very sensitive to the risks involved with what we are all proposing and what she is contemplating at this point, and there are some risks to it.
Diana:	But, to be very honest with you, I'll leave here today exactly the way I came in. I won't go home and bear my soul with him and I will be able to deal with these gut problems better until the next time. . . .
Steve:	You get hospitalized?
Diana:	. . . Or blow up in here [points to head].
Steve:	Well blowing up in here is what we are here for. But I'm concerned with the pressure you are taking on yourself. It's going to come out sooner or later.
Diana:	I guess I'm telling you I'm not willing to change things. Things are running. . . .
Steve:	Now we are getting to the crux of the situation. Did you hear what you just said? You are not willing to change.
Diana:	Right! OK!
Steve:	Now, you are not saying, "It's impossible." Now you are saying, "I'm not willing to do it." That's different.
Diana:	You know I'm not willing to pull out my "block" and have "my house fall down."
Steve:	But you are assuming the worst.
Diana:	Because my feelings are very close to the surface and I've got to keep a cap on them. Because, if I don't . . . .
Steve:	You're not keeping a cap on them.
Diana:	Yeah, I really am!
Steve:	No, you're not!
Amanda:	Except, here I think she is!
Steve:	I can't agree. I mean, I see what you are saying but I

can't agree.

Diana: I think you must see it, but. . . .

Steve: Well, I'm not that sharp, but if I'm seeing it, then others are seeing it.

Diana: Like I say, though, somehow I can be different. . . .

Steve: I mean, I don't even give a hoot how other people feel. I'm concerned for you.

Diana: No, I think you think other people know. . . .

Steve: I see how it affects you.

Diana: Because if other people were as sensitive to my feelings as you are, then everybody wouldn't come and unload all their problems on me.

Steve: But I'm concerned for you.

Amanda: Do they really? I thought I was the only one who attracted emotional cripples. This one pathetic soul. . . . I thought I heard the last of her. Doggone it! She got all sentimental at Christmas and called me up.

Diana: You see, but all these strong people have got a cap on their feelings. Can other people feel they can do this with . . . ?

Sally: Well, who said there are only two kinds of people in the world? The strong ones and the leaners.

Diana: So I'm a strong one. So I keep it to myself.

Steve: I'm concerned for you because I think you are kidding yourself when you say that you are handling it.

Diana: Well, I'm telling you in the next breath that I'm not willing to change things. I won't say six months from now I won't find a gun and blow my brains out because I've boxed myself into a corner. You know. I don't know what I'll do six months from now, but. . . .

Steve: See? Now you are saying you are not doing things out of a need for them as much as a need for yourself. You are talking about something different now: "I'm holding all this anger in because of my own needs, because I'm not willing to do anything else. Because, I deserve this. What else can I expect from life? This is what I deserve!"

Diana: It's not going to change! I don't mean to be presenting another problem, but I'm telling you, I'm going to leave here today and I'm going to go home and I'm going to do just what I've done. . . .

Amanda: Stop by the grocery store and go home!

Diana: . . . And my life is going to keep right on going. And I'm going to have these same frustrations and these same feelings. And I'll handle them! Sometimes I handle them better than at other times. Maybe I'm a first candidate for the "funny farm." I don't know, but. . . .

Steve: . . . But what else can you expect? That's what you are saying: "What else can I expect from life? This is it. I have no right to expect anything happy. This is it."

Diana: Right! You know I see prostitutes on the street. I see mothers that beat their children. And they've never seen a happy day in their life. Well, this is my lot in life.

Steve: "My lot. There's nothing I can do about it. I'm impotent. There's nothing I'm willing to do about it."

Diana: Because I'm not willing to do anything because it's fine for everybody else, my family.

Steve: I guess I'm being selfish right now. I'm not concerned with "everybody." I'm concerned with Diana.

Diana: But being a mother you think less about yourself. If I were the healthiest person in this hospital, my husband and my children would come before I do. That's just the way it is. You'll find mothers who want to do their own thing and find their own place. Terrific! Good! I'm not one of those and so it's more important that my children are happy and my husband is satisfied. He's got enough problems without. . . .

Steve: You used a different word for him, you didn't say happy.

Diana: Well, you know . . . well, we brought the fact up that maybe he's not happy. That maybe he has frustrations.

Steve: What am I doing now? Are you getting a little angry with me?

Diana: Well, you know, I'm just saying. . . . We are right back where we started.

Steve: *You're* right back where *you* started!

Diana: I'm right back where I started and it's not going to be any different. When I go home it's going to be just like it is! I'm not going to sit him down and say, "Hey!" Because I've lived with him thirteen years. I'm sorry!

Amanda: Don't apologize! I just think this is a decision you have made and you have the right to make.

Diana: And who knows. Maybe I will find a peace in it someday.

Sally: That's true.

Jane: There are many things that have happened in the case of cancer, and in 1975 I was given three months to live.

Diana: But Jane, don't you understand? I've been given six months to live! I've been given ten months to live!

Jane: But the thing is this. . . .

Steve: I think we are going back to try to support her again.

Jane: . . . And events changed. But somehow there's a case of stability where one does not have. . . . And I think it's your mental attitude also. So it didn't become an obsession with me. You remember I related to you how I felt about it.

Steve: I don't think. . . . What I'm picking up from you is that you are saying one shouldn't take away the hope. And I don't think that's what Diana. . . .

Diana: And there again! Maybe if I were fifty years old and my children were grown and my husband was getting ready for retirement . . . maybe I would look at this a whole lot differently. But I'm not! I'm thirty-two years old!

Amanda: I don't believe she'd look at it a whole lot different.

Jane: But you see the fact remains that you are robbing yourself of the possibility of. . . . Your mental state is such that it is not conducive to a change in your condition.

Diana: But my condition is better than it has been!

Amanda:	That it's stabilized, isn't it?
Jane:	So that is a hopeful sign. I'm not saying that you have to be morbid about it, but oh God! "Just because there's a temporary change that I'm going to live forever". . . . But I think it is a hopeful sign. I think it should give you some solid. . . .
Diana:	But I've been through hopeful signs. This is the third time, you know!
Jane:	I've had it a few times also.
Diana:	[sarcastically] You just handle it better than I do.
Steve:	You are a three-time loser and going down. Is that what you feel?
Diana:	Only each time. . . .
Steve:	"So why take anyone else with me? I may as well just suffer in silence." So it is a choice. It's a conscious choice that you refuse to do anything about your situation in terms of the relationship . . . in terms of up here [pointing to head] situations . . . even at an expense to yourself . . . your self-concept.
Diana:	*I get a feeling I must be rebelling against my decision.*
Steve:	Your decision is between how you said you feel and how you seem to feel.
Diana:	I guess that's why I'm hell-bent to get everybody to say how you do deal with it. . . . How do you deal with it? Because I haven't been able to deal with.
Steve:	But even when you hear how they deal with it, you don't accept it anyhow. That's what you say; that "it's not possible for me! I reject that! I won't do anything about it!" So you are saying that you want to hear how they are handling it? How we handle our frustrations about things? And on the other hand, you say, "I don't really care how you handle it anyhow."
Diana:	OK! And one of the people I have the most respect for in this room is Amanda because she is a very strong person. Apparently I am a very strong person. . . . And she's on top of her problem.
Steve:	She doesn't sound nearly as angry as you do.

Diana: But, you know, who's to say it won't rub off on me?
Steve: Everyone has a certain part of self that they show and a certain part of self that they don't show. And that's the *apparent* self. The word apparent is a key.

It was very significant that in the end Diana left open the possibility of behavioral change. Very early in session 8 (the next session), Diana verbalized that she had gone home and asked her husband whether or not he cared about her feelings. While, psychologically speaking, many interpretations could be made regarding the content of the following dialogue, the most significant aspect was that in spite of protests to the contrary, Diana felt somewhat comfortable approaching her husband regarding her feelings. Unfortunately, it seemed that he did not wish to break the conspiracy of silence nor was Diana willing to push the matter. The fact that Diana approached her husband was, however, a significant testimony to the potential effects of group counseling/psychotherapy with cancer patients. Diana had enough confidence in the support of her group to at least make an attempt, albeit small and somewhat unsuccessful, in the real world.

Diana: Oh! I will tell you I did go home and at dinner I asked my husband if he cared about my feelings. And, you know, he rolled his eyes.
Amanda: He says, "Diana, have you been drinking?"
Diana: Yes. He rolls his eyes and he said, "Of course! What are you talking about?" And then I asked him if he was aware of how depressed I have been at times. And he looks at me like "I am aware." He said, "I do notice." And he said, "I also know that it's something that it doesn't matter what I do, that you have to work it out yourself." So I didn't talk about it.
Carol: Diana, and he still loves you?
Diana: Yes, he still loves me. So, he is aware.
Sally: Well, I wondered how you could conceal it all.
Diana: So I don't conceal it. But what can you do?
Sally: It's just not talked about!
Amanda: People don't conceal things from people who love them very well. You're very perceptive about people who care, most of the time.
Jane: Maybe he feels that if he doesn't say anything, that it

is a better course. It is a better course for you. That you probably will come out of it.

Diana: But you know I felt very comfortable discussing it and then when I was aware that he was aware and I really knew he was, you know, we are in tune to each other's feelings.

Carol: You just wanted to hear it.

Diana: *Yeah, so I heard it and we didn't discuss it.*

CAROL

There are many different kinds of family systems. In Diana's case, a "young" family that comprises a husband and two, elementary school-aged children was presented. Carol presented a different family system. Carol was a widow. Her four children were young adults. The oldest was living on his own in California. The next two siblings, both girls, resided in Carol's home, although both were no longer pursuing formal education and were gainfully employed. The youngest child, a boy, was in late adolescence and was a senior in high school

In the first excerpt, Carol described her family system and the problems it presented.

Sally: Are all your children at home, Carol?

Carol: Well, I have three at home. My oldest is in the Navy in California and he's asked me to come out there to live. I don't want to move out there. If I move out there, he might get orders to the East Coast. And all my friends are on this side.

Steve: Plus, the fact is you've been independent and managed to raise your family without your husband over these last few years, you know. . . . You're so reluctant to give up that independence: "I am who I am and if I give up, then I'm, in a sense, giving in."

Carol: Well, another thing that bothers me too, Steve — both of my girls are working and they live with me. But they cost me money living with me. They are careless with electricity and they shower for twenty minutes, washing their hair. . . .

Sally: *Fifty* gallons of water!

Carol: And the laundry that's going. . . .

Steve:	And it's hard for you to confront them because it's so good to have them there.
Carol:	Right! And I love the fact that they are with me because it keeps me from being lonely. But they are really costing me a lot of money operating that house with them living there. And yet . . . well, I know that Sue could go on her own. She makes a good salary and she hopes to have her own apartment. But they both have dogs. And they've ruined my carpet! They've ruined my furniture! I have nothing left.
Amanda:	Do they pay room and board?
Carol:	I charge them $50 a month, but that's probably nothing.
Amanda:	Don't you ever say anything to Jane again! [laughter].
Carol:	And my grocery bill is just out of sight. And I eat like a bird at home, but I have to buy food. I don't buy dog food and I don't buy shampoo because I have my hair done and I don't buy any of the girls feminine things. Those things they buy themselves. And I don't buy any colas and all that stuff because I don't drink it.

One can begin to see the pattern of interaction between Carol and the three children that lived at home. It seems that the old nemesis, guilt, was at work again.

Amanda began to confront Carol as to why the two, working-adult children were still living at home. Carol shared some very interesting salary figures with the group.

Amanda:	Honey, if they had an apartment, they would drop dead the first month from expense!
Carol:	Well, my youngest daughter lived in one for six weeks and she says, "Mom I can't afford it. Can I come home?" So I let her move in.
Steve:	What would happen if you shared with them what you are sharing with us? What would happen if you had this conversation around the dinner table?
Carol:	"Oh! Mom, I can't afford it," and I told them. . . .
Steve:	Well, I'm not really hearing you asking them to move out. I'm. . . .

Carol: I told them this. I said . . . and I told them the other day when I got the $80 electric bill. . . . I said, "Listen! You girls have got to help me cut this down!" And I said, "If everything goes up, come July I'll have to up your rent." "Well Mom, I can't afford it!" I said, "I can't afford it too!" My telephone was $12, it's now $19. I've got four telephones; I only need one.

Amanda: This is really none of my business, and you have a perfect right to saying it's none of my business: Give me a range of their salaries.

Carol: Sue makes in the neighborhood of maybe $500 and Kathy brings home $350 [per month]. She works for the orthodontist and he's so stingy.

Amanda: Well, the $350 one has some justification, but not the other one!

Carol: And the older one works for the Civil Service and she has a part-time job and often she works three nights a week.

Steve: Between the two of them, if they were kicking in proportionate to their salary. . . .

Amanda: . . . It'd be more than a $100 a month certainly!

The therapist began to confront Carol with the reality that there was a strong possibility that she would not live very long. I wondered aloud if her children were aware of this dynamic and aware that they would have to care for themselves after her death. Amanda intervened, in her own way protecting Carol, but also trying to help Carol see the need to be more direct about her financial problems. I wondered whether or not Carol might be martyring herself so that her children would not feel guilty about the further burden that they were placing on her.

Steve: I was wondering, what would happen to you if you confronted them with the fact that you don't know how long you are going to be with them and what are they going to do when you are not here?

Amanda: You know, Carol, young people are so . . . they can't help, Carol, I'm sorry. They tend to be . . . they are sometimes thoughtless and they just might be so distressed if you really were quite honest with them. I think they might be uncomfortable but I,

	really . . . I think they would just be horrified maybe to feel that they had put this additional burden on you.
Carol:	Well, I believe they would too.
Steve:	But you don't want to put guilt on them.
Carol:	I don't want to put guilt on them.
Amanda:	No, No.
Steve:	But on the other hand you, aren't you martyring yourself?
Carol:	Yes, I am.

After proceeding to defend her children as to their need to live with her because of their own financial problems, Carol was confronted with the possibility that there did not seem to be a whole lot of honest communication between herself and her children. Carol allowed this confrontation to slip past without a response. The lack of response might suggest that honest communication was lacking and Carol was not interested in discussing this issue. She described the situation surrounding the money that she had inherited after her husband's death and her fear that this money might run out before her illness ran its course and took her life. Again, it was asserted that her children needed to be confronted in an honest fashion. Was Carol afraid that they might leave her were she to do so? Her answer was interesting, and at the end of the excerpt, Amanda shared what seemed to be an accurate insight: Carol was more afraid of an angry confrontation than abandonment by her children.

Steve:	It sounds like a situation where there's not a whole lot of honest communication back and forth. I think what Amanda is saying. . . .
Carol:	. . . And the money that my husband has left me is being drained because I have all these additional expenses. Everything goes up except my salary. And I have to go into my savings to take care of all this.
Amanda:	. . . And that's scary!
Carol:	It is scary, Amanda, and I think that is what bothers me. I don't know how long this money is going to last. Fortunately, my illness hasn't. . . . I mean I haven't had to pay anything for that. But my children are really costing me a lot of money.
Steve:	I think you are afraid that if you confront your chil-

dren in an honest fashion with the stuff that's come out here . . . that you're afraid they'll just say, "Well the heck with you!" and take off. And you'll have this big house by yourself.

Carol: No, they won't do that.

Steve: They wouldn't do that?

Amanda: I think she's afraid of an angry confrontation.

Carol's anger became more apparent as she described the situation with her youngest son. It illustrates the complexity that all parents know regarding raising teenagers in a changing world. Such child raising further complicated the course of cancer.

Carol: He has a car now. And when he bought it, it had 80,000 miles on it. I tried to tell him it's going to fall apart, but mother's the dumbest person on the block. They never listen to me. So consequently, the thing has already cost me $300 and him $200. And I said, "Larry, I'm not putting another dime of my money into that car." So I think I mentioned before at one of our meetings that he took the December Social Security [survivor's benefit] check and blew it. And so January, February, and March . . . I mean January, March, and April we decided he's going to be on his own. Well, he comes up with this idea. He's met a friend of his — a man he works with who wants to sell his Trans Am. And he's going to buy it! The man's going to buy a Corvette. So Larry's going to buy this Trans Am for $142 and he's going to use his Social Security money to buy this. I said, "Larry, look at it this way. You are going to have a $142 lemon." First he wanted to buy a big car. He wanted me to cosign. I said, "I'm not cosigning anything anymore for anybody!" I said, "They can go to the bank and borrow it just like I do." But anyhow I said, "This car's going to cost you $142." I said, "You can figure at $50 a month or more for gas." I said, "That's roughly $200." I said, "You are in a high risk insurance because you are a male under twenty-five." I said, "That's another $275." I said, "You won't have $300 to support a car." I said, "If you are talking about going to college," I said, "You need that money to go to college. That's what it's for!" He said, "Well, you said you were going to send me." I said, "Yes, I said that two years ago, but," I said, "things have changed. I may have to retire medically." And I said, "I can't afford $400 a quarter or whatever it costs to send a person to college." And at this point he said, "Well, Mom I'm eighteen years old. I can do anything I want." So I'm sitting here wondering, is he going to blow all his money on that car and then find out he can't pay it? Then they'll take the car away and he's going to have nothing.

Following Carol's soliloquy, the anger and frustration that she had with her children and her resulting guilt were addressed. Carol was made aware of the fact that she continued to defend her children's lack of responsibility.

Steve: Let me bounce this off you. In a lot of respects you sound like you've got Jane's problem, except instead of one child, you've got three of them. What I'm hearing in addition to your anger is a feeling of guilt in yourself that somehow you've failed him. And I'm also hearing something that's touching me. . . . Your unwillingness to allow them to take responsibility for their own behavior. And that is, "You either make it or you don't make it. And you can do whatever you want with your Social Security check. And if the bank comes and takes your car, then that's your decision."

Carol: Well, that's what I told him.

Steve: But you are not telling that to the other girls either. In the same sense the other girls are doing the same thing too. Like, what would happen if Cathy is only making $350 a month and she know she's got to go? She's either going to have to get a job that pays more or she's going to have to move out and move in with some other people and support herself.

Amanda: Carol, $350 a month is hardly minimum wage and she's crazy!

Carol: Well, that's what I tell her! But she's looking for

	another job. But nothing's come up yet.

Steve: another job. But nothing's come up yet.

Steve: I'm getting a little angry with your children, just sitting here and feeling your frustration. . . .

Carol: Well, I get aggravated with them too.

Steve: If she had to support herself, which eventuality exists anyhow, when or. . . . If and when you do die, she's going to have to support herself.

Amanda: She's never bought groceries; she's never paid a utility bill; she hasn't the slightest idea. . .

Carol: Well just in that six weeks. . . . She got a taste of it in the six weeks. But she just found out that she didn't have anybody.

Steve: Do you notice how you are defending your children?

Carol: Yes, I know I defend them, Steve. But I don't know how to. . . . I look at it like this. I've got a big house and I've got bedrooms that I'm not using. So they may as well use them. But on the other hand, they are costing me money living.

Steve: What you are saying to me, and, I think you are talking to them. . . . You are saying it to all of us and I think you are really talking to them . . . is that "either you kids start helping me support this place, or we are getting rid of this place, or you are getting out of this place — one or the other."

Carol: Well, I have told them that. In the springtime I'm putting the house up for sale. And I said, "When it sells, you do your thing, and I said I'm going to do mine." And Cathy says, "Can I live with you?" And I said, "Well, I'm not going to get a three-bedroom apartment." I said, "I don't need a three-bedroom apartment."

Steve: There's more guilt tied up in that one. When she says, "Can I live with you?" and you're trying to give her the boot and yet you want them around. So there's a fear: "If I do kick them out, will they come and see me? Maybe it'll be so good over there that I'll never see them again." But on the other hand, there's the anger of them taking advantage of you. And this is confused with the guilt and the martyrdom, which is the mother kind of thing that Jane was talking about. "I am their mother. I gave birth to them, it's hard to just. . . .

Carol: Well, I look at it this way too. They are all good children and I know they love me and they've been very good to me.

It is interesting, as Carol's tale unfolds, that the psychodynamic of guilt and the psychosocial implications of guilt become truly manifest in her case. A discussion of cancer and the possibility that Carol's having cancer might have been depriving them of a normal life with mother ensued. Out of her guilt, Carol shared how she had gone overboard with her charge cards in buying Christmas presents. One of her children came to her requesting more money for a ski trip and Carol had to say "no," stating that she was "sorry but it was not possible." The interaction of cancer and Carol's relationship to her children was explored in the following excerpt.

Steve: I hear words like "Sorry. . . . I apologize to them . . . I just can't do this any more." And I'm hearing the fact that you don't really think you have that much control over your life. The cancer aside, right now . . . that you are really controlled by your children.

Amanda: If you didn't have cancer, you'd still have these problems.

Steve: You'd still have these problems. And they are accentuated because . . . "I don't want to alienate my children when I need them."

Carol: But my cancer doesn't bother my children. I think they feel that I'm going to be here forever because I'm not bedridden.

Steve: I think what you are saying is you don't want to put the "guilt trip" on them and say, "You know, I'm not going to be here forever. And the way you kids are treating me, you are going to send me to my grave early."

Amanda: . . . Like people used to do. You don't want to do that.

Steve: You don't want to do that, but on the other hand, don't you have a right to be selfish in this case? Don't you have a right to live for yourself?

Carol: But all my life, Steve, I have been a very generous person . . . not just to my children . . . to my friends. In fact, I was overly generous when my husband passed away and I came into all his insurance money. And I gave a lot of it to charity.

Steve: You felt guilty about having that much money?

Carol: Right. And of course. . . .

Amanda: You are not the first widow who didn't handle insurance properly.

Carol: They say, "Don't look back." But if I had known that all of this was going to happen to me, I would have been. . . .

Steve: Let's not look back. Let's look at today. You are still doing it. Instead of giving away your insurance, you are giving away your life. You are giving away your self-control. And some of it's being taken from you because you don't have a choice. But the rest of it you are giving. And so, in a sense, what's happening to you with your children, you are at least in part responsible for.

Amanda: Carol, if you could distinguish . . . if we all could distinguish between being considerate and loving and generous and being a darn doormat, there is a difference. There really is a difference.

Carol acknowledged the need to be assertive with her children and related ways in which she thought she was dealing with the problem in a productive fashion. However, some of the group members were not convinced. Amanda was one of those members. She wondered whether Carol made idle threats that she had no intention of acting on. The group began to process the dynamics of Carol's interaction with her children.

Amanda: Carol, may I ask you something . . . and this is sort of in the category of Jane. . . . It's too blunt really for social conversation. . . . I would never dream of doing it if it wasn't this kind of a group. Do you make a lot of idle threats which you never carry out?

Carol: Yes, I really do.

Steve: And they know that.

Carol:	And they know that.
Steve:	And you know it. Is it a little game you play with each other?
Carol:	And I know too if my husband were living, everything would be different, because the children wouldn't. . . .
Amanda:	Of course, you can get yourself into an awful jam making threats and then carrying them out. You say, "Oh, Lord! Why did I ever say that?"
Sally:	Yes, you can?
Steve:	But on the other hand, what I'm hearing is that you are going to the other extreme.
Carol:	I've had to say no three times, and it's just the end of January.
Amanda:	And the world didn't fall in, and they didn't leave home.
Carol:	And they haven't left either.
Amanda:	And they hadn't stopped speaking to you.
Carol:	No, they still love me.

Carol was confronted with the need to live her life for herself; not having to feel so responsible for her adult children. She acknowledged that it was time to turn the tables and to think about her self. The group seemed to agree with her. Amanda shared a brilliant insight and awareness with Carol regarding the gift that Carol might leave her children if they were to be permitted to serve her and be somewhat responsible for her well-being as well as the other way around. Amanda shared that she had gained a feeling of worth at having been able to have provided that sense of responsibility for her daughter.

Steve:	I'm thinking that you have a right to live for yourself. That in addition to the responsibility to your children who are no longer children in the true sense of the word, you fulfill a large responsibility to them getting them to this point and you are not being responsible to yourself. Maybe this is a case where you should be a little more selfish.
Carol:	Well, I think it's time that I got to be selfish and thought about Carol instead of my children and all my friends.

Amanda: And, of course, I'm sure that goes . . . that does not come easily for somebody who's spent his life thinking of other people. And I seem to be talking out of both sides of my mouth, because I had just said a minute ago, I think it's more important to be considerate of other people than of yourself. But what I really mean is not to be so self-centered that you never think about anybody else.

Carol: Now it's time. I've got to turn the table and think about me.

Steve: So that produces a little uncertainty and fear too: "What's going to happen?" But I think Amanda was saying . . . and Sally was saying too . . . that the world isn't falling apart. You are able to say no and your children are able to take responsibility for themselves. And it's time for you to take a little bit out of life as to what you want.

Sally: Oh, these young ones!

Amanda: But, you know, really, Carol. If you can look at it this way. . . . If you can give them, really, the privilege of waiting on you and being protective of you, you'll be giving them something that they'll always remember. It'll be more than money because. . . . I remember my mamma. I used to think, "Darn just wait until I get grown. I'm going to have people waiting on me hand and foot." But Mama did us a great favor. She really did! By demanding. . . . I mean, she didn't say, "You go and do this. . . . " It just never occurred to her that we'd do anything else.

Steve: And as you look back on that, that gave you a feeling of worth . . . that you were able to do something.

Amanda: Greatest feeling in the world.

While there was no definite course of resolution to Carol's plight with her children (nor did she ever verbalize such a discussion with her children), it was comforting to know that when Carol died, shortly after the group ended, her children were with her to support her and she was able to die at home. Hopefully, such an interaction may have been facilitated in part by Carol's experience.

JANE

You know what the worst thing is? I'm not going to die of cancer. I'm going to die of an emotional situation. My son's going to drive me up a wall!

Jane

To this point family situations regarding three of the five core members of the group have been discussed. Amanda was found to have an only child. Essentially, she raised her daughter as a single parent due to being widowed. Diana had two young children in an upwardly mobile, middle-class, socioeconomic situation. It was interesting to contrast the unique dynamics of her family and compare them to the others. Also, Carol's situation as a relatively recent widow with three of four adult children living at home was examined.

It is interesting to note that four of the five women in the group were single parents. In addition to Amanda, Carol and Sally were single parents because of the death of their spouses. Jane was a single parent as a result of divorce. It is also interesting to note that of the five core members, Sally, Amanda, and Jane each had one child. Very often having one child entails more responsibility and produces more trauma than having many, for the parent becomes preoccupied with that child as the focus of existence. It is common knowledge that putting one's immortality (eggs) into one "being" (basket) is challenging fate itself. As such, there is much more personal investment in the outcome.

In earlier chapters Jane complained of the emotional stress of loneliness and her difficulties in dealing with the role she might be playing in being alone. She demonstrated profound feelings of anguish over emotional traumas and stated that having cancer itself was not as bad as having the emotional difficulties entailed in living with cancer. Jane's chief problem in life was her son. It was a problem in her life right up to the day she died. While this passage will show Jane beginning to resolve some of the struggles with her son, Jane had so much "unfinished business" with her son that it would have taken years of therapy to work through their difficulties.

Jane presented a unique situation to our group in that she was one of the most open members. She was so open that at times she monopolized the group. Prior to reaching the halfway point of the group, Jane was confronted about her chronic complaining. The group began to offer suggestions and foster insights regarding Jane's contribution to the problems with her son. It was difficult to ascertain whether or not Jane's perception of her situation with her son was being overdramatized. However, as with any other client, one can only assume that the perceptions are real for that person.

A similar communication difficulty existed between Sally and her daughter. However, Jane's situation remained the most dramatic and possibly the most traumatic as well. In the following excerpt, Jane introduced us to her difficulty with her son and the absence of family in her life.

Jane: I don't wallow in my cancer situation. I don't even think about my cancer. I think of my inability to cope with my son. That's the thing that bothers me: my inability to cope with my son.

Carol: Do you have any other person at all in your personal life?

Jane: No, I have no family at all. . . . I actually plead with him and put out these feelers and these subtle expressions that — "God! I really need you! I love you! I want you to be part of this! I want this to be a good relationship! And I can't reach him. And I can die. I think I'd rather die of cancer than of that.

Sally: But sometimes we have to loosen and let them go.

Jane: I have released. I never call him. And I've said to his girlfriend, "Please call me just so that I could feel that somebody really cared about me." If she called me, say just once a month. I would feel good. But they don't even do that. I feel such a horrible feeling of rejection and pain. There are different kinds of pain. There are pains that can be alleviated by drugs. You can take a person with cancer and give him all kinds of drugs. They can be terminal and they are not going to even feel it. But what are you going to do with somebody who has emotional pain? That's much harder to deal with.

Louise: Have you ever suggested to him some therapy? Has he ever had psychiatric help?

Jane: Oh, yes! But, there's nothing wrong with him! Nothing wrong with him! That's his consensus.

Sally: They never do see anything wrong with themselves. That's the bad thing.

The reader begins to get an insight into the apparent love/hate relationship that Jane had with her son. Also, note that Sally's self-disclosure alluding to the difficulties that she had with her daughter.

Through the first several sessions of the group, Jane made impassioned pleas for relief from the emotional turmoil caused by her relationship with her son contrasted to the process of cancer: the relationship being the more painful. About halfway through the group's life, Jane began to disclose some of the more significant aspects of her relationship with her son. The following excerpt typifies Jane's description of the relationship.

Carol: Jane, I want to ask you a question. If you don't want to answer it, just say so. Why do you give John the check every month? Is it part of his inheritance after your husband died? Do you feel you owe it to him?

Jane: No, it's a demand.

Carol: He demands it?

Jane: Right. It's a demand and if I don't have it. . . .

Carol: . . . You have to go get it.

Jane: I have helped him.

Amanda: I believe that's what Steve is leading up to: that whether you are doing it consciously or not, your actions are simply perpetuating a very painful situation.

Jane: They are.

Amanda: Now what can you do to make yourself face up to this? The worst person in the world to fool is yourself. And to fool yourself about your motivations, or whatever, you are just asking for trouble.

Jane: I'm scared. I'm scared of a lot of things he used to do. Like he tried to choke me. He tried to do other things. He beat me. He did a lot of things, and he knows that I'm frightened. He knows he can manipulate me and he does that. And I know that I'm playing . . . that I've got to take a chance in which I'm planning to very shortly, because he started to get some G.I. benefits. See, he was thrown out of the service and I was able to get an authorization to upgrade his discharge. So now he's eligible. He had a dishonorable discharge. Now he is eligible for G.I. benefits.

Jane's guilt began to manifest itself. She was confronted by Amanda regarding some masochistic aspects of her relationship with her son.

Diana: I have had a thought now that I'm interrupting you. What about your relationship with John when he was a little boy growing up? Can you look back and say, "I should have done something and I didn't do it, so now I'm going to make up for it?"

Jane: No. It's not a guilt feeling.

Steve: You know what it sounds more to me like? It sounds more to me like over the years in your relationship with John that he has come to expect Jane, or Mom, or whatever he calls you, to do things for him. And now, when you don't, he feels that he's entitled to this. And he gets madder than hell and takes it out on you.

Jane: That's right.

Steve: And I guess the thing that's coming to me is that you are.... I think Amanda said it earlier ... you are perpetuating the relationship.

Jane: I'm perpetuating, and. . . .

Amanda: You know, it's almost masochistic when you are punishing yourself.

Although Jane denied that she was feeling guilty, it seemed that some guilt was manifest. Jane went into a rather lengthy discussion and series of confrontations and interaction with the group concerning responsibility for her son's behavior. A typical example of this type of situation is illustrated in the following excerpt.

Steve: You said first he got discharged from the service for an undesirable discharge but you haven't allowed him to take the full responsibility for that because you went out and got his status upgraded and got it fixed up.

Jane: . . . Because he wouldn't have done anything. You

know what he said? He said, "There's a seven year
statute of limitations" . . . and his interpretation was
that if he waited seven years, nothing could be done.

Steve: But I guess if I had somebody like you that I knew
would do it for me anyhow, if I just raised a little hell
and scared the hell out of you, I guess I wouldn't do
anything either.

Jane: That's right.

Jane was asked to examine the relationship as her son might
perceive it from his subconscious. It was doubtful that she had ever
consciously entertained this possibility previously.

Steve: What I want to say is you've already given him the
check by going and upgrading his G.I. Bill status. It's
just one more in a series of events that you are continuing to do for him so that he expects you to keep
doing them. What's going on in here. . . . If you kept
doing things for me all the time, I'd have two feelings. One is I would come to expect it. . . . "You better give it to me or I'm going to be pissed and I'll
throw a tantrum" . . . . Except the tantrums have
grown up a little bit and have become beatings or
harassments or whatever. The other feeling I'd have
is, I would resent you. . . .

Jane: That's what I think he does.

Steve: . . . I'd resent you not allowing me to be responsible
for myself. So I'd get angry at you at that end because
I'd have all kinds of guilt tied up with being twenty-
eight or thirty or however old he is.

Jane: Twenty-five. . . .

Steve: . . . twenty-five years old and still being a "mama's
boy" and being dependent on you. And on the other
hand I'd come to expect it. And it's one of these
things that produces this kind of a *pulling* conflict
and this kind of a *pushing* conflict. You're becoming
the focus of that conflict. You have a role in it
because you allow it to go on.

The group began to support Jane by trying to give her alternatives for handling her situation with her son. Most of the solu-

tions centered on either Jane leaving or else taking legal measures to enjoin her son from harassing her. However, while Jane may not have wished to be harassed, the group missed the point: Her son was her link to immortality, and to fail with him would be the "ultimate" failure. After some time, Jane admitted that she had contributed to her present situation by having pampered her son in an attempt to absolve herself from the guilt of seeing her son as the victim of her poor marriage.

Amanda: But your pampering of him. . . . Is that what you've been doing? Your pampering of him. . . .

Jane: I think that I have contributed to it.

Amanda: OK! Now facing up to that and then wanting to change patterns of twenty years standing. . . .

Jane: I have created this to a large degree. But I can also say. . . . You see, my marital situation was such that John was a victim of it.

Amanda: So you are trying to make up to him.

Jane: No, John was very resentful. I think John actually would like to lash out at his father.

Carol suggested that, instead of lashing out at his father, John was taking it out on Jane. Jane acknowledged this possibility. Jane finally acknowledged her role and confirmed the group's suspicion.

Carol: He takes it out on you.

Jane: I'm a good scapegoat, because he manipulated me and I have pampered him. I have pampered him. He even has one picture, a snapshot, on the back of which he wrote, "Just finished twisting her around my little finger."

Amanda: This sounds terribly blunt, and it may be a little cruel, but it seems. . . . I feel like you have helped create this monster.

Jane: I have!

Amanda: . . . And you've got two choices. You can terminate it with perhaps drastic reactions or you can just say, "I'm stuck with it and I've got to learn to live with it!" Period!

Jane: But you see, I feel that that isn't really a. . . .

Steve: Which way?

Jane: The second way. . . .

Steve: The second one?

Jane: Yes, for this reason. I'm allowing this neurotic being to go on. I'm not allowing him to grow up and assume responsibility. And I'm stunting my growth.

Amanda: Well, it's a little late for both of you. You know, you kind of get past the point of no return. And do you all think that's wrong?

Steve: What I'm feeling is that Amanda is hitting it right on, I think, judging from the way Jane is interacting. . . . But, I have a couple of observations, for what it's worth. . . . One is that you keep covering up about how you feel about the thing with words. [to Jane] You talk. You just talk about it. I don't really know how you feel about it, because in some ways. . . . This is going to seem a little blunt too, but in some ways I think you "enjoy" the relationship. Some attention from your son, because of some of your own guilt involved, is better than not knowing what's happening to him or not having his attention. I think you are getting to the point where you are fed up with it, but I don't think we all still know how you feel about it because you talk about him being a manipulator.

Jane proceeded to tell the group how she felt about this relationship with her son. It was quite clear that she had suppressed considerable anger. Jane acknowledged the possibility that she felt very guilty about her anger with a son that she had deprived of a normal father/son relationship and that she was now depriving him of their relationship as she proceeds to die from cancer.

Jane: How do I feel about it? It makes me very angry!

Amanda: You just hurt from the bottom of your soul.

Jane: I'm angry at my lack of self-esteem — that I let him do this. And I'm not taking any real strong action! I hate. . . .

Steve: I think you feel like a failure to him as a mother.

Jane: That's right!

Steve: And there's some guilt with that: "If I hadn't done all this stuff, this wouldn't ever have happened." But you know what else I think? I think you still keep trying to make up for it by letting him continue — saying, "This is what I deserve."

Jane: I don't know. I don't know whether that is. . . . I would have to think about that. I couldn't really give you an answer. It could be and it couldn't be. Maybe it's a subtle feeling that I've got there . . . a feeling of guilt that I can't really identify.

Amanda: They are very difficult to identify.

Toward the end of the session, Jane began to decide how she wanted to approach the problem with her son. The group offered to support her efforts. They also reflected from their own experiences how difficult family problems were, especially considering cancer. In particular, Carol wondered how any child could be so cruel as to put his mother through the agony that Jane had endured (as though cancer were not enough). Jane tried to do some self-analysis by suggesting that her son was lashing out at his father through her.

Jane: Well, I'll tell you. I feel that I've got to do first things first. And as soon as I. . . . I've got to work on this. I've got to decide how I'm going to approach it . . . what I'm going to do. And that's it. And I promise you I will say nothing again until I have acted to tell you I've been successful.

Carol: That you've done one little thing.

Amanda: We'll have a party.

Steve: I want to back up a little. I heard a commitment to try to do something. I don't think that the group is saying that you have to do something or we are going. . . .

Carol: . . . We're not going to cut you off.

Jane: I'm not interpreting it that way.

Steve: We are saying we are here to support you in anything you try.

Jane: I'm not interpreting it that way. I have no feeling of animosity or anything like that toward anyone here. As a matter of fact, I love all of you and I appreciate

what you've tried to tell me today. And it's going to
be a great deal of, as they say, "food for thought." It's
not going to be something that I'm going to be casual
about.

Carol: What crushes me, Jane, is how your son and my son
or anybody's child could treat their mother like your
son treats you.

Amanda: Really!

Carol: Even though you have this terrible disease. . . .
That's something that you have to fight which is bad
enough. But to have this on top? How can he be so
cruel to you?

Jane: He's. . . . The only way I interpret it was that he was
mad at his father. Because when I came home from
the hospital after the last operation he said. . . . And
I didn't say anything to him because I never discuss
my physical condition with him. . . . He said, "I
guess you're feeling sorry for yourself and all you had
was superficial surgery." I said, "Superficial surgery?"
I said, "Then what would radical surgery be?" He
said, "Inside of you. But yours was on the outside of
you." So I told my doctor this and he said, "Send him
up here and I'll cut his testicles off and I'll tell him it's
superficial surgery because they are on the outside."
But he's very immature in a lot of ways.

Amanda: A lot of ways? I would say 100 percent!

Diana: You know, I hope my mother never gets in a position like this.

Carol: I'll bet she's saying you are the sweetest little girl in
the world.

Amanda: Some people are just very fortunate. They just never
have any difficulty with their children and I don't
know if they deserve any particular credit for it. They
are just lucky.

It was also interesting to note that toward the end of the above excerpt Diana shared that she hoped that her mother was never in a
position where she could abuse her. I suggested that in some respect
Diana was identifying with John, a person who would be within
seven years of being her age-mate.

The support of the group seemed to be pivotal in Jane's verbalization that she would begin to make an attempt to work through this problem with her son. Also, note Jane's anger about her son's insensitivity to the massive surgery that she had undergone. Two sessions later, Jane returned to the group sharing that she had made a start toward solving the ongoing problems with her son. It was a significant interaction, for Amanda took on the role of Jane's therapist and the two interacted in a therapeutic dyad in what may be seen as a further testimonial to the effectiveness of the group!

Jane: And now to continue with my current activity and current developments. I had crystallized my thinking. I met with my son on one occasion and broached the subject I found that, while there was displeasure which I anticipated, I wasn't physically abused. So that to me was encouraging. And I felt well. Now I'm writing a letter which is going to explain to him how I feel about him and why I'm taking this course of action. I feel that I have deprived him, by what I did in the past, of growth. And that I love him so dearly that now I want to give him his opportunity. But of course, I worded it a little differently. But it has given me such a good feeling. It has given me self-esteem. It has made me feel. . . . See I regard all of you with a great deal of respect and particularly when Amanda said — sat here and said. . . .

Amanda: Me and my big mouth. . . .

Jane: That was the best thing you could have done to me. When you said . . . when Steve said to you . . . "And how do you feel about it?" I'm not quoting it accurately but this is the essence . . . "And how do you feel about Jane?" And you said everything that I thought. It was about time I got this feedback. And I was listening to a description of a person I couldn't respect. And I said, "Well I'm not going to continue in that pattern!" And I did some thinking about it! And I was so grateful to all of you for telling me something. See, you never know how you appear to others and if somebody tells you . . . if you respect that person . . . there's no resentment. As a matter of

	fact, I felt gratitude.
Amanda:	I think that says a great deal for your generous feeling. I might not have been so grateful at the time. I might have come around to it, but I wouldn't have felt so grateful.
Jane:	And I immediately put things into operation and kept giving it and saying, "I'm not going to be this weakling." And if I love my son as I say I do, I'm doing him a great injustice.
Amanda:	And he may not believe a word you put in your letter now, but I'll bet he'll come. . . .
Jane:	That's right! He'll probably be angry. I can understand that. Here I am removing from him something that was very comfortable. Everything was done for him. No effort.
Amanda:	Isn't it grand you feel good about it?
Jane:	I feel very good about it.

Whether or not Jane's letter made a significant difference in her relationship with her son, it was important to note that at some point after her son received the letter, he began to demonstrate more interest in his mother's health as evidenced by increasing contacts with Cindy, the nurse practitioner in the oncology/hematology unit at the hospital.

SALLY

Sally's situation was unique enough to produce adequate stress, which, when suppressed, could certainly lead to the breakdown of the immunosuppressive system in support of the psychosomatic theory of the onset of cancer.

On several occasions during the course of the group, Sally mentioned that her daughter had undergone intermittent psychiatric care throughout most of her adolescent and adult life. Perhaps the following excerpt will "shed light" on what kinds of situations in her family experience might have led Sally's daughter into the need for psychiatric care. It also elucidates the tremendous amount of stress and suffering that Sally had to endure during the course of her life.

Sally: My first husband died when my child was twenty-seven months old. I married a second time when she was five, and that marriage lasted seven weeks. My first husband died of a coronary occlusion and the second died of a coronary occlusion. Of course, my second husband was in the kitchen when it started. He came into the dining room and fell. I ran to the telephone and called the ambulance, but by the time they could get there, of course, it was all over. And it was something else because the two boys that came on the ambulance were the two boys that came when my first husband died. Now I was there by myself again. I was there the first time by myself. They looked at me and they said, "Are you here again by yourself? And I said, "We got to do what we got to do here." That second thing. . . . I just kind of walked around in a daze, but I had a very understanding elderly man who I worked for, and he, in more ways than one, helped me through that.

Amanda: You felt just like he was standing by.

Sally: He was just sort of like. . . . He felt like my father to me. And I didn't go to work for a week. And he called me . . . he always called me Lady. . . . And he called me up over the telephone, and he said, "Now, Lady," he says, "I expect you to be on the job in the morning. You know, you do have a job to do, and you just come right on. You'll just be saved as if you are in Abraham's book." I says, "But I can't come." And he says, "But you'll be here!" I thought that was the last thing. I didn't want to see anybody. I wanted to shrink up, see. Well at five years old, my child didn't remember anything about her own father, but she loved her stepfather and she was so happy to have a father. And she had expressed to me, going to the store once after we were married. . . . She hoped nothing happened to this father. So she was devastated. She went into a little shell, too. She wouldn't discuss it with anybody. But she would ask me questions: "Is Dad in heaven?" "What do you suppose he's having for breakfast?"

You know such things as that. But anyway, as I say, there always seems to be a way provided for help that we are not conscious of. Maybe we don't realize it. At the time I didn't realize how kind that man was being to me. But in looking back, I see now it wasn't sympathy. It wasn't, "Don't do your job or anything else." It was a kind of a strength or something that he sort of put forward that you felt and you got, but nothing much was said about it. But it picked me up. It put me on my feet.

With the exception of some oblique references, Sally did not discuss her daughter again until the sixth session. During that session, Sally made apparent reference to the fact that her daughter had had an emotional collapse and that her daughter's doctors felt that the knowledge of Sally's cancer had "pushed her over the edge." Amanda attempted to support her and help her not to feel guilty, and the subject was quickly skirted. It was sad that during the course of the group, and to the best of my knowledge during the rest of her life, Sally never was able to forgive herself for what she "had done" to her daughter.

Sally: I couldn't tell my child. I just told her I was going to have a biopsy. I wasn't going to tell her what I was going through for anything in the world. But fortunately, my very best friend in the world was here from Birmingham and she found out I was going in the hospital. She teaches school. She teaches Mongoloids. And she says, "I don't have to go home." She says, "I'll stay with Sally for awhile." And she stayed ten days. And my doctor said that was one thing that happened to my child. Of course I'd never been sick. She's never been sick. She's never seen anybody sick.

Amanda: Sally, I don't believe that.

Sally: What?

Amanda: I just don't think that burden of guilt should be placed on you. You couldn't help it 'cause you had cancer, and to say that was the thing that contributed to your child's illness.

Sally: They said that it was the thing that brought it to the head. I don't know. Many contributing causes.

Amanda: I don't think that's fair!

Steve: You know as I look at you, I notice you are anxious. There are some fears. What are you feeling right now?

Sally: Well, it still comes back. It's still so real.

Chapter 4

DEATH AND DYING

Well at one point one of the heart and lung men, a specialist, gave us a book written by some popular [person] — I believe it's a lady doctor — who has written a book on death and dying, and we laughed and burned it. You know, we face this; we live with this every day. And sometimes. . . . Well, she hasn't been sick. You know, there were a lot of different interviews. And I read some good things about it. . . . But we didn't read it. But he really gave it to my husband so he'd understand me better. So I hope at the end of this we don't laugh.

Diana

THERE is the tendency to react strongly in one direction or another toward the possibility of imminent death. One way is to become depressed, isolated, and withdrawn from the challenge of life. Here Diana and her husband have chosen to cope with the fear of death in their lives and to imitate bravado by laughing in its face and tearing up the evidence. They do so by striking out in anger at anything that suggests the acceptance of death, even Elisabeth Kubler-Ross's book titled *On Death and Dying* (*see* Suggested Readings).

The fact that approximately two-thirds of people who contract cancer die from it further illustrates the significance of the ever-present awareness of death once one has cancer. It is one of the first fears registered when the possibility of cancer exists. Cancer is thought of in our culture as being synonymous with death.

Since, from an existential viewpoint, *Angst* (the pervasive, unconscious fear of death) is ever present, this awareness magnified by the prospect of cancer makes existence almost unbearable. One has the choice of either succumbing to the fear or of developing behaviors to counter the fear: behaviors such as "gallows" humor or death-defying acts. For instance in the case of Carl, shortly after he was given a relatively clean bill of health and told that his cancer was in remission, he proceeded to recklessly endanger his life on a motorcycle to the point of finding himself in serious condition in the hospital's critical care unit for almost a week. He had lacerated his

126

liver in three places as a result of this accident. It was almost as though his unconscious had sought an encounter with death to show that he could survive and master death, making his cancer seem less threatening.

The subject of death and dying was present from the very beginning of our group. It was present even before there was a group and was manifest in very many different ways during the course of our initial interviews. It was during these interviews and due to federal regulations that I announced that I was working with a group of persons who had "terminal" illness. My research was designed in such a way that I had to mention to each patient that this was a group of severely, critically, or terminally ill persons. It was interesting to note how different members of the group reacted.

Shortly after I introduced myself and discussed the nature of the group with Carol, the following interaction occurred.

Carol: You did mention one thing that bothered me about terminal patients. I have never considered myself as a terminal patient. I don't know how bad my condition is. Doctor Norris never said . . . he never told me. I was in the hospital in November of '75 for five days . . . then December . . . then January. And after three months treatment, I did very well and I wasn't on any medication whatsoever until September when I started losing weight and my appetite just went kind of down. So we decided I had been too long without the medication. So he gave me a shot of chemotherapy. Then he also put me on that horrible medicine that just set me back six months. I had a terrible reaction from it. I'm getting better, but I'm still not feeling like me. But hopefully by the time all that gets out of my system, I'll be good as new again. But really, I've never considered myself as a terminal patient. I do know that in January of '75, I was very, very ill, and they didn't give me much hope at the time, and I was under the care of Dr. Moriarity, and he put me in the hospital here for a twenty-one day treatment. And they put a tube through an artery which drained into my lung. And that did better than any. I think that sort of put me back on my feet again.

Steve: So the word *terminal* itself is. . . .

Carol: I never use it.

Steve: You never use it. Well, I'll try not to use it too.

Carol: Maybe some people do. Maybe they consider themselves terminal.

Steve: Yeah. The study is geared around severely, critically, or terminally ill persons, and so when I use that word, it's open to any interpretation that you want to use.

After that encounter, Carol related a statement implying her feeling about the finality of her cancer: "Well, I've sort of accepted my illness, and it really came as a blow. In fact, it came just a year after my husband's death and I really hadn't recovered from that at all. And all of a sudden all of this [was] found in my head, and I thought, "Oh! Gosh! God is really after me." But I've learned to accept it. He plans for everything and for everybody. So I've just accepted it."

Faye was interviewed and decided not to join the group when she found out that all of the potential members had metastatic, incurable cancer. Although she also had metastatic disease that had been diagnosed incurable, she alleged that she was "cured" and had her cancer under control. She did not want to be in a group with persons who were dying. After asking me the questions: How does one know when one is terminal? Faye answered her own question: "I wouldn't want to know it! No way! I don't think the Lord intended us to know when we were going to die. I mean we are all terminal, we know that. But to have an idea of when it's going to be, no, I wouldn't want to know that."

The subject of death and dying manifests itself somewhat differently in Jane's initial interview. After going through a standard discussion regarding some of the ground rules for the group, — Jane reacted to the use of the word *terminal*, preferring the use of the word *incurable*. She continued to elaborate upon the whole usage of both words. She stated that if one was thought of as terminal that person might as well get into a bed and wait to die. When one uses the word incurable there is room for hope. To my mind, it is another means of repressing the awareness of death for the cancer patient.

Jane: See, I don't like the word terminal.

Steve: Yeah, you don't, huh?

Jane: No, I prefer to use the word incurable.

Steve: OK, let's . . . well then. . . .

Jane: You see, I think psychologically it's a better word.

Steve: OK, fine, yeah, I guess it would be, and I don't. . . .

Jane: See, because that leaves room for hope.

Steve: OK.

Jane: As soon as you say to a person you are terminal, get me my obituary. I don't feel terminal. And I know that I can hang on long enough until there's a breakthrough.

Steve: Well great, great! OK! So you would prefer when I'm talking to you I use the word incurable. Fine. Well, anyway.

Jane: See I think it's a good word to use for any of those patients because you see a lot of these people are not advanced emotionally to the point that I am and have not accepted it. As soon as you say terminal to them, they're wasting away. They may as well get into bed and wait to die.

Steve: That's a good point.

Jane: When you say you're incurable, so that leaves room for hope. "Well gee . . . maybe tomorrow there's going to be a cure for me and I'm going to be living." And I can hang on. But with *terminal* I can't hang on. I'm just waiting to die.

Steve: Well, I anticipate this very thing coming up in the group.

Jane: Well, Steve, don't forget that these are scared people; so you want to choose your words very carefully. You don't want to create more anxiety.

In another case Dave was interviewed. Again the standard introduction regarding the group and ground rules once in the group dictated by research design were presented. Part way into the interview, Dave wondered aloud whether or not the people in the group had a terminal illness. I replied that they did. Again it was a case in which I knew Dave also was suffering from terminal cancer. His reply follows. It illustrates the tremendous amount of difficulty he had with death in general and how this had become more magnified in denial as death became more imminent.

> That is the only part that is going to disturb me. When those particular individuals open up. I know I had some adverse reactions to one death a couple doors down the hall from me last trip into the hospital, and this is very unsettling to me. I still haven't really recovered from it in my own mind. It's justified, I suppose, but for about two weeks thereafter I was dismissed from the hospital, I was having some pretty bad nightmares concerning that. When you are close to it, it sort of shakes you.

Dave knew too.

SPIRITUAL ASPECTS

> Well, I feel that I haven't fulfilled my purpose in life or God would have taken me three years ago. I feel that He wants me to do something, maybe to help Diana or to help this group or help someone in my office. Well, just last week we had two women come down with cancer of the breast. So I feel that He's not ready for me. But when that time comes, I'll go. In the meantime, I'm going to love each day and live the best as I put my feet on the ground every morning thanking the Lord for another day.
>
> Carol

The spiritual component of death was manifested verbally and/or nonverbally by every member studied. Each member of the group expressed her spiritual concerns from many levels. The maintenance of hope, the purpose of life, the meaning of suffering, and the meaning of life were just some of the issues directly addressed highlighting this spiritual component. Any group leader or counselor who works individually with cancer patients must be prepared to be open to that person's perception of God, death, and afterlife. Moreover, some research has shown that the more religious one is, the less anxious one appears in the face of death. It seems, at least from observation, that this generalization held true in our group. It seemed that Diana, who was the angriest with God and who professed the least religiosity in the traditional sense, also had the most difficulty and frustration resulting from her confrontation with death throughout the course of her disease.

Suffering is a topic that emerges in any discussion regarding spirituality. Victor Frankl has developed an entire therapy (logotherapy) based on the theory that one can grow and understand oneself in a spiritual context only if one has developed this growth through a process of suffering. For the cancer patient, existence and suffering are practically synonymous. The suffering occurs at many levels. Suffering occurs when mini-hopes are shattered by X-rays and discouraging interpretations. Suffering is incurred with each debilitating bout with cancer and the loss of control over one's existence as dependency on others increases.

Suffering increases proportionately. Most of the suffering discussed to this point has been connected with mental anguish. However, one must not overlook the obvious suffering that accompanies chronic pain. There is suffering from surgery, radiation treatment and its after effects, and the side effects of chemotherapy. Truly, if Frankl is correct, the cancer patient presents so much suffering that any growth arising from it would certainly lead to an altered state of consciousness and transcendence that should be tantamount to bliss. In theory such may be the case. In reality, existence may be sheer agony with little time to reflect on the good that comes from such suffering.

Suffering occurs at another level. Suffering occurs each time a cancer patient looks into the eyes of loved ones. Thinly veiled attempts to humor the dying patient are often given away by the glistening of eyes and wavering of voices. The greetings and the hugs communicate messages that in effect say "I must hold you closely now for I may never hold you again." Suffering includes the working through of "unfinished business" as children, spouses, and other loved ones confess aloud previously secret concerns and pains that have been known to both the patient and communicator for years. Suffering includes the knowledge that every anniversary, every birthday, and every holiday may be the last for the patient. Selfishly, loved ones hang on to the hope that the patient may live on for many years, while unconsciously they pray that death may be quick and merciful. Not only does the cancer patient suffer, but those around him often suffer as well.

Such suffering returns guilt to the forefront of our discussion. Guilt is insidious throughout the entire cancer process. The cancer patient feels guilty for making those around him suffer. The survivors feel guilty for selfishly wanting the cancer patient to exist at almost any cost in order to preserve that person's presence. On the other hand, as the disease progresses and becomes more debilitating and incapacitating for the patient, the hope that death is quick and merciful presents guilt at another level: "How can I wish someone I love dead?" The suffering-anguish-guilt complex is subtly perpetuated even further as the survivors begin to thank God that they themselves do not have the disease. There is no conscious: "I'm glad that it's she (he) and not I." But unconsciously, all of us wish to survive and few wish to give their own lives in exchange even for loved ones. It is a rare person who does not see life as precious, even at the expense of another on occasion.

By the second session the whole concept of suffering and sorrow was manifest in an interaction between Louise, Carol, and Amanda.

Louise: I'm very weak, but I think everyone in our condition should take today and forget about tomorrow. Of course, I know there's going to be a tomorrow if we live but still make the fullest, make the best of what we have today because we might not have a tomorrow.

Carol: I have a plaque on my desk and I keep it where I can see it every day and people really love it. It says, "I'm not afraid of tomorrow, because I've seen yesterday and I love today." And that's a good way to live. A lady gave it to me when I came back from the hospital. She decoupaged it for me.

Amanda: I think all of us will survive. What, your husband died and mine did. . . .

Sally: Mine died when my child was twenty-seven months old.

Amanda: We have all known people who have had great sorrow and some of them have picked up their lives and gone on and others have continued to mourn. Now, its' my personal conviction that you have to work at that. The human spirit just bounces back, no matter. And when you find people still mourning after ten years and bursting into tears every time the dead person's name comes up, you can just put it down; they really work at that job. And I think that's something about us. We could either try to live normally knowing we are going to have low spots and allowing for them. So what, we have them. But we just don't work at being a cancer victim.

Carol: I feel that I have *suffered* more in mourning than I have with this disease. It took me a long time to

recover from my husband's death. I just couldn't
believe it happened to him. But like you say, I didn't
dwell on it. I had to live for my children.

Guilt and suffering are close companions. On closing this discussion about spirituality and death, it is important to note that persons who are dying often harbor hostility and anger toward God. However, in our society, anger is not generally encouraged, let alone anger directed toward God. Therefore, suffering is further compounded by the unconscious guilt felt by one who feels anger with one's God. The persistent feelings of futility at arguing and bargaining with God and the subsequent anger of failure in negotiations come full circle as guilt is presented for not being happy with the life that one has had. Questions such as "What if I had only done this differently?" or "Why haven't I done this?" sometimes arise providing further guilt for not having lived life to its fullest and thereby not having had the most productive existence. Therefore, one has effectively dishonored the covenant between one's spirit and God. Guilt piled upon guilt brings about a sense of depression. Without encouragement and loving support, the cancer patient flounders not only in the hopelessness and fear of the disease, but in suffering and guilt that complicate an already tormented existence.

THE PURPOSE AND MEANING OF LIFE

In therapy there are two questions one asks the client that will provoke silence and deeply emotional introspection: "What is the purpose of your life?" and "What is the meaning of your life?" Whether one's suffering has either organic cause or psychological cause it is nevertheless real. From all suffering toward growth, the questions of purpose and meaning of life are paramount.

Each of the group members addressed the issue of purpose of life uniquely. At the beginning of the sixth session, Carol shared a near-death experience with the group.

Carol: Monday I thought I was about to meet my maker because I didn't think I'd come out of it I was in such pain.

Amanda: Oh! I'm so sorry.

Carol: So they want to put me back again in February for another dosage hoping that it would take care of this.

Amanda:	Have you ever had radiation?
Carol:	No, I've never had it.
Steve:	Carol, when you are having the physical symptoms, when you are having the physical pain, what kinds of thoughts are going through your mind?
Carol:	Well, this time I really thought that I was dying. It was so severe and it just wouldn't ease up. And when I felt it coming on, I grabbed for my pain pills right away. But it was much too powerful for that pain pill to do any good. And I really thought that I was on my way down and that I wasn't going to come out of it.

Sometime later in the discussion, Carol shared that her close encounter with death had caused her to rethink retirement from her job. While Carol had many close encounters with death, this was the most dramatic. She began to share her anxiety about this particular experience. Carol hinted that her purpose in life was finished. She saw her life coming to an end and her responsibility and chief role (meaning) in life as being maternal. With her children grown, her maternal obligation was finished and she could accept the possibility (reality) of her death. Amanda rushed to support her out of her own anxiety. Carol as much as said that she was ready to die. Carol was the first to die shortly after the group concluded.

Steve:	Carol, I hear a lot of anxiety, particularly this week. And I know that there's been. . . .
Carol:	Right! These last two weeks have really been sitting on my mind.
Steve:	It's just been an awful time, like sitting on pins and needles. I kind of hear you asking the group, "Where am I?" You know, "Give me some feedback as to where am I?" And I'm wondering, to help us know where you are, where do you see yourself right now?
Carol:	Well, I think I'll see tomorrow but whether I'll be here in six months, I don't know.
Steve:	OK. You are thinking about that right now. And when you think about whether "I'll be here six months from now," you say that in a very matter of fact way. But I'm sure that that's very emotionally laden.

Amanda: Well, it has to be Steve! Nobody can talk about dying casually. And if they do, then it's just put on. I don't think that's a genuine attitude.

Steve: I guess what I'm feeling here is that a minute ago I felt all of you were asking for a place to kind of explore those feelings and on the other hand saying that you all feel that way. I lost the thought. That's why I'm a little confused now. I guess what I'm saying is that here is a place where we can try to explore that because you've all shared that you have similar thoughts.

Carol: Well, Steve, *I feel that my purpose in life is finished.* My daughter that lives with me is going to get her own apartment in April and my son gets out of school the end of May and he plans to go on to college. Whether he does or not, I don't know. And my other daughter is working and I'm at the point where I may have to retire. What am I going to do? My life is getting kind of blah at this point.

Amanda: Carol, your life is not over!

Sally: No! It isn't!

Carol: Well, what am I supposed to do?

Amanda: Well, honey, you can do all kinds of things . . . active, energetic, on committees and all that kind of thing. And people say, "Well what are you going to do?" And I say, "I'll think of something" because I want to enjoy so much and I don't have to get up every doggone morning that rolls around. And I love it! And I think you will too! But, of course, if you don't feel too well, that has some effect on it. But, by and large, I think you can just have a grand time and do all the things you've never had time to do before. I'll tell you, I felt so guilty when people caught me in the grocery store at 10:00 in the morning. I thought I should apologize for being there because for so many years I had to do the marketing in late afternoon or on the weekends. So you sort of develop a whole new approach. I had worked for so many years I really had to sort of develop a new attitude, but I loved it.

Carol: Well, if I have to go back to my house if I'm by myself, I can't take care of it. And it's a long way to. . . .

Still later in the session, the group's support of Carol was confronted. It was their anxiety about death and dying that was causing them to remove the stress of discussing this subject from Carol. Carol was deeply moved by the group's support and reported that there were tears in her eyes. Amanda suggested that she may be projecting her own attitudes regarding dying onto Carol. Crying and expression of feelings were encouraged. However, it was shared with the group that while there was a need to cry and to hurt, it was important to keep discussing feelings. Amanda shared an experience that she had with a friend of hers who died and that person's accepting attitude. In dealing with her own death, Carol then shared efforts by one of her sister's to come and live with her and the problematic nature of the generous offer. Similarly, she shared her perception that the problem of her pain and suffering was intruding on the natural development of her children's lives.

Steve: I'm just feeling for Carol right now because I'm feeling that we're giving her the kind of support in the group that you are all saying you don't like in the outside world. If you would try to explore some feelings that you are having on a thing because of how other people might react, you don't get into those and share them. And I guess I was reacting to something, Amanda, that you said awhile ago, and that is there's not a big need to share the feelings and stuff because somebody's going to cry. And I wonder if that's fair to Carol or whoever happens to be talking about how they are. . . .

Carol: . . . tenderhearted and it brings tears to the eyes.

Steve: Yeah, I know. And I guess what I'm saying is we don't want to set an atmosphere that encourages just crying and stuff. I see where you are coming from, but on the other hand sometimes just letting the feelings out so they are out in the open where you could share them . . . I agree with you. We know how she's feeling, and we can feel that. But we are doing the same thing to each other in the group that you all were telling me is being done to you on the outside.

We are not letting the group be a place to vent and get this stuff out and work with it.

Amanda: Well, I'm sorry if I gave that impression but I think I was feeling very protective of Carol because I'm putting myself in Carol's position. I just repeat. I am reserved! I don't like for people to get too close. I'll determine how close you get, not you determine how close you'll get.

Steve: I agree. But what I'm hearing is that you are saying that for Carol, too, and I'm wondering if she needs the protection.

Amanda: Well, maybe that's where I can be wrong. I am projecting my own attitudes onto Carol, and maybe they obviously are not for you and I shouldn't try. But I don't think. . . . If I gave you the impression that if you break down you are weak and all that kind of thing, I'm sorry. I didn't mean to. But there are enough things that you can find to do, even if you don't feel too well, which can help time pass rather pleasantly and you can pick up a lot of things you haven't had a chance to do before.

Sally: That's true. But as I said, I sort of picked up what I wanted to do gradually, you know . . . I feel it's so much as to descend on her all of a sudden.

Steve: That's where I was too. I don't know if we can work it through in the group, but I think it's important for Carol to share where she's at in the group. And I could see the tears coming. And I guess what I wanted to say to you from where I am. . . .

Amanda: Maybe you need to. . . .

Steve: That it's OK if you need to cry — that you can cry in here and we are going to still work. We are going to work through the tears. We're not just going to leave you crying. And I was very concerned about your feelings of uselessness and your feeling of "I might as well just give it up if my life is over; if my need is over," instead of this anxiety about "is it going to be six months or six weeks or a year," and that you need to talk about it.

Amanda: You know something Carol. I have had . . . well, one . . . I've another friend. She died with cancer. I felt, when people reported it to me, they were mixed in their reactions. Some were horrified and some thought it was lovely and thoughtful. I thought it was lovely. She happened to be a very affluent woman. And special things of hers that had meant a great deal to her, she gave to her friends because she said, "I want you to have it." And I thought that was simply lovely. Now I don't mean for you to go around dividing up your possessions, but I thought the way she managed it was just simply marvelous. It was a very accepting attitude, not morbid. I was kind of glad to hear about it.

Carol: One of my sisters in Minnesota asked me to quit working and come live with her. I don't want to sell everything I own and just have a suitcase full of clothes and just go from one sister or brother like my father did. I have a friend who lives in Florida. She and I were in the service together, and she wants me to live with her. I love her very much, but she talks so much. I'm afraid that she'd get on my nerves. I mean I don't want to put all my belongings in one suitcase and just shuffle from relative to relative. And I don't want to intrude on my children's lives because they are young and they kind of want to have their young friends over and they don't want mother sitting in the living room with them.

The essence of suffering and the subsequent search for the purpose and meaning of life is summed up succinctly, as was often the case, by a very forthright Amanda: "What I believe you are saying is it's not just the pain that made you think of imminent death, but it's all these other decisions that all of a sudden you can't put off. You feel you can't put them off any longer. And you are just sort of overwhelmed by them. Then you just kind of have to sort them out and say, "I don't like that alternative; let me think about this one a minute." But don't . . . it's just like giving all your money to your children, don't do it."

While Amanda approached the process of searching for one's purpose in life and making decisions, she just could not resist one more effort in supporting Carol toward not giving up and hanging on to her life.

LOSS OF CONTROL: DEPENDENCY

One of the fears that all of us have, and it is particularly pronounced in the cancer patient, seems to be the fear of loss of control and subsequent dependency on others. This fear was alluded to in the previous section where Carol discussed her sister's offer for "asylum" and her fears of intruding on the "normal" development of her children and that it was beyond her control to do anything about the letter.

In the same session, the subject of loss of control was approached when the question was posed as to whether or not Carol was feeling as though she was running out of alternatives. Amanda reacted strongly to the prospect of loss of control in her life in the following excerpt. This excerpt highlights anger as a reaction to the fear of loss of control that the cancer patient typically feels. Put yourself in their shoes, and you will get some small idea of the terror that grips one at the thought of existing totally dependent on others for survival and nurturance.

Steve: Carol, I wonder. Are you beginning to feel like you are running out of alternatives?

Carol: I don't know, Steve. When I found out that I was getting 2,000 mg. instead of the usual 12 or 1,700, I knew that something was more wrong than they were letting me know.

Steve: So you sense that there is more going on than you are being told and that adds to the anxiety. You'd almost rather know.

Carol: And I have never been so ill as before this last treatment. It's because it was such a heavy dosage.

Steve: And then when your sister and your friend invite you to sell everything, and come live with them and your doctor's talking about a medical retirement, you begin to wonder. . . .

Carol: What's left?

Steve: "Am I just going to be a piece of flesh that's going to be shoveled around here?" I think you get. . . . It's that fear, loss of control, you're no longer in charge of your own life. And, Amanda, you reject that vehemently. I mean I can just see that if you felt that you were losing control, that would be enough.

Amanda: That would really undo me!

Steve: That would push you over the edge.

Amanda: It sure would! I'm used to running things, not being on them.

Steve: And I think Carol's saying the same thing: "I'm used to being vivacious and doing what I want to do, even with the cancer. And now I'm beginning to feel some people are holding back on me and I'm losing control. They are treating me as a child — as if I don't have any say in what happens to me."

Amanda: Yes, the one thing that sends me up the wall is to be treated as if I didn't have a grain of sense.

PLANNING FOR THE FUTURE

Diana: But what I'm saying is that other people our age are living right now. They are raising children and looking towards later years, and I can't do that, not realistically!

Amanda: That's right, Diana! Other people your age are planning for the future and what lies ahead. And you can give lip service to it, but down in your heart you wonder if it's going to be. I mean, you feel like it's not going to be.

Diana: OK, that's what I meant.

Amanda: And it has to solve a problem any way you look at it. And I think, personally, you would be a blooming idiot not to face up to it realistically.

One of the guiding principles of Alfred Adler's teleoanalytical therapy involves the concept that one is pulled in the universe toward final, fictional goals. Thus, one acts out according to perceived inferiority or superiority that is determined by one's fantasy of those fictional goals.

For the cancer patient the final, fictional goal might be seen as humiliating defeat at the hands of an unmerciful adversary in the form of cancer. What type of self-concept might one have who is being pulled into the future, and to some degree, whose life is now being governed by the erosion of self toward an end of "nourishment" for the disease? One can only feel helpless and used in such a situation. Anger, bitterness, and frustration begin to yield to resignation and even martyrdom. Difficulties in planning for the future are obvious. The erratic course of cancer, with a pattern of attack-remission-attack, leaves future planning speculative at best.

In the following excerpt the group was discussing those situations of hurt in life that time is supposed to heal. Diana responded to the concept of time healing. In the attempt to explore the difficulty in planning for the future, the concept of growth and suffering resulting in added meaning to life was verbalized by Sally. It is interesting that this verbalization occurred at a time when the group was having difficulty discussing problems of planning for the future.

Diana: But time doesn't heal what we've got. We haven't left it back there. It's something we live with every day.

Steve: Which makes it difficult to look too far ahead, but it also makes it difficult to look too far back. The kinds of things that Sally's talking about are things we can't keep looking back on or dwelling upon, which is what you are saying. And the kind of thing you just talked about, which makes all of you unique, is that you can't plan too far ahead or you get in trouble that way. So what we're all saying is that there's got to be a way we can make life more meaningful right now.

Amanda: You know Diana. . . .

Sally: Problems! When you are in the middle of them it's terrible! And we are in one right now of course. I don't know how we are going to get out but I can say one thing, just from my experience. In the past you have a terrible problem, and it seems like hell! And you are going through it. And this and that and the other . . . and you are resentful, and you have a lot of other feelings about it. But once it's over with, and you can see a little bit of life, you can see if you just analyze the situation, the good that came from it — what you have learned from it and it seems like it puts you one step . . . and it fortifies you to meet something else or to help someone else.

The issues of dependency, loss of control, loss of function, and planning for the future are intertwined in the following excerpt. Amanda shared the frustration of the erratic course of cancer and planning for the future. The *he* that she alluded to was her oncologist.

Amanda: What's ahead? I don't mean tomorrow or the next day. I don't think they know that as far as specific times are concerned. But, as he said, everything begins to be involved and then everything begins to go including all the vital organs and so on. But he said I do not believe in putting people in the hospital and letting them stay forever and ever. He mentioned about visiting nurses and so on. And, so you know, I'm a compulsive list maker and planner. If it happens before 1977, this will be true and so on. And that was a really very comforting thing to me. But, as Steve said, I can still stay in control. I can still stay in my own place. I'm not dependent on anybody. I don't have to be the poor mother who has to go up to Boston for somebody to look after her. I won't be a burden on anybody.

Steve: I guess another thing I'm feeling, too, is the pressure, you know, the looking at the alternatives and trying to decide; the running out of alternatives and trying to avoid the loss of control; the depression, the fear, the scariness of the death experience you [Carol] had on Monday; and all these things coming together and almost wanting to know. I'm getting the feeling it would almost be better to know that "at this date I'm going to run out of time and that the alternatives will take care of themselves."

Sally: Everybody would like to know that, Steve.

Amanda: Then you'd know exactly how to plan. It's that business that you plan for six months and it turns out to be a year. So then you move it up and you plan for a year and then it turns out to be two years. And I think, I believe I mentioned this. My child said this: She said that it gets to be a burden when you have your life sort of scheduled and all of a sudden the time limit is altered.

For the cancer patient with an incurable prognosis, planning for the future also included anticipation of an afterlife. While the concept of afterlife was not attended in this group, at least not in so many words, those who are inquisitive about unconscious dynamics may agree with the assertion that there is the unconscious innuendo of impending death and afterlife suggested in Amanda's recollection of an experience in Rome. Carol responded to the unconscious dynamic verbalized by Amanda, stating that going to heaven was her one goal in life.

Amanda: I just think Rome is terribly depressing. I've only been there once. But we were on the roof of the hotel and drinking champagne, and the swallows were circling, and I could see St. Peter's Square. And I thought, "You have died and gone to heaven!"

Carol: That's my one goal in life!

The difficulties in planning for the future have yet another dimension. Cancer patients seem to want to have the physician give the prognosis. In this prognosis, the cancer patient would like to, in the case of incurable cancer, have an idea of life expectancy. Physicians are justifiably reluctant to make such predictions. On the one hand there is the issue of the self-fulfilling prophecy. According to this philosophy, the suggestion (made by a strong authority figure) that a patient may die in a year may predilect the patient to die at the appointed time when such may not have been the case under other circumstances. The power of the Shaman to place a curse and have an otherwise healthy person die at an appointed time is a prime example of the dynamics of the self-fulfilling prophecy at its extreme.

Of course, making a prediction that one has a finite expectancy with metastatic cancer may serve as a motivator for one to fight for life and prove the establishment wrong. Persons who are independent, strong, struggling, and determined to not accept authoritarian proclamations will often respond well to such a challenge. The doctor says you will die in six months, and the patient says, "I'll show you! I'll live for six years!" Such seems to have been the case with Amanda. In the following excerpt, Amanda shared the utterances of her physician's prognosis; the orderly and realistic steps that she went through in order to prepare for her final days; and the disappointment (and yet happiness) at the doctor's errant prediction. Maintaining dignity and a healthy self-concept, as well as the issue of hope, are all touched as the group wrestles with future planning and life expectancy.

Amanda: Well, originally when they did the surgery, it never occurred to me that that would be the end of it. It's just like taking out your tonsils. You've done it, period! That's the end of it! I began to see there was a percentage. Statistics! And it didn't look like it made too much difference what kind of treatment you had. Roughly 50 percent of mastectomy patients don't have an ordinary life expectancy, which puts a very different slant on it. And then when Doctor Maste told me . . . when was it? Well, about two years . . . I'm really not supposed to be here today . . . about two years ago, that I had just about reached the end of the line, it never occurred to me that that wouldn't be true either. And here I am. I think maybe it's a different policy on both sides of the hall. I believe the surgeons say you got so long and they just don't. . . .

Jane: You know I had never asked a doctor what my prognosis is because I think it is unfair to ask him. . . .

Amanda: I wanted to know!

Jane: And expect him to answer that. He can't answer it because. . . .

Amanda: He could give me an educated guess!

Jane: Because so many new chemicals, so much new medication like yours is coming out on the market, and you don't know when there might be a breakthrough.

Diana: But, like I was told twice — and it's kind of totally destroyed part of me because I fully expected to die — they said I was going to, and so I didn't.

Amanda: Well, I think what irritated me was I rearranged my life when it apparently was not that necessary. In fact, I chided Doctor Maste that he made me give up my career prematurely, and that's exactly what happened.

Steve: So, I could imagine, as you tell that, that it would be very frustrating for a person like you, who is extremely well organized, to have something that isn't very well organized.

Amanda: I rearranged my life on the premise that that was accurate information including giving up the job at the speech school and so forth, and here I am still! Now, I take claim. I'm sorry I don't have to worry about the heat and are we going to close or not close school . . . I'm not primarily responsible any more!

Steve: I guess I'm just wondering to myself, you know, that it must be difficult to have plans all made out and find out you have to keep rescheduling all the time. . . .

Amanda: Right! Because, as I told you, I'm a compulsive list maker. So I sit down and say, "Now if I die before 1976 I'll have this to leave to Amanda. If I die before 1977, I will have to spend some of that and so Amanda won't get this money." But, hells bells, it looks like I'm going to be here too long!

Steve: Your exit isn't well timed.

Amanda: Well, I just can't stand such disorderly acts!

Steve: I wonder if it's possible in the planning down to the days like that that the planning could become more important than the living.

Amanda: It couldl! It could! Except I don't spend an awful amount of time on it.

Steve: You just work it over sometimes in your mind.

Amanda: Yeah, well any person. . . . You've got to arrange your financial affairs to get the most return from what little money you have and to spend it so that you can enjoy reasonable standards of living without. . . . I mean, I'm going to do without everything!

Jane: But you could do this without even having a condition such as. . . .

Amanda: Yeah, but people don't!

Steve: Jane, I think that one of the things I'm feeling in the group is that this is a common frustration, even for yourself, even though you say that it's not. I guess I'm

	hearing that it is. Each member of the group deals with the lack of structure in not knowing a little differently.
Amanda:	I think maybe you have just put your finger right on it and it's a thing that basically is bothering Diana. Of course, ordinary distress of leaving your children and your husband and not having the kind of life you expected to have. . . . *But it's just not knowing!* You get all set for one thing and then they pull the rug out from under you. So then you get set again and they pull it out again. And you just think, "Well should I believe them or shouldn't I?"
Steve:	I guess I hear the way that you react to that frustration is by maintaining order and dignity and maintaining your self-image.
Amanda:	It beats falling apart!
Steve:	And I guess the way I hear Jane dealing with that is saying "Look maybe something's just around the corner! I'm Jane! It's not going to happen to me!"
Jane:	Yeah!
Amanda:	You see, I don't have that kind of hope! I really don't!
Jane:	I really feel that. I'm very optimistic about a lot of the strides that are being made. I do a lot of reading concerning medication that chemotherapy patients get or, for that matter, the type of treatment that cancer patients get. And I'm very optimistic.
Amanda:	I think I'm an optimist too, and I pride myself on being a realist.
Jane:	I think I'm a realist. I know that eventually this life of mine is going to end.
Amanda:	Yeah, even in your own heart, and when you say eventually, you mean about a 1,000 years old.
Jane:	I'm not evaluating it because if I were interested I would say to Doctor Norris, "How long do you think I'm going to live?" I'm not interested. I think that when the time — when it's ready for me to leave this world — I can leave this world.

PERSONAL EXPERIENCES

During the course of our group, one of the group members

shared a particularly moving, personal experience with death. We have already heard Sally's series of horrible coincidences in her life in which both her husbands died from similar circumstances five years apart. As she recalled, the death of her second husband with the same ambulance attendants, the same disease process, and occurring at almost the exact same place in the same house was a *déjà vu* experience that almost defied reality.

Early in our sixth session, Carol was sharing her close encounter with death and the almost unbearable pain. It was during this session that Sally revealed her own personal experience with the death of her mother from cancer. The following excerpt will enable Sally to share her experience with you.

Sally: But you know I saw my mother. . . . In fact, I was holding my mother when she passed on, and she had cancer, and she had gone through the tortures of hell for seven years with it because she passed on in 1943, and you know how long ago that's been . . . and they didn't know much about what to do then, and they had given her radium and that was all. They didn't have all these "chemos" and everything. Well, the only kind of pain killer that would relieve her pain in any way was codeine. And she just fought like a tiger to keep from taking that codeine until she would go to bed at night because she didn't want to be a drug addict. And I used to beg and plead with her. I'd say, "Well mother! For heaven's sakes! If you are in pain, honey, please take it!" Well, that didn't do any good. But she was like you [Carol]. We had to have a practical nurse the last three years of her life at home. But she was up and on her feet, and she would get in such excruciating pain she'd get up and go to some other part of the house. [My father was retired at the time and I was living at home.] . . . My husband was overseas and just the practical nurse was there, but she'd go off somewhere because nobody would bother her by herself in the bathroom. She just didn't want somebody to see the pain.

Amanda: Well, I think that's good! That's considerate of other people, and, you know, I feel strongly that you should be. . . . I mean being considerate of other people is far more important than expressing your own feelings. I know we [to Steve] don't agree on that, but I feel that way.

Sally: . . . she went about 11:00 at night. We had a small sofa on one side of the living room and another one over on the other side. It was in December. She died on the 29th of December, and my father had a big fire in the fireplace, and I went over to sit beside her on the little sort of a loveseat, and I asked if she thought she would be comfortable if she got over on the other sofa, and I put the bed rest on. She decided maybe so, and then she looked at me and she said, "You know, I'm going to leave you." But she said, "Don't worry about it." So I took her, helped her when she got up, held her by the arm, and took her, and she sat down on the other sofa, and I put the bed rest on. And as I started — I had this arm under her head to lay down — when I was going to get it down, she gasped and her face before was just nothing but wrinkles in pain. And I remember I said to her, "Mama do you know me?" And she shook her head this way [up and down]. And I said, "Are you alright?" And she shook her head [up and down] and that was the last of her. But just when the last breath left her, it seemed to me that her face just all cleared up. And I mean it was relaxed looking and, you know, you didn't see the pain. And I'll tell you, we had been up and she had suffered so, and it was just a matter. . . . I know I felt great relief. I felt like she was out of all that pain.

IT'S ALL RELATIVE

As with many situations in life, cancer places circumstances in positions of relativity. Two features were prominent during the course of the group, and it is appropriate to share them at this juncture.

Prior to one of the sessions I was having lunch with Carol in the hospital cafeteria. As I recall, I was on one of my ten annual diets. (I have lost 300 pounds in the last 10 years.) Thus, I was eating boysenberry yogurt accompanied by celery sticks and carrot slices brought from home. I suddenly became aware of Carol eating her cottage cheese salad. Immediately, I was overwhelmed by a feeling of nausea. Contemplating this feeling, I began to realize how paradoxical it was that in sustaining her own existence by eating, Carol was feeding the cancer that was consuming her body. As I became more aware of the paradoxes of survival and the progress of cancer, I sensed my own anxieties about the whole subject of death and dying. I became aware of the fact that all of us feed potentially pathogenic organisms that could ultimately destroy us. The question of living and dying is one of relativity.

I can also recall a different circumstance during the course of the group. Carol was absent from the ninth session. She was being hospitalized and the group was preparing for the announcement of her death, especially in the light of her close encounter with death she had shared with us during the sixth session. At the tenth and final session Carol was present, bathrobe and all. She was still alive! It had been discovered that she was "*only*" suffering from diabetes. The group cheered wildly and congratulated Carol on being alive. Leave it to Amanda to verbalize what was being felt by all: "But isn't it absurd that everyone was so delighted that Carol had diabetes?"

It's all relative.

ACCEPTING REALITY

But to look at it realistically, though, I'm going to die from this because science isn't going to find a cure. They may be able to help my children, but they are not going to be able to help me.

Diana

It was during the eighth session that the action of introspection was most manifest. It was during this session that the subject of death and dying was extensively "worked over" by the group. The expression *worked over* is used as opposed to the term *worked through* (a psychoanalytic term), for none of us ever works through our own death until the moment of final reckoning (if then). It was during this session that Diana shared with the group the fact that she had burned her copy of Kubler-Ross' book entitled, *Death and Dying*.

Diana: I had a heart and lung specialist who gave me a very short time to live, gave us a book by the doctor lady. . . .

Amanda: That Elisabeth Kubler?

Diana: Right! *On Death and Dying.* We laughed and burned it in our fireplace. Maybe now that I have hindsight I feel that maybe we were afraid to read it.

Amanda: I expect you were.

Diana: Rather than the boldness we felt at the time, I really think we did laugh and we did burn it. *But I really think we were probably afraid to read it.*

Diana shared her fear to read it, suggesting that her laughter was a bravado in the face of death.

In the following excerpt, the group discussed the reality of the prognosis that accompanies metastatic cancer. Diana and Jane tacitly seemed to accept the reality that most persons with this type of disease die from it.

Jane: I went to a class that we had at the Unitarian Congregation about four years ago about death and dying and that was rather. . . .

Amanda: They are not really the best ones to teach you about death and dying.

Jane: And in that group, there was a woman who had cancer, and she subsequently passed away.

Diana: That's the trouble. Subsequently, most everybody you know who has cancer passes away. Thank the Lord that none of us in here passed away during the group; it would just floor me.

Jane: No! But she had . . . her's was terribly metastasized, you see. . . .

Diana: I can't pronounce that word.

Amanda: Now, Diana, you know, subsequently everybody passes away!

Jane: Everybody passes away, and I have always accepted. . . .

Diana: Yeah, I can't say "Ma . . . " How do you say it?

Amanda: *Me-tas-ta-sized!*

Jane: I always accepted the fact that I was going to pass away eventually.

The following excerpt occurred just after Diana had given good feedback to the group regarding the help the group had given her. She stated that she still was afraid to die, and everyone discussed the reality and acceptability of that fear. Also in this excerpt, Amanda shared that there were some good aspects of cancer in that it gives one time to tie up loose ends. The group continued to verbalize the realities of death and dying and the depression that this manifests in real life. The group was confronted with the fact that, even when things appear to be sailing along, there is always the reality of death to fuel depression and despair.

Diana: I still feel like I'm just as afraid. I don't want to die any more today than I did. . . .

Carol: Yesterday!

Diana: Yeah!

Amanda: You know, I don't think anybody wants to die. If they do, then they are really sick.

Carol: I don't want a slow long death.

Amanda: Nobody wants that. We all have it figured out. We want to go to sleep and not just wake up. That would just be great. But unfortunately, that doesn't work that way all the time. But it seems to me that it's not a question of saying, "Well, I'm not afraid," because we are all afraid.

Carol: I think we all are.

Amanda: Because it's unknown when we are going. But there's a difference between normal fear and absolute terror. And that's what I hope I can always avoid . . . that terror. One thing I think it's beneath my dignity. I'd rather people say, "Oh! She's so gallant," rather than say, "She's scared to death"!

Carol: I still like what you said once that you want people to say she makes a beautiful. . . .

Amanda: A beautiful corpse!

Carol: I said that in the office the other day. They said, "Carol we don't want to hear that!" So I said, "Well, I don't want you all to come view my body and say, 'Oh, doesn't she look peaceful?' I want you to say, 'Doesn't she make a beautiful corpse?' And they hit me on the head.

Amanda: That's an odd sense of humor.

Carol:	They didn't like it, but I enjoyed joking about it.
Amanda:	Well, on a purely practical basis, since we are on the subject of death and dying, has everybody made a will?
Carol:	I have!
Sally:	I have!
Amanda:	That's one good thing about this! It gives you plenty of time to catch up on your loose ends. You can get even with a few people.
Jane:	When I was told I had three months to live, this was in 1975, I said to the doctor, "Couldn't you stretch it to two years? There are a few things that I want to take care of."
Diana:	Well, that doesn't seem to have disturbed you that they gave you X number of months to live. Yet Cindy and Doctor Norris think that because twice in my life they've said you've got X number of months to live, that that accounts for part of the reason I am like I am today. They said I've been told too often I'm going to die.
Steve:	When you say part of the reason you are the way you are today, what do you mean?
Diana:	Well, I don't know. . . .
Amanda:	Well you are just so conscious of death!
Diana:	Yeah, or I get. . . .
Jane:	She gets so alarmed!
Diana:	Well, I'm thinking when they said . . . it was last August when I had lost control — you know my nerves were just shot — this is what they said. They felt that I was told I was going to die so often that it accounted for the anxiety. Like I go along fine and all of sudden I hit rock bottom and sometimes I can feel it coming on. I can actually feel the depression. I can feel it coming on me, and even though I can rationalize. . . .
Amanda:	You know what it is, but you just can't dispel it.
Diana:	Yeah, but I can't stop it.
Steve:	Sometimes you feel the depression coming on, and it just makes you anxious. Really anxious. Uptight.
Diana:	And then I begin to have symptoms in my body that

something is wrong, and it's really . . . there's
nothing wrong but nerves. So Jane handled it. I'm
not thinking psychologically. Somewhere back in
my brain I store things like this little baby out here
who had her hair. . . .

Amanda: Her hair shaved off?

Diana: Yes! She probably has a brain tumor and is getting
cobalt. Well, OK, I'm storing that back here, and
days from now I'm going to think about it.

Sally: You know when you need it, it'll come to you.

Diana: But when I don't need it, it comes to me!

Sally: You've got something stored that's good maybe. And
you think, "Well, am I going to keep this?" I think that
the time comes that you really need that, maybe.

Diana: But Sally, I've stored things I don't need.

Steve: Are you saying she stores those kind of negative
events so that when things are going pretty well she
reminds herself of what might be the depressant?

Sally: No, I think this may be a way out or something. I
thought maybe she'd store it up there.

Steve: Oh, to help her? I was thinking something else. I was
thinking that you store them and when everything's
sailing, you remind yourself of the apparent reality.

Amanda verbalized another reality. Not only does the cancer patient have trouble accepting the reality of death, but so do those who
minister to the patient: chiefly the oncologist and nurse practitioner.
Amanda said, "But do you know who else had more to talk about
death and dying . . . because I had jokingly said, "Now listen. All I
ask of you all is just let my time and my money run out
simultaneously." And Cindy and Doctor Norris both of them said,
'Oh, Amanda!' Just like everybody else on the street, you know:
Don't talk about *that!*"

The following is a rather lengthy excerpt that is illustrative of the
conflict that reality poses for the cancer patient. Diana had been
sharing the difficulties that she and her husband had been experiencing in order to crowd the normal expectancy of a marriage through a
lifetime and compressing those experiences into a brief period of
time. This was dramatized by excessive purchases of, for instance, a
Lincoln Continental, a mink stole, and a house somewhat beyond

their financial means. Amanda confronted Diana and the discussion
ensued. It is a powerful look through the eyes of cancer patients.

Amanda: What are you doing, Diana? Are you just trying to
dull the pain?

Diana: Could be.

Carol: Yeah, that's a good one.

Diana: Could be, but I'm very jealous inside as my husband
goes up in his job, and he makes a good salary, and
his potential is even greater. OK, I want us to go to
Atlanta and get to Cleveland or Chicago and go to
get to Bridgeport. I want to be able to enjoy the
money he makes because . . . thirteen years
ago . . . we got married and our dreams were so
small, and he went to school and to college, and he's
educated to do what he's doing, and he's good. But I
want to be able to share in that. We had our children
early so that they would be grown and we would still
be young enough to enjoy this.

Amanda: You've got something to hang on to.

Diana: No! I'm not going to live that long! I'll probably not
see my children grown!

Amanda: Diana, can you bring yourself to look at it like this:
"OK! So I may die by the time I'm thirty-five, and
there's nothing I can do about that. Period! But I
fooled them twice in seven years; so I'm just going to
try to shove that to the back of my head and just go
on."

Diana: But somehow I can't do that! I hear what you are saying, and I want to do that. Even the things that Jane
said about not being afraid, being able to accept it
and look at the medication that hasn't even been
passed yet. You know, there is hope. But like on the
questionnaires, one of the words was hope. Hope is
a joke to me. I wish I could feel the way that you feel
and the way that you feel but somehow. . . .

Amanda: You just can't do it.

Diana: I can sugarcoat it, and I can say you know, "OK, I feel
that way today," but I really don't.

Amanda: Well, I just think it's like telling somebody with a broken leg to get up and walk. If you can't you can't.

Carol: I feel awful today, but I'm looking forward to the springtime.

Diana: Somehow I don't feel the future. I can enjoy the things you got planned, but that's like signing up for a year at this figure salon. I think, "No! I can't sign up for a year because we may be blowing our money on a year."

Amanda: Let me tell you. I felt that originally when they first told me that I got a year and a half, two years at the most. So I would think, "No I better not do that." I even thought about renewing magazine subscriptions. This just shows you. I mean I feel if you just give the human spirit a chance, it just doesn't stay down. I've bought way too much Christmas wrapping paper because I forgot I had some. And I really laughed out loud when I said to myself I can use it next year. And I thought, "Well, hello!"

Diana: On good days I can say that and on. . . .

Steve: You say you don't feel for the future. Is it you don't feel for the future or you don't want to feel for the future?

Carol: See feels that she's not going to have a future.

Diana: Yeah!

Steve: Is it a conscious choice or is it just a feeling as you think about it right here?

Diana: I don't know. I'm thinking that for so long I've been told by people that I have great respect in doctors — to live today.

Amanda: *But Diana, there's a difference in to live today and eat, drink, and be merry for tomorrow you may die.*

Steve: Are you saying to her that when you try to force a lot of things and crowd them into a short time span, that's an added pressure?

Amanda: It's a kind of frantic thing. Yes, I think you could be pressuring yourself without realizing it. Grab quick! Quick! It's going to get away from you!

Steve: And in the hanging on like that, there's a frustration of never catching up; never moving quite fast enough; that it's just getting out of reach from you.

So it's kind of a damned-if-you-do and damned-if-you-don't position.

Carol: If you don't have faith in the future, Diana, why are you going to Weight Watchers® and why are you going to the doctors?

Diana: [sarcastically] It's cheaper by the year! But you know. . . .

Carol: You are talking about tomorrow and tomorrow is the future.

Steve: When you hear Carol ask you that question, what do you feel?

Diana: I don't know. I just, gosh. . . .

Steve: What's your impulse?

Diana: My impulse is to agree with what she says, but I know deep down inside that. . . .

Steve: Your resistance won't allow you to feel that way. But your impulse is to want to feel that way. Maybe not resistance. Maybe how you perceive reality.

Diana: It's really like looking for a job. You know, as really badly as I wanted a job because I felt like I needed to do that, always in the back of my mind, I thought, "How can I ever assume the responsibility of a job?" Not because, you know, they are expecting me to be there and I can't do that. I could never get into a long-term thing because most probably. . . .

Steve: As I hear you say that I feel your anger right here. I wonder if in being realistic, in that sense, if you are really helping yourself or if you are not just agitating yourself further?

Carol: Diana, you are so full of life today. You are not going to die today of cancer.

Diana: No! But even as good as I feel today, even as good as I feel, and I'm really taking some positive steps in my life, I think that I'm only on a ride. Because I've fallen off so many times just when I thought I had it all together, just when I thought my life was begining to mean something, that I really had it all together and I really felt like the cancer was in remission and finally I could look to the future. And it came back! And it didn't come back little! It came back bad and I fought it! And I fought it! And I guess that's when a complete defeat came. And I can't get, I can't. . . .

Steve: I wonder. The reality probably is pretty hard, I mean, not probably, it is pretty hard. But that if in choosing to perceive that reality today like that, each day, if that is not self-defeating?

Carol: Diana, I have felt. . . .

Steve: Kind of, I didn't mean to interrupt you, but I'd kind of like to hear. . . .

Diana: I don't really understand what you mean.

Steve: That's what I thought. I'll just come back to it again. I didn't mean to interrupt you Carol.

Carol: I have felt worse these few weeks of February and all of January than I have for many, many years. But I don't feel that I'm on my death bed yet because I can still put my feet on the floor every day. If I can make it through the day,

Amanda: But you did a few weeks ago.

Carol: Yes, I was really sick in January.

Sally: I told Cindy it was mighty hard to get out of bed this morning. You know, you just don't have to have cancer to feel bad. And I could hardly get up. I could hardly get in the bathroom. I could hardly get my bath.

Amanda: Oh really, was it this morning?

Sally: Yeah, it's been that way a lot in the last few months.

Carol: I have trouble moving too, but I make it.

Sally: I don't have any energy and it's just hard to get going. During the day you want to do something but you can't hardly get around. I don't know what it is. I don't know what you are worrying about.

Amanda: I'm always tempted to say, "None of your blank business."

Diana: Can you be worried and not know what you are worried about? Can we subconsciously. . . .

Amanda: Don't you think we can suppress things though; pretend that we are not worried about this specific thing and so it breaks out in another area. It's just like saying, you know, like children can't tell you where it hurts sometimes. They'll say, "My throat hurts," when actually it's their stomach that hurts.

Sally: Mine used to say, "I hurt in all my pieces!" "Where do you hurt honey?" "In all my pieces, Mommy."

Steve: I guess I was wondering, to come back to Diana a little bit, that in looking at the reality every day. . . . Like right now looking at the reality and saying, "What's the use" . . . if that isn't self-defeating, because it stirs up all the anger and bitterness. And each time it's a little more.

Diana: But you see somehow I will fall back on some of the things I've said last week. Somehow in all of this, most of the time I'm able to put — to screw a top on it. And I'm able to suppress it. And I only voice it here because I feel like this is what primarily we are here together for. But most times, it never leaves me, and in the midst of really feeling good, that black spot comes into my head.

Amanda: You are just like the cartoon, you know, the little black cloud hanging over your head.

Diana: And so you know you cannot talk about it. And I really feel good today but realistically, it's even like this morning. As good as I felt, the positive steps I've taken, I still . . . it's still there. I still think about the probability when it comes back. You know they say I'm in partial remission. I've been in partial remission most of my life. So it's good now, but it's going to come back.

Amanda: You really can't permit yourself to enjoy. . . .

Diana: Because I did enjoy it!

Carol: And it came back.

Diana: And it came back!

Amanda: And you got fooled and betrayed, and you haven't forgotten it.

Diana: Right! Right!

Amanda: It's hard to forget, literally, whether it's a personal relationship or you made a stupid mistake yourself. But if you really had a deep sense of betrayal for whatever reason, it's very hard to get over it.

Diana: But I can't seem to get a firm foundation.

Carol:	You'll be all right.
Steve:	I guess I'm wondering if Diana feels like she'll be all right. I know we are trying to give her support. . . .
Diana:	What do you mean, if I'll be all right?
Amanda:	All right mentally?
Steve:	I think Carol was saying you'll be all right in terms that I think she was trying to be gentle and say you'll be able to cope with it. And I wonder if you feel you will be able to cope with it?
Diana:	Oh, I feel like I'm coping better today. And it's been, it's nearly been a year; nine months in April it came. Well, it's been a year because I began to get sick in January. I'm handling it better today than I did at the beginning. But I'm not going to be foolish enough to think it's not going to come back, because it is.
Amanda:	Well, I think that's just being honest with yourself.
Diana:	That I was foolish enough nine months, a year ago, to believe it would never come back. Everything I believed in, every fiber of me, I could argue with everybody in this room because I knew it would never come back because everything I believe. . . . If positive thinking could keep something away.
Steve:	So right now you are still feeling the anger and bitterness of having had that belief and then having it come back.
Diana:	Yeah. So now I'm not going to be foolish enough to think that again.
Steve:	So, are you saying you are not going to be foolish enough to allow yourself to experience some sort of joy and happiness? That it's always going to be present? But the reality is it's going to come back again after partial remission? Are you saying "I'm not going to allow myself to experience a whole lot of happiness in the interim?"
Amanda:	You know, Diana, it sort of reminds me of somebody who has been bitterly disappointed in love, and a girl's been wild about a person, and he's let her down. So she says, "I will never run that risk again. I will never expose myself to that again." And conse-

quently she deprives herself of a great deal of personal happiness. And I think that kind of thinking may be governing you at the moment, and maybe you should be brave enough to take the risk.

Diana: I don't know, you know, right now, Amanda, I'm not. . . .

Amanda: Because I think you would be happier, not because it's upright or a fine thing to do. I just think you would be personally happier.

Diana: But, you know, I fell nine months ago and I fell hard. And it still hurts bad. And I feel like now that I have to be realistic about this thing and you know. . . .

Amanda: You have a right to be realistic. You are talking to the original realist.

Jane: But that was nine months ago. You had no idea that there would even be a partial remission, and this has come to pass; there is now partial remission.

Diana: Sometimes I think it would have been easier nine months ago to have died than it has been to live with this.

Jane: Well, I have lived with a radical mastectomy which. . . .

Diana: Let's not compare, honey! Let's not compare what surgery we have had!

Jane: No, but I just want to tell you how easy it would have been, and I live alone, for me to have given up.

Diana: I haven't given up!

Jane: You see it went to my liver and it went to my bones, but with the new medication I've got, it is now stable. I had no idea that this could come to pass.

Amanda: But you never were afraid to die, you see. And Diana's always been afraid to die.

Steve: I wonder if Diana doesn't feel like, "Look, Jane, maybe you don't know. You can't know how I feel because of our age difference. You've had the opportunity to have these experiences whether they've gone right or not. I haven't." And so I think what she was saying a minute ago is, "Don't try to compare yourself to me."

Jane: No, I guess. . . . The only thing I wanted to express was the fact that I was not looking for this kind of a change in my physical condition and it came about.

Steve: I guess what I'm hearing from you, Diana, is that you did expect this kind of a change in your physical condition and it didn't come about. And in addition to being angrier than hell about that, you are not willing to take the risk that Amanda was talking about to experience today with relative happiness.

Diana: Well, there again, like we said last week, everything's OK! You know, everybody, everything's OK! And I'll go home in a few weeks, and I'll be my happy, cheery self, and Mother and Daddy will be happy, and we'll all be happy.

Amanda: But you are just stiff when the day is coming when you won't be. . . .

Diana: Well, there again, I'm going to put it this way: I'm not going to kid myself into believing it's not going to come!

Jane: Well, I think you are right. I think you are exactly right about that.

Diana: And I don't go around with a long, moping face. And I will leave this room, and I'll be just like I was when I came in.

Steve: Amanda, I think what you are trying to do here is say to Diana, "Maybe there is a way you can deal with the reality and accept it and still free yourself up to be relatively happy today."

Amanda: I hope I can get that across. As I say, "I'm the original realist." My husband used to say, "She'll make you lie because she just pins you down." So I can quite understand that part of your feeling. I just hate to see you make yourself unhappy by. . . . I mean, you know it's coming. I know it's coming. But I just can't live today thinking what's going to happen tomorrow. I just can't do that.

Carol: Enjoy today!

Steve: Amanda, is that what you feel some of the writers mean by acceptance of the reality — that it frees you

	up to. . . .
Amanda:	I think it does. I really think it's quite liberating to be accepting of reality; not pessimistic; not stupidly optimistic; just say "OK, this is the way it is." And I always have to bring the church into it. But I remember our minister making a statement. And I have quoted him a thousand times. He was talking about somebody losing a relative: "Every experience can be redempting." Now, it's not going to be if you don't let it be, but it can be. And I'm not saying that you should develop any marvelous, beautiful, saintly character because of this. I'm just saying you can use this experience not to deprive yourself of every drop of happiness to which you are entitled. But just say "OK, that's the way it is!" Accept that. But I'm going to accept the other part of it too. I'm still here and I'm going to enjoy it!
Diana:	I guess I'm stupidly optimistic. I hang on to those two words. I was stupidly optimistic.
Amanda:	I think we can be! I think we can be! We fool ourselves! The worst person in the world to fool!
Steve:	I wonder if your reaction to that and the anger and the bitterness you carry around with you and that you are gracious enough to share with us here isn't defeating your enjoyment of the things. . . .
Diana:	But maybe I need more time. Maybe. . . .
Amanda:	You may need more time. You may need more time.
Diana:	Maybe this will come about. Right now maybe it's coming about and I'm not even aware of it right now. Like I say, I know things are better but, like I say, everything I believed in was totally, well, thrown back in my face; my face was just literally. . . .
Steve:	Like somebody stuck a boot right in your face.
Diana:	Yeah! Yeah! Everything I believed in, everything I preached and shared. . . . And everything, all of a sudden, was just thrown back at me. Everything! It's like everything I said was lies, but I believed it.
Steve:	Almost like you wanted to scream out, "You liars!"
Diana:	And so now I'm a. . . .

Amanda:	You may really have hit upon it. You just need more time.
Diana:	And, you know, definitely this new turn of events with the new medication things are better.
Amanda:	You know something, Diana. This just occurred to me. This was borrowed from a psychologist friend. Not you (to Steve)!
Steve:	I heard that: "Not you!" I'll remember that.
Amanda:	Well, I mean I'm not accusing you. But, actually I felt at the time, "Oh Lord!" But I really think it's true. When very bad things happen to us . . . you have to go through a period of mourning. And maybe you are just coming out of that period of mourning. And it's very wrong for people to try to suppress it. You do that a lot when there's been a death in the family. You try to cheer them up and just let them cry. Let them be. Just get it out and let them mourn. And maybe that's what's happening to you — that you really are coming out of it and it's good that you had that. It kind of cleanses your whole system.
Steve:	I guess my concern now is that you don't really mourn. I think that my concern is that as you mourn; that even now with the anger and the bitterness, and as you accept the reality of the time limitation, you just don't know how long. My concern is that if you keep putting off finishing that kind of mourning and accepting the reality, as Amanda says, without overoptimism or without overpessimism but just, "This is the way it is." The longer you put that off, the shorter time span you have to enjoy the things that you and Dave seem to be working so hard for.
Amanda:	Diana, we are going to save you if it kills us all!
Diana:	OK, I understand what you are saying. But, it's like last week. I said I hear everything you are saying. But things are good the way they are; so I'm going to leave them this way. But maybe in my own way even now, even through this year, this ventilation. It's like *I read the journal and I tore it up and I threw it away because I have grown and matured from the*

girl who wrote that.

Jane: Isn't it great that you recognize that?

Diana: I was very disappointed that I had those feelings. Now maybe tearing it up and throwing it away is suppressing it. I don't know. But somehow in my own little uneducated way I'm plowing through this: by the things I do; by the things I believe; maybe by the literature I read; I don't know. But I'm plowing through it. And it's not easy! But it's something that I'm going to have to do. And I'm not saying that the things that are said here don't go back here [pointing to head] and they come at the right time. They come and they help me, just as sometimes I store the bad things and they come at a time I don't need them. So you know I feel like, even though I'm being realistic, I'm going to make it. You know, I'm thirty-two. I don't know if I'll live to be thirty-five, you know. But maybe the day will come when I can make long range plans again.

An important ingredient toward accepting reality is the ability to maintain some hope. In the face of imminent death, hope must be maintained even though it might be a flickering ember, for hope is the thread of life that forms the fabric of one's faith and spirit.

Chapter 5

CANCER PATIENTS AND THEIR
REACTION TO TREATMENT

I hope that through this, that if nothing else happens, this paper you are going to write . . . that the doctors are going to hear it. I know what I went through for so many years. And if meeting together can help some other young woman to not go through what I had to go through because there was nobody who could understand, nobody I could talk to, *nobody*! . . .

Diana

T HE discussion of symptoms and treatments is a phenomenon characteristic of all self-help groups. To some degree there is safety in discussing one's aches and pains and complaining about the "system." Cancer patients are no exception. During the earlier sessions of the group, symptoms, comparison of scars, "war" stories, doctors, nurses, and treatment modalities were major themes, whereas other shared experiences were verbalized more in later sessions. As the group matured, the discussions became more personally relevant and more intimate in nature. More emphasis was placed by the group members on the psychosocial, psychological, and familial aspects of the course of cancer.

Several observations are worth noting before discussing the problems with treatment in more detail. First of all, the subjects that received the most attention during the course of the group were those dynamics of cancer, including discovery, fear, cancer symptoms, comparisons of cancer to other diseases (i.e. heart disease), identification with others having cancer, and the acceptance of cancer. All of these subjects can be grouped under the broad category of one's discovery of cancer and the effects of such a discovery.

Chemotherapy received much attention as well. This was not surprising, as most cancer patients who have been diagnosed as metastatic have to suffer with chemotherapy.

Another subject receiving much attention was the subject of the oncologist. Many reactions to the oncologist included looking at the oncologist as a Shaman, hoping for a magical cure; anger with the oncologist; and difficulties in trying to relate to the oncologist as a human being instead of just relating to the role of physician. Interestingly enough, in the course of fifteen hours of group therapy, the subject of radiation therapy was discussed on only three occasions during the first two sessions. Furthermore, regarding complaints surrounding the treatment and cure of cancer, usage of the word *terminal* in describing cancer patients was definitely inflammatory. One reference was made to dynamics of surgery. One reference was made to the clinic staff during an initial interview. Occasional references to surgeons were made as well as a reference to psychiatrists.

In several cases a general animosity was manifest. Such an attitude was not surprising in view of the fact that for most cancer patients stimulation from the outside world involves something painful done to them by a professional. It would be difficult to imagine having strong positive feelings for persons who, however softly, are still participating in one's death. Treatment is often palliative and while the patient may not be familiar with that word, he understands that the professional community gradually exhausts its "tricks" until there are no more in the bag. The patient must ultimately face his end. Such an outlook would certainly generate bitterness. The attitude might be, "Why, Doctor, do you pretend to be saving me when you and I both know I'm dying?" Yet there is the hope that the "magic" of technology executed through the hands of entrusted professionals will work this time! The relationship between the doctor and the patient might be analogous to the relationship between alcoholics and their spouses: "If we can just try this for one more day *maybe* we'll find that it works. In the meantime, a cure is just around the corner!" With the alcoholic, recovery is possible. With incurable cancer, recovery defies reality.

During most sessions, if an atmosphere of warmth, openness, trust, and caring is created, the client(s) will reveal those facts that are most significant to them. Being a counselor, one is more interested in what is not being said than in what actually appears to transpire verbally. Helping to clarify, interpret, and reflect about things of importance is where the skill of the therapist is involved toward uncovering unconscious dynamics of behavior. Thus, the omission of verbalizations is as significant as the commission.

For instance, during the group's life there was not one verbalization regarding nurses, social workers, clergy, psychologists, and/or counselors. This points up a real problem with regard to the treatment of cancer patients. Either these professionals are not available to incurable cancer patients, or if they are available, they are not making a significant impact in the delivery of services. To any knowledgeable person, these professionals are available to cancer patients in most modern medical facilities. However, it is apparent from this small sampling that such professionals must become more concerned with making a more significant impact in the care of metastatic cancer patients.

I HAVE CANCER

Discovery

> Still, with all the diseases in the world, I never thought I would come down with this one. And when the doctor told me what I had, I said, "You've got to be kidding!" He said, "No! You have it. . . ." I couldn't believe it! I couldn't believe that it happened to me! And now, why not? I'm no different from Mary or Sue or whatever.
>
> Carol

Carol couldn't believe that *she* would be a cancer victim. (Incidentally, the use of the term *victim* is a man's feeble attempt to anthropomorphize cancer, giving it "body" and "mind" so that it can be conquered and the multi-headed "dragon" will be slain.) This statement seems to be exemplary of the shock at the discovery of the disease. Even when shock is not professed, the fact that one has cancer still is sobering.

Jane: I was not shocked when I learned about it.
Carol: Well, I just thought I was going to die of old age.
Jane: I have a strong history on the paternal side. Everybody died of cancer. But somehow it was another side to me. . . . I never thought about it. And to this day, I can't understand why I didn't get cancer insurance. I could have done many sensible things.
Carol: Oh! I know! Gosh!
Jane: Somehow, I preferred to shut that out of my mind. I

think that's what I did. I recognized it perhaps subconsciously that I was a high risk.

In addition to the shock of the discovery of cancer, a process reported by some of the cancer patients in the group was that of anticipatory grief. In this case the one being grieved for was the patient
herself.

> **Sally:** I was just trying to go . . . trying to make it, see, but I
> felt. . . . I mean I really condemned myself to begin
> with and, then I felt, "Well, that's not right!" You see,
> to condemn myself, considering I was doing the best
> I could do, and if I couldn't do any better, there was
> no use to *"grieve over spilled milk."* Heaven help
> you, you got to face the situation then the best you
> can! So that's the way I felt then. But I would. . . . I
> mean it does. . . . You know it distresses me.

Certainly, anticipatory grief follows the shocking reality that one
has cancer. The reality of the discovery and its association with the
strong possibility of death couples to produce a feeling of horror that
might be akin to psychosis. Almost universally the response is the
following: "This cannot be happening to me!" Such an attempt to put
distance between the harsh realities of life in one's existence produces
a psychological strain like no other in this awareness.

> **Steve:** Well, when you talk to yourself, if I can ask, what
> kind of things do you talk to yourself about out loud?
>
> **Amanda:** Well, I really haven't done it in quite a long time. *I
> think when you first discover you have cancer, that's
> something you just really have to rear back and say,
> "Wait a minute! What's happening to me?"*
>
> **Carol:** I couldn't believe my ears when the doctor told me
> that!
>
> **Amanda:** You really feel like they are talking to somebody
> else. And there again I go back to the basic makeup
> of people of whether you are born that way, wheth-
> er you acquired it deliberately, or however you ar-
> rived at that point. My technique, most of the time in
> any kind of a situation is, "OK! What are the facts?
> What do I want? How do I get there?" And when you
> can line it up like that, then you can sort of handle it.

Steve:	Are you saying that's the way you are coping with it today?
Amanda:	Yeah! Sure is!

Fear

Earlier fear as psychodynamic of cancer was discussed. In the context of the patient's reaction to treatment for cancer, it is interesting to further examine fear as it incorporates in context with reality.

Fear occurs at many levels. For example, some cancer patients fear the struggle. On occasion, several of the members verbalized the desire to allow nature to "take its course." Several of these persons also felt that the nature of their treatment was often experimental and, because of this feeling, they were being used as guinea pigs. In the following passage, Jane took exception to this notion and verbalized wanting to be a "guinea pig," in order that what is learned from her treatment might be used in treating others. Diana and Amanda both verbalized their fear of being treated in this fashion. Such fears are compounded by the sense of hope given with each new treatment. On the other hand, there is the feeling of relinquishing life's grasp as each mini hope is dashed in failure. The rise and fall of emotions accompanying this pattern of treatment is almost more than the human spirit can bear.

Jane:	Why do you say you're sick of it [treatment]?
Diana:	The struggle. Everytime you come into the doctor's, the possibility of there being something else; finding it somewhere else. . . . You know, eventually, you know, I want to say, "I'm through! I'm going to *let nature take its course!*"
Amanda:	Well, maybe it falls down to this, Diana. Any sensible, rational person is going to do anything within reasonable limits. *But I draw the line at being a guinea pig!* Maybe that's what we are really talking about.
Jane:	You draw the line at being a guinea pig?
Amanda:	Uh huh!
Jane:	You know, that's exactly what I said to Doctor Norris. I want to be a guinea pig!

Amanda:	You want to be one?
Jane:	Yes!
Amanda:	You see, I don't want to be one!

Another example of fear in context is the fear of verbalizing what is known unconsciously. While the oncologist has many difficulties in making predictions with regard to the prognosis of cancer, particularly in metastatic cases, for the cancer patient with metastatic disease death is certain. The unconscious knowledge is often repressed with the hope that treatment might bring resolution and reprieve. In actuality, there is little satisfaction with a treatment that only continues to produce pain and suffering. Therefore, the cancer patient is at complete odds with himself regarding whether or not to allow nature to take its course or to keep fighting. When a physician makes a prognostication, it can have the effect of either allowing the cancer patient to let nature take its course and die at the appointed time "designated" by the doctor or it can serve as an impetus to fight against any one person having that much accuracy and influence regarding one's demise. Thus, there is fear that the oncologist will be right and a fear that he will not be right. While such fears are not explicitly stated in the following interaction between Jane and Diana, the astute reader will notice the subtlety of the dynamics.

Jane:	Last year I was given three months to live, and I'm living. And I get along pretty well. I have no physical impairments. Nothing hurts.
Diana:	And I think it's tremendous! And I look at Carol and I look at Amanda, and you and right on! Because, you know, you're vocal about it. And, you know, I'm living and I feel fine. I've got this garbage in my lungs, you know; but yet I can't . . . there's something in me that can't be satisfied with just treatment. I want to be completely healed. I want to be like other girls my age. I want to go out and play tennis; I want to be able to go out and take vacations and go and drive a car.
Jane:	Can't you play tennis?
Diana:	No! Well, because my lungs never healed.
Jane:	Well, I've got the same thing. I've got cancer of the pleura.

Diana: What I'm saying is I can't do the majority of things that girls my age do.

Jane: Well, not every young woman plays tennis.

In a later session, the dynamic of fear, suggested subtly in the foregoing passage, is more explicit. It is probably a function of the fact that by this time in the group, members were interacting in the *action* phase in terms of group dynamics. (Phases of groups are discussed later.) The freedom of open expression is obvious and as such is a sign of growth in the group. In the following passage, Sally expresses the sheer terror of the discovery of a spot on her lung and the interpretation of its significance to her. She discussed her interaction with her oncologist. Significantly, as the group moved to support her, all of the members began examining the terrible reality that no one is claiming to cure the metastatic patient. Rather they are trying to maintain the patient in remission for as long as possible in order that the patient might enjoy a "normal" life expectancy. It was during the interaction excerpted that all of the members verbalized their awareness of the stark reality facing them, letting down the hope/denial mechanism for coping with their disease. This is the one brief interaction of unmasking during our entire group in which this reality was addressed in such a unanimous verdict.

Jane: You know, I've always had the feeling that somehow I could overcome these conditions and they never alarm me that much. Even when Doctor Schmidt . . . do you know him? He's an internationally renowned thoracic surgeon. He gave me a very bad prognosis. It didn't seem to bother me because I was Jane Harding! And somehow I was going to get better. And when he saw me the other day, he looked at me and he didn't believe I was alive.

Sally: In November, I went to see Doctor Maste just for my routine check. . . . He spoke about this spot on my lung. Nobody had ever mentioned this spot on the lungs. But somewhere I heard it. . . . And I thought I'd ask him . And I thought. . . . Well, I agonized over it a week. And then the next week, I had to go see Doctor Norris. . . . He says the X-ray's all right and the other blood work's all right, blah, blah, blah

	. . . And he said that spot's all right.
Amanda:	There's that spotting game! Out damn spot!
Sally:	And I'm telling you what then! Doctor Norris came out and I asked Doctor Norris about it and I'm telling you, all of a sudden I got so frightened. . . .
Amanda:	Your voice wouldn't even work.
Sally:	You know that I got out of there and I didn't ask Norris . . . and I was half way home and, I thought. . . . Well, I agonized. I did call up. And I just agonized with that thing. I sat here one day in a meeting, and I was in just such a turmoil. . . .
Diana:	In here [pointing to stomach]?
Sally:	Yeah! Just about to croak! I mean, I couldn't hardly think about what was being said. I was just thinking about that darn spot, that spot and if it was a reoccurrence. And I thought I had gotten myself all reconditioned and if a reoccurrence occurred, I could take care of it. But I was just frozen. I went through all the holidays with that thing and when I came back, boy, I got my can in to Doctor Norris and I said I was wondering about that spot. "Well, what are you wondering about that spot?" And then I told him *what a spot I'd been in all the time.* . . . And if he didn't ream me out from stem to stern because I didn't call him back if I was that worried. He explained to me that that spot was there when the first X-rays were made . . . in any event, before I ever had the surgery. It was probably a scar from an old thing and all this. But I'm telling you, I just put myself through the charges of hell! Terror!
Amanda:	Oh, yeah! Literally terror!
Sally:	What little activity we had to do. And there was my daughter and the family. . . .
Diana:	And you didn't tell anybody, did you. You didn't tell anybody. You carried it in yourself.
Steve:	This is the first that you've shared that with our group.
Sally:	That's right.
Carol:	And this goes back to Christmas time?

Amanda:	Before Christmas?
Carol:	Oh, before Christmas!
Steve:	I wonder how you are feeling now that you've shared it with us.
Carol:	You're not afraid anymore. . . .
Sally:	I couldn't say I'm not afraid anymore because if I went up and Doctor Norris said to me something about that spot and there is a reoccurrence and we are going to have to do surgery, I don't know if I'd be afraid or not.
Steve:	How do you feel right now; right in here?
Sally:	I feel all right. I don't have any particular reaction, other than when she mentioned fear and then terror. What a terrible experience it was.
Diana:	OK. I've lived like that for seven years.
Sally:	In other words, when she said, "Well she's up," well, gosh, when you tell me that, you can imagine that I felt like my whole world was starting to get back together again. So I guess that's the way Diana feels when she's on top of it. But then if you get something. It may reoccur. There's going to be something else to "knock the rug out from under you," but still. . . .
Amanda:	You know this Doctor Gates was quite honest with me the other day. I guess he was honest. I don't know whether they are honest or not. They think they are being honest. . . . That he didn't make any bones about it. He was talking about various types of treatment, and I said, and I think this is true, that "you all do not really claim that people may hear it differently but you don't really claim that anything you are doing for anybody is going to cause a cure. It may come as remission." He says, "That's right!"
Sally:	That's right! Doctor Norris said, "Don't let anybody fool you!"
Diana:	Well, they say we'll never be cured, but we can spend the rest of our lives in remission. Never would we be considered cured.
Amanda:	Well, if you have an ordinary life span, I would con-

sider it the equivalent of cured.

Another dynamic to be examined here would be the aloneness/loneliness series of behaviors exhibited by the cancer patient. In context, an excellent example occurred during session 10. Here the ladies in the group were seeking a genteel manner of expression regarding their prognosis when confronting their families. They furtively searched for diplomatic ways to interact with those with whom they wished to be close, so as not to experience the rejection of forced loneliness and isolation. At the same time, they preserved their aloneness with the cancer by using synonyms for cancer itself. Thus, there seemed to be a fear of offending others and causing rejection while at the same time needing people in opposition to a desire to be alone with the awful reality.

Amanda: Well, it seems to me that one of the good things that all of us have gained, and it's true in my own case. . . . You just don't talk about your aches. It just bores the heck out of people or else it scares them to death. And if it's your own family, they get all anxious and unhappy and worried. So it's kind of nice to be able to talk to people very openly and matter of fact; you know, that delicate way of saying a malignancy.

Jane: To say what?

Amanda: A malignancy, instead of just saying c-a-n-c-e-r, cancer!

Sally: Well, I have a friend who won't even mention the word. She refers to it as "C-A!" Yes, she does! Now this is the truth! And she's so scared . . . and she's a good bit older than I am. . . . And she's scared, absolutely afraid that she's going to have one; which she may or she may not. She's already in her 70s. I wouldn't think that she would.

Amanda: I think she's past that.

Sally: But that's the way she does. She's just that ticky about it . . . or whatever you want to. . . . I don't know the proper word to describe it, but she refers to it as "C-A." If I'm sitting somewhere and somebody else mentions it, she goes, "Shhh!"

Amanda: But it is good to be able to talk about it. Pills you are taking. . . . Does it make you sick or doesn't it make you sick? Or how do you feel? I can talk to "little" Amanda pretty much except that I don't think it's fair to burden her a thousand miles away with saying, "I don't feel good." What the heck can she do about it? So it is kind of nice to be able to do that. I really wouldn't want to go on indefinitely talking about my illness because I get bored with it myself.

Jane: I enjoy talking about my illness because, first of all I don't feel sick. For the benefit of all. . . .

Amanda: You said that once and then you just kept on talking about it.

Jane: Well, I was repetitious.

Diana: I haven't said I'm not going to do anything; so then when I do it. . . .

Sally: What you say you're not going to do you are going to end up doing.

Jane: I want you to know that I am forty-nine years old!

Steve: There's kind of a. . . . Were you going to say something?

Diana: It's just trivial.

Steve: I was going to say that in addition to being able to talk about cancer in the group in the safety of the group and not feeling like people are going to reject you or be particularly afraid, there comes a sense of support with that. It's . . . like I feel what Diana was saying, was that even though she may not see Amanda in the group again or Sally, maybe we won't get together as a group again. . . . But she'll carry this kind of support with her for a long time. She has shared some of herself with other women who have cancer, who are faced with the same fears and the same concerns and the same frustrations, and that's the basis of support. I'm not alone.

Amanda: Of course, intellectually we know we are not alone. I tire of people using that delicate term malignancy. I have a friend who has really a nice personality, and it's so sad because she's really very bright. . . . And she has to have somebody live with her. . . . And this particular person is the woman who stayed with her mother who had the same problem. So I really think Sadie is homesick and wants to go home, and I'm sort of involved because I have to look after her affairs . . . insurance . . . so people don't cheat her out of any money. So Sadie tells me her health is extremely poor and that she's going to have to go back to Tampa in two weeks. I said, "Let's get you to a doctor first." "Well I know what it is." "Well what is it?" She said, "I have a malignancy." "I thought you were telling me about a malignancy." And that turned her inside-out. There's not a doggone thing wrong with her. And she says, "I know what it is. I have a malignancy. It sounds impressive."

Symptoms

Often discussions focused on symptoms. Such discussions were more typical during the first three sessions. It was interesting to notice the different themes covered within the broad, descriptive term *symptoms*.

Members would utilize the group sessions as opportunities to verify their symptoms: comparing theirs to those of other members of the group. In effect, this was a way that group members tested their normality relative to other persons in the same predicament. It is sort of like coming out of a midterm examination with a borderline grade needing a *C* or *B* just to stay afloat in the course. At the end of the midterm, members of the class congregate to compare notes regarding their accomplishment and position relative to other members of the group. Such is the comparison dynamic in a group of cancer patients.

Carol: Diana, do you find that your energy is kind of blah at the end of the day?

Diana: No. I don't allow myself to rest much. You know, it's different for all of us. And I guess I'm a very strong person. That's my opinion of myself. . . . And I guess I want to live up to what people think. So, you know, my mother and I are leaving next week for Israel for eight days. And you know, I'll make it with the time to spare, as far as going the trip and all. . . . But being tired is a weakness and I just won't accept weaknesses. This is for myself now! This is for me!

Carol: I find that by the time I come home from the office I have to lay down.

Diana: But I don't work either. I'm home all day.

Amanda: Oh, yes, you do!

Diana: But both of my children are in school and I really, you know . . . I can pace myself.

Notice that Diana tended to exhaust herself mentally in an effort to deny the deterioration of her stamina. Also, she seemed to overcompensate for her physical inadequacies by crowding life into a small space as if to validate her vitality. Such crowding produces further fatigue causing further overcompensation. Ultimately, this results in mental exhaustion. In Diana's case, she related later that she had spent some time in the hospital for "mental exhaustion" the summer preceding our group.

The next excerpt finds the group discussing their perception of reality versus society's perception. The high drama of cancer, treatment, remission, and cure and life and death as portrayed in the media, contrasts sharply with the perception of the group members about the course of their own disease. Society's eulogy for cancer in pictures contrasts sharply with many of the cancer patient's own experiences, producing an anger. Suffering with cancer is not always an act of heroism. Societal expectations that one be heroic in the face of this horrible reality produces much dissonance between how one *should* be versus how one *is*. Listen to the frustration expressed.

Diana: I wonder. . . . I've been this way for so many years, and I wonder if anybody else has this problem. I cannot sit and watch programs about people who have cancer. . . . And invariably they die, and/or they are miraculously healed, or something like this.

Amanda: More than likely they are miraculously healed.

Diana: But anyway, and I was wondering, is it just me? Is it one of the things that go to make me up? Or does it bother other people to watch? You know, I'm not even interested. I'll switch the stations around or something like that because it really bothers me.

Carol: It doesn't bother me because I'm perhaps hoping to learn something. . . .

Steve: We're just going to stop it here for a second. OK. Is there a way you could put that, that might help? A different way. . . .

Carol: You mean to help somebody?

Steve: Well, she's really asking anybody in the group what kinds of feeling do you have. . . . Correct me if I'm wrong, but I hear you saying, "What kinds of feelings do you all have . . . do we all have when we watch movies, hospital movies, doctor pictures, and to see cancer patients who die heroically or miraculously recover?" And what I heard in there was anger. And it really turns you off. It's not so much . . . and correct me if I'm wrong. It's not so much you can't watch it because you're repulsed by talking about it, but it's like a fairy tale and it really turns you off.

Amanda: I'm inclined to agree with Diana. I had a great difficulty voicing reaction before it was really pinned down. I suspected it, but didn't really want to. And I carefully avoided reading articles on cancer, which was stupid and careless. But once they said, "Kid! You've got it!" Then the act of facing up to it. . . . I'm like you. Those are just movie-type entertainment things that I don't think. . . . They are kind of boring. I don't think it upsets me. I don't really think that. And I'm more inclined to read articles about it now than I did before because they seem to have a little more scientific basis, a little more basis in reality. But entertainment type things I really. . . .

Diana: But you know somebody else. . . . Even when we were taught at the beginning and we shared our cancers and what treatment and all this. A lot of times I can listen and I can . . . that symptom will. . . . And you know, maybe that's the TV programs and all . . . is that if I sit here and talk about it long enough, I'm going to get worse. . . . Or my shortness of breath is going to increase.

Amanda:	Or don't you think we are all sort of susceptible to that kind of suggestion?
Diana:	I don't know. I know I am. But I don't know if everybody else is or not.
Amanda:	I think lots of people are.
Steve:	OK, here's another group point. We've got to get back to you because I don't want to cut you off.
Carol:	Well, no, I was too. . . .
Steve:	Amanda, you can say it's something personal for you?
Amanda:	I just said I wouldn't read things about cancer before it was actually diagnosed because it was a form of avoiding. But once I confronted the fact that I had it, then I don't mind reading about it. But it bores me . . . drama based on it.
Steve:	I just don't like this. . . .
Amanda:	I'm sorry! I spoke in an editorial way for so many years. It's hard for me to get out of the eye.
Steve:	We're going to run into this problem until. . . . It takes a little while to get educated to making more personal responses. I know that even here I was talking about how we all feel. "We this". . . . And I'm not trying to make it as a put down, but trying to make it so you can get more out of it for yourself . . . and that Diana could. And I liked the way you looked over at Diana after awhile trying to catch your eye with your feelings. And that's what we're trying to do. I want to get back to you [Carol]. I did not mean to cut you off. What were you trying to say? Because I think it is important for Diana to hear this. So, do you want to come back with that again?
Carol:	Well, what I said could help. I like to watch that type of program because it helps me to understand my disease and understand why this happened to me.
Steve:	Are you possibly saying that you don't resent the fairy-tale-like type of presentations in some of these shows and movies, like *Marcus Welby*?
Carol:	No. Because I'm sure that somewhere they must look at some records to find accurate information.

Sally: I was just going to say that. . . .

Steve: Are you talking to me now or are you talking to Diana?

Sally: I'm talking to Diana about what she said. I mean, she said she gets kind of affected. My mother had cancer and we discussed it. We looked at the whole thing for an hour and right at the last. . . . I don't like it [shows etc.] in the first place. I didn't like it before I knew I had cancer because it was not entertaining to my mind.

Diana: Well, when I had my breast cancer seven years ago and they had these self-help programs that people put on, Foundation People. . . . And my doctor was totally against that. He didn't want me to have any part of that or have the women come in and show me how. He wanted me to have nothing to do with that. And I was twenty-four years old. And I guess there have been times when I begrudge not being able to wear a bikini. You know, not that I might have, but it's just that I couldn't. That decision was taken away from me. And sometimes the movies or even *Love Story* destroys the feeling within because we live with that every day, and I don't know. . . .

Amanda: Do you think documentary-type things are more acceptable than things that are written just for drama because it speaks in "Walt Disney-type stuff"? I've heard it said one time that *Time* and news magazines like that always seem very authoritative until they got on something you happen to know something about and you know how wrong they can be. And I think that may apply to this kind of thing, you know?

Diana: I remember reading a magazine. I can't think right now if it was *Redbook* or *Good Housekeeping*, but one of them. It seemed like they were dwelling on cancer and a young mother dying. And I finally wrote them and said, "Stop this!" We can't even get a good magazine without having some big bold thing about having cancer and how bravely they lived and all that! Hogwash!

Amanda: To me cancer is no longer synonymous with death and I'm not scared of it. I feel that there are problems aside from lung cancer, which to me are much more difficult to cope with. Because I have this confidence in Doctor Norris and all the drugs that are available. But I don't. . . .

Diana: Well, does it bother you to watch a TV program? Or suppose a movie and the heroine has cancer?

Amanda: No! Because I know it's not real and I realize the origin and I know why it's being done. There are a lot of people who like this gory stuff. They get some kind of kick out of it, you know. It's a morbid kind of thing and it doesn't interest me at all. And so I'm able to separate reality from fantasy.

Pain is an obvious problem for the cancer patient. The anticipation of pain exists constantly. In addition, there is the stigma imposed by our society regarding relief from pain. For example, our society seems to value suffering with pain and does not seem to value the amelioration of pain with narcotics, such as morphine. This attitude further stigmatizes the whole process of having cancer to the point that the cancer patient, while having pain, still feels dependency and loss of control as a result of having to take pain pills. In the following excerpt, Carol discussed pain and the need for pain pills with Amanda. Because there was more pain, Carol was concerned that her cancer might be spreading. Thus, the elimination of pain would serve a two-fold purpose: (a) It would serve to allow the patient to live his life to the fullest of its potential without the constant fear and suffering from pain, and (b) it would also serve to quell much of the anxiety about the course of the disease when the patient already knows the prognosis is incurable.

Carol: If mine spreads somewhere else, I want to know that. I want to know. I don't want to hold anything back. For a whole month now I've had to live on pain pills because I've had such terrific pains in my stomach. So I'm thinking, "Maybe it's spread in there." But Doctor Norris says, "No!" But I feel that something is not right because I've never had to live on pain pills like I have this past month.

Another symptom that the members seemed to discuss quite readily and frequently were the side effects from chemotherapy. The use of chemotherapy is intended to kill cancer cells with toxic chemicals. The only problem with this mode of treatment is that in the process of killing cancer cells, often otherwise healthy cells are indiscriminately killed. Further compounding the problem is the breakdown in the body's immune system, clotting ability, and production of other blood cells, both red and white. Another difficulty is that many of the chemicals used in treatment are irritating to the stomach and intestines, causing nausea and vomiting. The following excerpt illustrates the almost matter-of-fact way in which Carol discussed the side effects from her high dosages of medication. It is illustrative of the type of side effects verbalized. It is such side effects that further traumatize cancer patients to the point where the treatment is almost worse than the disease. As end stage approaches, cancer patients may welcome death as relief from their suffering from not only cancer but the treatment as well.

Jane:	First of all, I was going to ask you: Did you complete your chemotherapy last week?
Carol:	Yes. Monday evening.
Jane:	Did you do all right?
Carol:	Un huh. I did better this time than I did before. I feel much stronger this time than I did before.
Jane:	Were you nauseated?
Carol:	Always. The second day it would catch up to me. This time they increased the dosage to 1,700 and I had been taking 1,200. And the fourth day my room was swimming. But they gave me a pill for it, and it was all right. And I just lost my meal twice.
Amanda:	I'm so thankful I've never had to take them. I have a little kind of a queasy feeling but never where I had to throw up.
Carol:	I'm scheduled to go back the 14th of January for the third series, and hopefully that will see me through '77.
Amanda:	That'll be a nice Christmas present.

All persons like to feel special. The cancer patient is no different. He wants to feel that there is something unique about the condition that can be identified and even boasted about. There is not much to boast about when one has cancer. Often there seems to be a need to search for some peculiarity of organicity that sets one off from the rest of society. Such a feature marks the person as unique in the world, thus still having importance. In the following passage, Jane had discovered that her urine had a peculiar characteristic unlike the urine of many other breast cancer patients. Her urine was more peculiar to leukemia patients. This has made her somewhat of a celebrity in the oncology unit. Jane was very excited about her good fortune to receive all of this attention from professionals. Notice the humorous banter between therapist and patient.

Steve: I'll bet you'll have the best ones [urine samples]!

Jane: I have special urine and I just want you all to be impressed that you are not to describe me as an ordinary individual but as somebody who is unique!

Steve: Isn't that terrific!

Diana: We knew you were special!

Jane: I always felt that all my life I knew that there was. . . .

Steve: You really missed your calling.

Jane: But I could never find out why. And I finally found it is my urine.

Steve: Isn't that terrific! You must have gotten lucky. How did you find out? What lead you to it?

Jane: Doctor Norris found it.

Diana: How did those subjects get. . . ?

Jane: Leukemia patients. And I am weird because I am a breast cancer patient. And I'm not suppose to have it.

Carol: Cindy asked if she could have a sample of my urine. I said, "You can have it all!" And they were running a test on every patient who came through there to see if there is something in there that would show up. And you're the one it showed up in.

Steve: Aren't you something!

Jane: I always knew I was special.

Steve: Are you girls ready for this? Now you're going to have to pay close attention to this. That's a real "pisser" [laughter]. No, I think that's very informative to share that with us.

Carol:	What are they going to do now that they found this special thing?
Jane:	Well, the only conclusion that I could come to. ˙. . . You know, loquacious Doctor Norris. . . . The only conclusion I could come to with my very fine mind. . . . I do query him about certain things. . . . I said, "In the case of cancer you have this multiplication of cells and if these cells produce this, does this also happen in the case of a pregnant woman who is also producing excessive cells?" And he said, "Yes." But it was not of any significance. The only conclusion I came to is that it might be a very simple thing that might have some import in other areas which are not now current. So listen I just want you to know. . . .
Steve:	We're getting to know more and more about you.
Jane:	I was getting tired of giving a specimen and they kept telling me everybody was doing it and everytime I came I'd have to give a specimen.
Amanda:	They're doing some type of experiment.
Jane:	I said, "Why do you want this special stuff of mine?"
Steve:	They are probably selling it on the black market.
Jane:	Well, you know, I'll tell you; I'm just something very special.
Carol:	Well, I'm happy that you are in our group.
Steve:	You ought to collect a vile and frame it.

Finally with regard to symptoms, it is important to note something that may or may not be obvious to the reader from other excerpts. Cancer symptoms place severe limitations on the patient. His mobility is cut down. Dependency on the medical system is increased to the point where the cancer patient must either decide to follow the treatment regimen religiously or die. Such feelings of dependency and loss of control lower self-esteem and self-concept. Physical activity becomes curtailed. Such curtailment ranges from the obvious, as in the case with amputation, and the sublime, as in the case of sexual dysfunction and emotional lability. Surely the reader can identify excerpts throughout this book which highlight the tremendous amount of pain and stress that these courageous people incur throughout the horrible course of the disease process. If in fact the opportunity exists for growth through suffering, the cancer patient has more than ample opportunity toward such growth.

The following excerpt illustrates the give-and-take flow of a discussion surrounding symptoms and side effects. It is interesting to observe the significance of body image and the maintenance of one's own vanity and narcissism in the face of cancerous destruction. It is also noteworthy that Diana was willing to go to the extreme of drug abuse, ostensibly to lose weight. One wonders if such abuse was also used to quell the terror. The group members fantasized drug use and discussed the relative merits of such use as if flirting with a seductive escape.

Diana: Would you believe Carol has diabetes on top of everything else? That's been one of the reasons she's been feeling so bad.

Amanda: Good heavens!

Diana: She just looks like a new person — feels good and the whole business. They are giving her insulin.

Amanda: It would seem like some of these drugs would counteract each other.

Diana: They said that it's in her family and that the cancer probably. . . .

Amanda: My golly!

Jane: Well, her diabetes might have aggravated a lot of her other conditions, and now that they. . . .

Diana: Well, they say that her other condition aggravated her diabetes.

Steve: Diabetes?

Diana: Yeah, right! That she probably would have had it anyway.

Jane: She's probably had diabetes for a while, but never complained about it. It was only recently by accident that she said to Cindy, "I can't see too well at certain times," and that's why I thought that maybe she's had this diabetes and it has aggravated conditions. And now that she's getting the insulin, one of the other things might lessen. You don't think so?

Amanda: Who knows! I'm amazed I haven't heard nothing on routine blues. . . .

Diana: I just haven't. . . .

Jane:	Well, they found something very strange in my urine. I have a condition which is peculiar to leukemia patients.
Amanda:	But you don't have it?
Jane:	And I don't have leukemia and very rarely do people with breast cancer get it. So they keep watching me. And at one point I had to fill 2 gallons of urine and they had to send a man over in a taxi and get it.
Diana:	How did you do that? It must have taken a long time, 2 gallons.
Jane:	Yeah, I had to keep it in the refrigerator.
Diana:	Isn't the weather nice outside today?
Amanda:	I'm kind of thinking the same thing. It's cold. Oh, Lord!
Diana:	Well. . . .
Amanda:	That's not what you had in mind.
Diana:	No. There has to be better things to talk about.
Amanda:	Well, tell us about your Weight Watchers®.
Diana:	It's fantastic! I lost 3 pounds!
Amanda:	Well, then they have sort of relaxed their requirements.
Diana:	They totally revised it.
Amanda:	I went on it once. I've still got the stuff.
Diana:	So, anyway, I told Cindy, "Why didn't you tell me about this nine months ago?" And she said, "I did, but you weren't ready for it nine months ago." And I'm sure she did. When I think how badly I've complained. . . . But I feel so good. I really feel very good, even though sometimes I leave and I tell you I'm not going to do anything you suggest or anything, for some reason I know it helps.
Amanda:	When you go down one size you'll feel perfect!
Diana:	Yes, but you know. . . .
Amanda:	That is the most satisfying thing, to be able to put on a dress that just looked tacky — tight before and now just looks great.
Diana:	Anyway, I'm not going to talk today. So I'll feel just as good all the time in here as I do before I come in and after I leave.

Jane: I know that I've got to lose weight. I have this very beautiful imported long dress and I got it on and tried to pull it up and tore the zipper.

Diana: You should go to Weight Watchers. You'll eat so good. You'll get plenty.

Amanda: Lots, lots more than you are accustomed to eating.

Diana: I wanted Doctor Norris to give me a diet pill; you know, that's the easy way out. He said the only diet pill he knew about met once a week. I don't know. I think it does you good. There's more satisfaction in doing it this way than doing it out of. . . .

Jane: I once induced a doctor to give me an amphetamine . . . you know, that's what these diet pills are . . . and I couldn't wait for that thing to wear off. My heart was palpitating. I felt awful. I wonder how these kids take it? How do they become addicted to something that feels so terrible?

Amanda: It makes you feel so bad.

Diana: I'm a firm believer that there are many adult women, men too probably, that have a drug habit just as bad as the teenagers do only the teenagers' problem is written about. I have been on as many as ten a day!

Amanda: Ten a day of what?

Diana: Diet pills. Amphetamines. My tolerance. . . .

Jane: Didn't your heart beat rapidly?

Diana: Everything, everything moved fastly, but I had to have it for self-confidence. I can remember if I was going to make a telephone call, I'd take one.

Jane: It was so awful!

Amanda: Oh, come on Diana!

Diana: No, that is the solemn truth!

Jane: I could not wait for that to wear off.

Diana: I took it. It's been since I had cancer; the second time it's been since. I could go into this guy; he wore these gorgeous Italian suits with the shoes. . . .

Amanda: I guess so. You were paying for it.

Diana: He didn't care how much I weighed. Did not care how much I weighed. You know, you pay him and he gives you your prescription. Then I quit cold turkey.

Amanda:	Then what happened?
Diana:	Didn't have any withdrawals, really. Then I found my lung cancer.
Jane:	Then they what?
Diana:	Then they found the lung cancer. And I haven't been back on any since. I couldn't clean the house. I couldn't do anything without them.
Jane:	What about this drug that Freddie Prince was taking? I understand that it produces terrible depression. Now why in the world would anybody take that?
Amanda:	Deliberately court depression?
Jane:	Yeah! Why would anybody? . . . and very deep depression? I can't imagine anybody wanting to feel that way.
Amanda:	No, if I was going to take something, I would take something to make me feel good.
Jane:	Something like heroin. Something like heroin.
Amanda:	That doesn't make you feel good, does it? We used to have a bookkeeper . . . in the first place I could not have paid her medical bills because she was running to the doctor every five minutes, and in the second place she could discuss with you any kind of tranquilizer. "Do you use this? Do you use that?" I said, "I don't know what you are talking about. I have a bottle of aspirin in my medical cabinet; that's all." But it seems to be a tremendous crutch for many people.
Diana:	And they are real easy to get if you want them bad enough.
Amanda:	And the money they put out for it.
Jane:	Yeah. Even if I wanted to get it, I wouldn't know where to get it.
Diana:	It wouldn't be hard.
Jane:	Where is it? What do you do?
Amanda:	Don't tell her; she'll go get it.
Diana:	You could find somebody if you look hard enough. Sure you could.
Jane:	I know how to be a hooker because all I'd do is walk up and down the street, but how do you get pills?

That's a different thing.

Comparison, Identification, and Pride

Just because heart disease is the number one killer . . . you say it happens instantly! Heart attack is fast; they're gone. And what we got is slow. It's eating away.

Diana

The above quote by Diana illustrates further difficulties regarding "prestige" and cancer. Unlike the case of a fatal heart attack, cancer is a painful, slow process that eats away ones body and soul. It undermines one's entire existence in the process of self-destruction. Oftentimes the cancer patient seems to wish that, given the choice of diseases, heart attack would be the disease of choice. A heart attack would enable the patient to die quickly, cleanly, and efficiently without prolonged suffering. The "great American death dream" is one in which one either has a stroke or heart attack and dies peacefully, instantly during one's sleep. Imagine being a cancer patient and not being able to die in the proper way. It is "un-American" to suffer a prolonged death.

On the other hand, the cancer patient has had the opportunity in recent years to identify with some very famous people as role models. The following excerpt shows Diana's ability to identify with Betty Ford and "Happy" Rockefeller and their battles with breast cancer. Such "coming-out" of famous personalities who have had cancer seems to serve to instill a sense of pride in cancer patients who can identify with these persons. Thus, while on one hand the cancer patient wishes to die neatly and efficiently and be as little burden on anyone as possible, there is still a sense of identity, albeit reluctantly and angrily, in being members of a select group.

Diana: But You know something else . . . something else I've noticed along with so many articles on cancer now because Ford's wife and Rockefeller's wife. . . . In reading short novel fiction stories they will use examples . . . like spread the cancer. It always blows my mind why they have to use that.

Acceptance

Well, Steve, intellectually we all know that there's nothing fair about life. If it was, everybody would have enough to eat; everybody would be warm; everybody would have a good house. So we know this intellectually, but emotionally we just don't accept it. It hits you! You just say, "It's not fair!" Well, what right do you have to expect everything to be so fair?

Amanda

The above quotation acknowledges the acceptance of the fact that one has cancer and tacitly acknowledges the fact that it is incurable, at least for Amanda. However, Amanda verbalized a feeling that seems to be typical of cancer patients. That feeling is one of resignation. There is nothing fair about being the one in four persons who contracts cancer. It is a sense of frustration that while at the same time one accepts that he has the disease, there is a pervasive anger about its unfairness.

Acceptance is very difficult. If a person were to accept the notion that he is dying, he would truly have to give up living. This is often the case. Colleagues and associates who have worked with persons in the moribund stage have often stated that when a person really and truly *accepts* that death is imminent, the will to live is often lost and the person allows himself to expire. One psychiatrist, in a macabre, humor-like fashion, relayed as to how she had become known as the "death angel" on the cancer ward. Oftentimes she would approach people who were dying. They would tell their deepest and darkest fears, dreams, fantasies, and failures. Often within twenty-four hours, the confessor would be dead.

All the group members were aware that they had incurable cancer. While each was aware that the time line of the prognosis was uncertain, many of these women knew that at any moment their cancer could permanently interrupt their lives. When persons are on chemotherapy and other forms of cancer treatment, there is always the awareness that one's life can end within a twenty-four to forty-eight hour period.

Such an awareness of the imminence of death takes the cancer patient through a cyclothymic range of emotions: from hope to futility; from optimism to pessimism. However, fear and anger are ever present. As stated by Amanda: ". . . it's just not fair!"

In the following excerpt, the question was posed to Diana as to how she appeared to be able to accept cancer and to live with it. Anger and frustration were touched upon. However, both Diana and the therapist accept that anger, frustration, and bitterness are pervasive and ever-present. Even at this writing, it is not certain that one could ever develop techniques or skills (nor would I want to) that would take away the vital energy necessary to maintain anger, fear, bitterness, and frustration. It is this vital force that fuels perserverance that the cancer patient might live to his fullest potential until life's end.

Steve: Diana, how does it feel when you hear, "That's just something you are going to have to accept and live with?"

Diana: I don't know. I'm a young woman who can do anything that my friends do. Only they can do it because they are healthy and I can't because I have cancer.

Steve: That's just one part of a lot of things that add to it.

Diana: It adds to everything else.

Steve: It adds to the fact that you experienced cancer and you talked about the difficulties of encountering people who don't know how to handle you with the disease — that they either back off or give you some kind of solicitous-type of sympathy. We've heard the looking at your children and trying to talk with your husband about these things, and we've also heard about talking with your parents, and I just feel a lot of things produce a slow burn.

Diana: But I don't see how we can talk about it . . . bring it out in the open here . . . but I can't see solving it. It's going to be this way. It's been this way for seven years.

Sally: Let me ask you. . . .

Diana: And you know I'm not going to look my mother in the eye and tell her to cool it or to. . . .

Amanda: Shut up?

Diana: Yeah! You know, I can't do that.

Steve: It seems like there's not a solution but maybe the exploring of it and looking at it from this perspective with your group can help. You say, "Well, I just have to accept it and deal with it." But I get the feeling that you haven't accepted it and dealt with it. Because the anger is still there; the frustration; the bitterness.

CHEMOTHERAPY

Chemotherapy is the use of potent drugs to fight cancer. As explained earlier, chemotherapy in and of itself can be as debilitating and emotionally excrutiating as the cancer that it treats.

An interesting coping mechanism observed during the course of work with these patients was the displacement of fear regarding cancer and chemotherapy by preoccupation with expertise in the treatment of the disease. Jane was one person who spent much time doing reading and research in the area of chemotherapy and nutrition. She was quite verbal and very intelligent; these factors facilitated comprehension. It is certain that she posed many problems for her oncologists with her facile command of knowledge in the area. The following excerpt demonstrates some of her concerns. It is excerpted from an initial interview prior to the beginning of the group.

Jane: Now a person can have cancer and become very depressed and that depression may not exactly relate to his cancer. He could be unhappy because of his cancer. But it could be exaggerated also because of some other condition. And I talked to Doctor Norris about the value of nutrition. I said, "Here we are being fed these highly toxic drugs. Nobody questions me to say what are you eating." If these drugs are that powerful that they can destroy the cancer cells or control them, they are undoubtedly doing damage to my healthy cells. I must compensate in my body with high-quality nutrition. I can't do it on junk foods. Now, I talk to patients and they are eating McDonald's® hamburgers. They are eating all of this junk food. I feel that also has to be incorporated; that has to become a part of this entire picture . . . the mind is a focal point; the attitude also controls how much progress I'm going to make.

Steve: So you would see a need for some nutritional guidance or a dietitian with some expertise in biochemical functions as a helper also on the team, in helping the cancer patients. That's certainly something to explore in the group and perhaps to explore with the staff at some point in time. It sounds like you've been pushing that for a while.

Jane: Yeah, I have. I noticed in a report that Doctor Norris and Doctor Gates were doing work on nutrition and the effects of the chemotherapy patient.

While Jane was interested in the relationship between nutrition and chemotherapy, Amanda presented a different picture. Amanda's initial interview seemed to communicate much resistance and fear when faced with the prospect of chemotherapy. During our first session, Amanda discussed her treatment with hormone therapy. While hormone therapy does not qualify as chemotherapy per se, there is a fine line between the patient's interpretation of the word *chemotherapy* versus *hormone* therapy. In this case, hormone therapy is the lesser of two evils. In the following passage, Amanda took the fine line and made it into a major highway to differentiate her willingness to cooperate with hormone therapy versus her pronounced objection to chemotherapy.

Amanda: I am under Doctor Norris, but I am not. . . . I don't think I'm technically in *chemotherapy.* I'm on *hormone* therapy because I flatly refused to take chemotherapy. I am an early retiree from a right-demanding job, which I thought I would miss, but I don't miss at all. I'm a widow and I have one daughter who lives in Cambridge, Massachusetts. So I live alone. But I have a lot of relatives here, which is a help. I've been here since 1970.

Steve: *When you say you can't take chemotherapy, you mean your body won't?*

Amanda: *I'm just not going to do it. Period!*

Steve: *Have you tried it?*

Amanda: *I'd just as soon be dead as. . . .*

Steve: *What is it you're taking?*

Amanda: *I take hormones.*

Steve:	*What kind?*
Amanda:	Well, I've been on three. I have had the female hormone, then I had the male and now I'm on. . . . I'm right in the current swing. . . . I'm having something that is fairly new in nature, which seems to be quite effective.
Steve:	How long were you on the male hormone?
Amanda:	I can't remember.
Steve:	Very long?
Amanda:	Oh, about eighteen months.
Steve:	And you're so beautiful. You don't project any. . . .
Amanda:	. . . side effects from it.
Steve:	May I ask where you have your cancer?
Amanda:	Breast cancer.
Steve:	Amanda, why did you so strongly object to chemotherapy?
Amanda:	Because every . . . it may be quite unreasonable, but my position is that it is my life and I will decide what happens to it. And when they told me that the information would be put on a computer and that would determine whether I would go on hormone therapy or the other, I said, "You just said the wrong thing to a sixty-year-old woman. No computer is going to decide what happens to me!"

It is interesting that by the conclusion of the group, Amanda did finally consent to the utilization of chemotherapy, if that prospect were to become necessary as dictated by the course of her cancer. Presumably, the effects of being in a group with people who were undergoing chemotherapy and of seeing that they were able to function and survive (leading relatively productive lives) were influential in the reduction of Amanda's resistance and cooperation with a regimen of chemotherapy.

To reiterate, the side effects of chemotherapy are often more physically and psychologically traumatic than the cancer itself. Witness the following passage.

Carol:	Now this doesn't bother me at all, but last October they put me on two new capsules. I'm telling you I had such a terrible reaction I thought I was going to die.

Amanda:	So did I!
Carol:	My whole legs went numb. My buttocks and all in my stomach were just as numb. I was bent over with pain. I have never been so miserable in all my life, and it's just now getting out of my system where I'm feeling myself again. But they didn't tell me I was going to react like this to it. My hair . . . when I brush it, the sink is just full of hair. I have never had this problem before.
Amanda:	You see, the thing I object to about the way patients, specifically chemotherapy patients, are treated is the fact that when you come in and are examined, I always felt like a guinea pig. I did not feel as a complete human being.

Chemotherapy was the treatment modality discussed most often. While radiation therapy and surgery were mentioned on occasion, chemotherapy seemed far and above the most traumatic aspect of cancer. It seems that recovery from surgery is painful but that it is generally a time-limited pain. Chronic bouts with the side effects of chemotherapy are often demoralizing and debilitating. The following section is a rather lengthy excerpt regarding a spontaneous discussion by the women in the group comparing notes on a number of treatment modalities with chemotherapy as the central and most painful issue.

Diana:	I think I would have lost all of mine [hair] if I would have stayed on the drugs they were injecting into me, but those were the ones I couldn't continue with. So when they took me off of those, then I was just taking. . . .
Carol:	How long were you on that?
Diana:	I had my first treatment the 28th of May, but. . . .
Carol:	Did you go up to the hospital for it?
Diana:	I came to the clinic. They give it to me in my left arm, but I was on one type. . . .
Carol:	Oh, that one about killed me!
Diana:	Well, it did me too, but it did clear up my left lung, the fluid. So the middle of August they put me on Andriamycin®, and I'm on Andriamycin now. And

that's when my hair came out, after the first treatment of Andriamycin. In a week's time I was bald. I just combed it out.

Amanda: Well am I the only one here who's had any cobalt?

Barbara: I had radiation.

Carol: I've never had cobalt.

Barbara: I had five weeks radiation.

Amanda: Yeah, that's what I'm talking about.

Barbara: I had that.

Amanda: Did it make you ill?

Barbara: No, it didn't make me sick. I was working at the time. I'd come take my treatment and go to work.

Carol: Well, I had my radiation, but this is just the medication. I had a treatment in November, then in December, then I had to go back in January. And usually three months treatment like that makes me sick for the whole year.

Barbara: With your first treatment, did it affect your mouth?

Carol: Yes.

Barbara: I've had a lot of sores since I came home.

Carol: But the treatment I had in November, I didn't have any symptoms, except the second day I was a little nauseated. But I didn't have any sores. And usually before as soon as I got home, my mouth was just full of fever blisters. But I didn't have that this time.

Amanda: Well, Carol, are you saying that this is the only treatment you have? You go in for five days and then you take nothing in between times?

Carol: Right, nothing in between times.

Amanda: That sounds convenient.

Sally: I had side effects, and then I was put on a male hormone. You can't use them as a primary medication, but I could use it after I had the other medication.

Carol: Diana, what type of treatment were you on? Cobalt?

Diana: The first time, and then the second time chemotherapy. And then this time — it started again in April — hormone treatment.

Sally: I had a hormone treatment done last year, but I've never been sick.

Diana:	I don't know if I'm a male or a female anymore [laughter].
Carol:	Diana, you're priceless.
Diana:	But you know, you've been on male hormones before, but I know it's just the thought of it. I make up more; I dress more. See how feminine I look?
Carol:	Yeah, but last week you were very, very feminine. Today you're just casual.
Diana:	Yeah, but you know I kind of have a tendency to overdo the makeup. Sure, you know what I am.
Amanda:	Well, when you're sixty-one, you don't really care anymore, Diana.
Diana:	No, but listening to where the places it [the cancer] is . . . [Carol] "Don't you know you're not supposed to be sitting in this room? Haven't people told you that Grandmother Elizabeth had it there and died and your Aunt Susie had it?"
Carol:	I was supposed to be dead by Christmas of '74 and here I am. Christmas of '76 and I'm still here.
Diana:	I mean it's just unreal that you're sitting up and making rational conversation!
Carol:	I may not be here next Christmas, but I'm going to love today and I'm going to enjoy it.
Louise:	Carol, did you ask or did you want to know how much time you had?
Carol:	They told me. When I came out of surgery the first time, I had forty-eight hours. They were just amazed that I recovered so rapidly, and then I wasn't responding well to the chemotherapy all through '74 and the doctor said, "You'll never see Christmas of '74!" And I did. But in January of '75 I got very very ill, and they put me here in Emory, and they gave me the 5,000 cc. through an artery directly into my liver and since then everything's been working beautifully.
Amanda:	Louise, we said last time they are mighty free with their predictions!
Carol:	But I never listen to them anyway.
Louise:	Well, I insisted on the truth to find out where it's going.

Amanda: I don't care where its going just as long. . . . I don't
               think I really want to know how much time, how
               long do I have. I don't believe I could really face up
               to that. I know, all things are possible with God, I
               know that. . . .

Carol: If mine spreads somewhere else, I want to know
               that. I want to know; I don't want to hold anything
               back. For a whole month now I've had to live on
               pain pills because I've had such terrific pains in my
               stomach; so I'm thinking maybe its spread in there.
               But Doctor Norris says no. But I feel that something
               is not right because I've never had to live on pain
               pills like I have this past month.

While chemotherapy is a big problem for the cancer patient, Jane
asserted that chemotherapy and its side effects were still more
desirable than the ultimate cause of psychosocial death for cancer
patients: loneliness.

Jane: I really feel that . . . you know how I feel . . . that
               now with chemotherapy there are so many wonder-
               ful combinations that do not make it a fatal thing
               with someone with cancer. I don't think anyone with
               cancer is a fatal case.

Carol: I don't think so too!

Jane: I don't really think so. You know what kills them? I'm
               a victim of what kills them, and it's not cancer.

Carol: What is it?

Jane: You. You're going to die of longevity.

Carol: Yeah, I know.

Amanda: It's not cancer. There are many other contributing
               causes to the medication they give you for it.

Jane: It's not the medication. There are certain emotional
               situations which stir the body in many ways which
               contribute to that. It isn't cancer per se that does it. I
               think if they did a study, *they would find that more
               people died of loneliness than died of cancer.*

As seen before, Diana was an angry person about life in general.
Here she was being angry with chemotherapy.

Diana: Well, you know we are all on medication. And I guess it's because I've had it longer than anybody else in the room and I haven't really known how to deal with. Thus far I haven't done real well. But always in the past it was hidden. All the surgery I've ever had, and everything. This time it's beginning to bloom out all over and I'm tired of people telling me . . . "well, just be thankful you're alive!" Is this alive? Is this worth being alive? Is it? And I haven't even scratched the surface on the medication I admit. But I don't want to spend . . . and maybe I'll live to be eighty years old. . . . I don't know. But say I've got a year, I don't want to live that year obese with all the side effects I'm getting from this medication. There's more out of life than this!

Jane, the ephemeral optimist, offered Diana support with encouragement regarding chemotherapy and other forms of cancer treatment.

Jane: But with chemotherapy they can remove your pituitary gland. They can do many many things. I don't think any longer that anybody who has cancer has to say it's synonymous with death; it's synonymous with pain. It isn't! And instead of you thinking or worrying about all the things that you are worried about. . . . You are beautiful. You are intelligent. You have so much to look forward to. Alright! Maybe you don't have two breasts! But that doesn't do anything to your brain. Your relationship with your husband, with your family, is good. And that's what I would be concerned about. And I wouldn't continue to project what's going to happen! Am I going to live until the age of 100?

As the sessions progressed, less and less was said about treatment. The phenomena of the group moving into action was such that the members focused more on feelings and situations in life that were causing emotional stress as opposed to comparing symptoms and notes on chemotherapy. From time to time, chemotherapy (hormone therapy) would be altered for any given member of the group. Pharmaceutical companies are always developing new experimental medications for the treatment of cancer. Due to the fact that the cooperating institution where the group was being held was also a teaching and research facility, many patients were asked to be subjects for research with new medications. Of course, each new medication brought the rejuvenation of hope. As such, this hope brought a new burst of optimism toward the future. Perhaps all hospitals and all oncologists treating chemotherapy patients should periodically switch agents if for no other reason than to the psychological effect of creating new hope for whatever period of time.

Carol:	Is that what they said you were in: partial remission?
Diana:	Complete would be if the tumors were gone and they are not. But he's satisfied if they stay there, that they can keep watch on them.
Amanda:	Who's that? Doctor Gates?
Diana:	No, Norris.
Amanda:	Norris? Then you are not on any medication.
Diana:	Oh, yes! Indefinitely on medication.
Amanda:	What are you taking now?
Diana:	Cogest. . . .
Sally:	Corgestrun®?
Diana:	That's right.
Jane:	Is that what you are on?
Diana:	Yes.
Jane:	That's a male hormone. That's what I'm on. It's the most marvelous medication.
Amanda:	A hormone?
Jane:	It's a male hormone.
Diana:	This isn't a male hormone. He took me off of that. This has only been out two months, and it has no masculine hormone in it.
Jane:	Then that's different. That's what they told me about Upjohn. As a matter of fact. . . .
Diana:	Upjohn is a brand name.
Jane:	Upjohn, the pharmaceutical company, told me about the medication I'm taking — that it's one of the few that has no trace of estrogen.
Amanda:	Jane, I just have to ask, how did you get in conversation with Upjohn about it?

Jane:	Because they were supposed to send it to K-Mart and they didn't. Something happened to the computers, and so I called Upjohn because I needed it and they were wonderful. They sent it by taxi.
Amanda:	Heavens above!
Diana:	Shows what you can get done if you talk to the right person.
Jane:	That's right.
Carol:	Are we on [taping]?
Diana:	Yeah.
Jane:	And they charged K-Mart. They didn't know me from a hole in the wall, but you see I'm so impressive [laughter].
Amanda:	Nothing wrong with your self-concept, is there?
Diana:	See how close we've gotten in just a matter of a few weeks.
Amanda:	You see what you've [to Steve] done?
Jane:	You remember how I came in here a cowering, sad little soul?
Diana:	This has to be different than what you were taking. . . .
Sally:	Are these pale green tablets?
Steve:	Baby blue?
Sally:	Baby blue. $30 for. . . .
Diana:	No, I get 100 for $17.
Amanda:	I'll have to ask them if it's the same thing they gave me. And if it is, I have some left over and you are welcome to it.
Diana:	OK. But if it's only been out two months, have been on this since. . . .
Amanda:	Just since September. It may not be the same thing.
Diana:	She said that there were some other medicines in the works that hadn't gotten through the red tape that are good.
Jane:	Do you know the name of the pharmaceutical company?
Carol:	Maybe they'll find one for me.
Diana:	I don't know.
Sally:	I don't know where they. . . .
Jane:	I read the inserts and I know everything about it.

| Diana: | Just people who have bad colds can give you this whole terminology, no? |
| Jane: | Well, I like to be a doctor! I read that stuff. I know all about it. |

RADIATION THERAPY AND SURGERY

Curiously, radiation therapy and surgery were discussed minimally throughout all initial interviews and the life of the group. Regarding radiation one can only surmise that this phenomenon was due to the fact that only one of the members of the group, Barbara, was actively undergoing any kind of radiation treatment. The other women in the group were treated primarily with chemotherapy.

With regard to surgery, the fact that surgical treatment was mentioned on only a few occasions suggests that either surgery is too traumatic to recall or that the aftereffects of surgery are minimal compared to other emotional and physiological problems generated by cancer and its general treatment. During the course of the group, no patient had to undergo surgery. Therefore, the anxiety and fear of not surviving surgery were subjects not discussed. Presumably, such discussions would be more prevalent in a group of persons who had just discovered that there was a possibility that they had cancerous growths in their bodies. It would be interesting to assemble a group of such people to examine the dynamics in similar detail to the group described in this book.

In the following discussion, Carol and Barbara compared experiences regarding radiation therapy. Carol's treatment had occurred about two years prior to the group's meeting.

Carol:	The cobalt?
Barbara:	Yes, the cobalt to just that area. So then they started in October.
Carol:	Did you lose your hair?
Barbara:	No, I didn't lose it all. It thinned out a lot.
Carol:	Well, I have.
Barbara:	You did?
Carol:	My hair got terrible. It thinned a lot when I was on those two drugs they injected.
Barbara:	I was as bald as Kojak.

Carol:	Is that right?
Barbara:	I was wondering how long it took you to grow it back? It's just. . . .
Carol:	It's reversible. Whenever they stop, it grows back.
Barbara:	Somebody I saw not so long ago had lost all their's and it had been five or six months and it was about out like this. And the hair had been straight before and it was coming back sort of curly. It was all over her head. And just the way it was cut and styled she just looked lovely. So you got some more? It was worse because I was so bald.
Carol:	But it does come back.
Barbara:	It's a couple of weeks since this has started; so I'm getting excited over that.
Carol:	Well, mine came out in various spots, but I never lost it.
Barbara:	Mine came out in a week's time.

During the beginning of session 2, the only other reference to radiation therapy during the life of the group was made in an exchange between Diana, Barbara, and Amanda.

Diana:	If you'd have worn it [a wig] last week, we wouldn't have known.
Barbara:	Of course, the people who knew me before see my hair's gray and this is brown.
Amanda:	Well, now I'll tell you, I had a new man do my hair not long ago, and he said, "What color is your real hair?" I said, "I haven't the slightest idea." It's been so long.

Notice that Diana and Amanda made a marked attempt to comfort Barbara and to assure her that she was still feminine. So much sexuality and self-esteem is tied up in hair and the presence or absence of hair for both men and women. In Western society, supreme degradation of a human being punished by any social group is associated with the shaving off of hair. The warmth and caring of Diana and Amanda were very moving.

One reference to surgery is noteworthy because it was one of the few references to the subject. It was a discussion by Amanda of some of the side effects of the surgery (and radiation) involving her arm.

Sally: I don't know. I just told Steve I haven't been in contact with anybody who has had the same type of
surgery that I had since I left the hospital. So I really
don't know.

Carol: A lady in my office just went in for breast cancer.

Sally: It wasn't that I couldn't use my hand or my arm, but I
had such a bad time. So that was why I couldn't. I
took my exercises myself. I was glad to get in this
group because it's a subject I wanted to discuss.

Amanda: Well, I can tell you my experience. I was operated
on in August of 1973 and I was back at work the 1st
of October, I think. And then I had to have cobalt
therapy. And I would come first thing in the morning
and then go straight on to work. So it didn't really
slow me down.

Diana: What's wrong with your arm now?

Amanda: Well, now, I don't know to tell you the truth. This is
the second time it's happened. The first time I was
still under Doctor Maste, and he thought it could
have been some radiation damage, and they sent me
up to Doctor Hopkins and . . . Anyway he assured
me that my arm was functional in their terms. The
fact that it was a nuisance he was sorry about. But
neurologically speaking, it was functioning.

Diana: And it finally got better?

Amanda: You see what happens? It just dangles from my hand
and I can't lift it, which means I can't grasp things. I
have no fine motor skills, which is really a nuisance.

Diana: Is it due from the surgery?

Amanda: They won't say. They haven't been able to pinpoint it
so it has to be associated with the surgery.

Diana: Is it only that side where . . . ?

Amanda: Yeah, and now it's happened again. It happened this
summer when I was in England. First there's a lot of
pain and the next morning it's just limp. So that's why
I'm going to the rehab people. Doctor Norris thought
it would be better. I don't know if there really is
some damage from radiation. But why would it
come and go. Seems so wrong. You see people all

crippled up with arthritis.

Diana: Amen!

One of the key ingredients to treatment is the relationship between the patient and his physician. Throughout the course of treatment, the rapport and trust established often seems to help the patient maintain hope and sanity in the face of adversity and pain. Much has been written of late regarding the patient-doctor relationship. As society focuses more and more on the quality of life and human values, particularly with regard to long-term survival with incurable diseases and chronic physical conditions, the medical community has increasingly come under criticism regarding the apparent tendency toward treating the patient as an organism instead of an entity.

Such criticism, while being fair, often fails to take into consideration the tremendous amounts of strain and pressure on staff personnel. Physicians, nurses, social workers, and chaplains all become intertwined, not only in roles, but in their own social systems and the patient's own family system. As if to underline the patient's perception of lack of concern for his value as a human being, it is significant that during the course of this group, with the exception of the mention of physicians, surgeons, and oncology unit nurses in the outpatient clinic, no mention was made of other hospital personnel. This fact existed in spite of the experiences of the cancer patients with long-term and intermittent hospitalization. Surely such an observation cries for attention, for while we continue to spend hundreds of millions of dollars on searching for a cure for what may be many diseases, the quality of human life eroded leaves one's spirit and soul naked in the face of overwhelming odds against survival.

Cancer patients seem to have an awareness of the difficult responsibilities faced by the physician. In her initial interview, Jane seemed to voice a thought reflected in many conversations with other group members.

Jane: . . . because when I come here, and I do respect Doctor Norris, and I'm cognizant to the fact they have a very good program. But he cannot be concerned with every one of my needs. Now, he treats me very adequately on the basis of medication. But there *are other needs*. And perhaps these needs can be fulfilled by other qualified people.

As the patient-doctor relationship progresses in the treatment of cancer, the physician is often placed in the position of being prognosticator. As such he has tremendous psychological influence regarding the patient's self-perception and maintenance of the patient's will to live through the dynamics of hope. One person interviewed for group membership but not able to join shared an awareness of the uncertainty yet maintenance of hope influenced by the doctor-patient relationship.

> **Gene:** I don't know whether I'm going to live a year, two years, five years. The doctor mentioned — he might have been very optimistic — but he mentioned up to eight years. So that's a pretty good time when you have a cancer, I guess. Although I hope the treatment I'm taking might. . . . I guess there's a possibility it might stop the growth completely. I don't know, there is that possibility, from what I understand.

Along the same theme of making predictions, one physician, the same one discussed in the previous paragraph, was shown to have some compassion by Carol as she discussed some of her difficulties in making plans without a firm prognosis.

> **Carol:** Well, I asked Doctor Norris today; I told him I had a lot on my mind. And I said I'd like to know just where I fit in this world. And so he told me that my liver was doing well and he was pleased with the prognosis. He said you're not going to die from that mass you have in your stomach. He says, "We'll have to take care of it somehow. So I can't tell you you are going to live six more months or a year." He says we don't know that anymore. So he says, "Just take each day and do the best you can with it." And I said, "I haven't been able to work full-time since October." And he says, "Well, let's wait until February and see how we come out with this next treatment and see what the next dose of chemotherapy does to that tumor and then we'll decide whether or not you should retire." And he said, "Can you retire financially?" I said, "Well I don't know. I haven't looked into it to see.

The same oncologist viewed with some compassion was also the source and focus of anger and frustration, especially during the early sessions of the group. It seemed that the oncologist is the focal point regarding perceived deprivation and dehumanization. Often the anger of helplessness in the face of imminent death and disease seemed to be projected onto the oncologist. Amanda seemed to reflect this anger in the following excerpt.

Amanda: Well, I'm for pointing out something the doctors can get from these tapes that will be of more benefit to other people. The medical profession as a whole, it seems to me, tends to take it for granted that you know a heck of a lot more than you do. And on the other hand, if you take any liberties at all and don't say, "Yes, whatever you say," they find that rather threatening, I believe. It seems to me there should be a middle ground somewhere. I don't blame them for not wanting to sit down and talk to somebody who never shuts it up and just goes on and on and on. And that's not what they are here for. If you want counseling, go someplace else and pay somebody to listen to you.

The reader will notice Amanda's confusion. For at the same time that she was complaining that the medical profession seemed to take patients for granted, she seemed to defend their right to do so; some other professional should be paid to be sensitive. Such a response would seem to be typical of the ambivalence regarding suppressed affect that cancer patients exhibit.

Later in the same session, Carol, Amanda, and Jane interacted in a dialogue regarding their frustration with oncologists and the difficulties with making predictions. Amanda's and Carol's chief concern seemed to be planning for future events. Significantly, Amanda appeared to be angry with the fact that she had planned her life according to the predictions insinuated or implied by her physicians and was frustrated with the fact that life was not going according to her plans. She was still alive while, allegedly, having finished her "business."

Amanda: Do you feel that maybe doctors are a little free with their predictions? For instance, you were told you had six months, three months. In a way I think it's proper that you get some warning. I don't want anyone lying to me or sugarcoating it. But I wish they wouldn't be so. . . . Jane was saying. . . . You know, she came in and didn't know and wasn't told. And I went in and I was told the bare facts. I was told the statistics in my particular case and what other people . . . and for my age there is no reason for me to be alive now. But here, they just threw a fit. They wouldn't begin to say I had X number of . . . because they don't know.

Carol: Right! They don't know! Well, when I went into surgery the second time, the doctor told my children. . . . He didn't tell me. . . . He says, "Your mother is very ill and it's doubtful that she'll make it through forty-eight hours." But I made it! And then when I was very sick all through '74, he told me, "You'll never see Christmas of '74." And I'm coming up on Christmas of '76. They don't know.

Amanda: I just decided I'm caught between a pessimist and an optimist [laughter].

Carol: I just take each day!

Jane: I have never asked. I've never asked because I didn't think it was a fair question.

Carol: Doctor Norris has never told me that I had six months or two years.

Jane: I didn't think that the doctors could actually predict with the drugs they have now. There are so many combinations that if you don't respond to one combination, there's another combination that can be used. Like, for instance, I was doing very poorly after a while on the combination of drugs that impressed you so much; I was developing very severe side effects. And then I was changed to this drug now and it's made all the difference in the world. They are great.

Amanda: You are illustrating exactly what's happening. It never occurred to me I wouldn't get well. After the surgery I felt, "That's over and done with!" Of course,

I never heard one yet say they didn't get it all. But that's beside the point. And then when it recurred and the specific predictions were made about my life expectancies and I planned my life accordingly and I retired earlier than I would have ordinarily. . . . And I'm glad I did! I'm having a grand time! But it never occurred to me I'd still be here. But here I am. I'm just taking a day at a time.

Later Amanda shared her anger and wondered aloud regarding the credibility of what cancer patients are told by their doctors.

Amanda: Well, you see, Steve, I don't think anybody can really understand if they haven't had it. And that may be one of the problems with the medical profession. So as far as I know, none of the doctors in the clinic is a recovered cancer patient. And you just simply are told a story. You have to walk in the other fellow's shoes.

The medical community admits that some doctors have difficulty with the dynamics of diagnosing cancer. It's not so much a question of technological expertise as it is a denial on the part of the physician. The denial seems to come from a compensation for the loss of power to heal the patient in the face of incurable cancers. Rather than verablize concern that the patient may have cancer, the clinician, for one reason or another, will occasionally miss or, more frequently, understate the diagnosis. The cancer patient must then search until he finds a doctor who is comfortable enough with cancer and verbalization of a diagnosis of cancer or until one gets into a system of less personalized health care, such as a large medical center, where a rather distant medical person "pronounces the sentence." Removed from the intimacy of the relationship with one's family physician built over a period of years, such a dispassionate and circuitous route toward diagnosis and treatment generates anger and bitterness toward the entire health care system. This anger seems justifiable to the patient, and is. Such laxities and oversights intentional or not, are unconscionable and need remedy. It is certain that the group would have agreed, as evidenced into the following excerpt.

Carol: When the doctor told you you had it. . . .

Diana: I went six months into the doctor every two weeks and they kept saying, "There's nothing wrong with you." But *you know* when *you know*!

Jane: I went eight months and discovered this lump in my breast. I went eight months having the doctor tell me I was neurotic and that what I had was fibroid mastitis. I did not have cancer. There was no suspicion. After eight months there was a change in my breast and he suggested a mammogram, and that? Two doctors concurred that it was a fibroid mass with no suspicion of a malignancy.

Amanda: I just don't think those mammograms are worth a hoot!

Jane: That's right! And I talked with the man who developed it who tells me it is not entirely reliable. Well, at any rate, I don't know how certain doctors can function as experts when there is a mass in my breast, which I, as a layman, indicated some cause for suspicion, and my breast was getting smaller. And even though they told me I had nothing to worry about, I said, "I want a biopsy."

Amanda: Well I'll have to be a little more understanding. I was hearing what I wanted to hear. But it was right here in the clinic. So I've been coming ever since Bob's there. . . . And I've made it my duty to stay as well as I could. But I found the lump and then when they said, "The mammogram's negative!" Hallelujah! I went right on about my business. I even told them at one point, "I'm getting ready to go on a trip; so don't give me any bad news." He obliged. He said, "There's nothing wrong."

As Amanda suggested, there is always the possibility that Diana and Jane heard what they wanted to hear. However, personal knowledge suggests that in some cases, doctors fail to diagnose cancer in early stages or refuse to consider the possibility of such for one reason or another.

Diana discussed another subject relating to her anger with physicians. Her discussion also points out unusual dynamics that further interfere with decisions not only regarding oneself but also one's children and the prognosis for the onset of cancer in those children.

Carol: Wouldn't it be a beautiful day when they find a cure for all this and they just give you a shot like they do for measles or whatever?

Diana: See, that's it. My two little girls have a 99.9 percent chance of having breast cancer.

Amanda: I'm sure they do. Isn't that something! Of course, my husband died of cancer and then when they told me I had it, my first thought was, "I want my daughter here to be examined right this minute." And she checked out all right. Her chances are down, but it was not inevitable.

Diana: In fact, one gynecologist in Dallas suggested that my children have their breast tissue removed.

Amanda: Oh, no!

Diana: Yeah, it's that!

Carol: But they say the disease is not hereditary.

Sally: Oh, I question that. My mother died of breast cancer and there was a strong cancer strain on the maternal side.

Carol: No one on my side of the family has ever. . . .

Sally: There must be. . . . Maybe it's not hereditary, but there is certainly a strong predisposition.

Carol: There must be something in the genes that are passed on.

In a later session, Jane described the ordeal that she went through before one of her doctors finally had the "courage" to definitively diagnose and treat her cancer and then only after much persistence on her part. Of course, people like Jane seem to present a clinical picture of an hysterical personality with hypochondriacal overlay. However, whether or not her personality was one of preoccupation with her bodily functions and organic processes, nevertheless, from her report at least, it would appear that the medical profession "dropped the ball."

Jane: Well, I think I have reason to be angry also because I had discovered a lump in my breast and my doctor kept telling me it was cystic mastitis. And after eight months it had been misdiagnosed. And after eight months I noticed a change and I had a mammogram, which indicated a fibroid mass with no suspicion of a malignancy. But there was this change in my breast. What I read was cause for suspicion. I was dimpling. And I insisted on a biopsy and I had a surgeon that was fairly aggressive. I was very angry, and, of course, I was much older.

Amanda: Jane, was it the doctors here?

Jane: No. It was an internist in Atlanta who was very highly regarded.

Amanda: Sue him for malpractice!

Jane: Listen. He had sent me to the surgeon and the surgeon was reluctant to appear as witness, his excuse being it was probably in my bloodstream. But I still have questions in my mind, since he was a general surgeon and performed this biopsy. How do I know that he didn't cut into the tumor tissue and spread it? Because it had not metastasized to my lymph nodes. There was nothing there. I was given an 85 percent chance of doing well. And three years after that, it metastasized to my pleura and then to my liver and. . . .

Amanda: Well, don't you think, Jane, that at some point you just have to say, "That's over and done and there's nothing I can do about it?"

Jane: That's exactly. . . .

Amanda: There's nothing I can do to change that. Now I've got to look at things from a different point of view. You could drive yourself to the nuthouse.

Jane: I subscribe to the fact that I've got to accept what I can't change and I accepted it. But I felt that I had every reason to be angry because I had pointed out to him that I should be regarded as a high risk. My mother had died of breast cancer and there were certain other. . . .

Amanda: Well, he just made a dang mess and you be sure not to go back to him.

Jane: There were other details that should have indicated that. And when I subsequently went to see him about three years ago . . . what am I talking about, a year ago . . . three years after it happened, I said, "You know, please don't do to any other woman what you did to me. If somebody tells you that they should be regarded as high risk and there is a mass there which is not clearly benign," I said, "a biopsy should have been performed." So he said, "Well, I can't be cutting people all the time. There's a danger of death from anesthesia." I said, "Now you know very well that that is remote with comparison of dying with a cancerous mass." He said, "Well I showed poor judgment."

Steve: So Diana's not the only one here who's angry.

Jane: Right! I was angry. But of course I can understand Diana 'cause Diana's much younger than I am.

Cancer patients are still people. They hunger for warmth and intimacy. The doctor-patient relationship is no different from any other human relationship. The exception seems to be the barrier imposed by medical dogma. In the following excerpt, Jane showed her sense of humor regarding her relationship with her oncologist and how gratifying it was for her to get an emotional response from him.

Jane: But, you know how I really feel? I said to Doctor Norris . . . and with his usual animated looks, he looked at me and I said, "You know, I really feel very deeply about this. I'm very scientifically oriented and I feel if you ever can't cure something that you felt you wanted to experiment with, and that something like a rat or a cat or anything like that would not be sufficient, and you needed something alive," I said, "I really want you to use me. I really want to even if there is an element of risk." And I got a smile out of him.

Diana: You did?

Jane: Oh, I almost dropped dead.

Carol: One time I got a smile out of him too, and I couldn't believe it!

Jane: He doesn't smile very much.

Carol: He does not!

The difficulties with difference in perception are echoed in the following quote. Here Amanda relayed a moment of tenderness and warmth by the same oncologist, Doctor Norris, who had been the subject of discussion throughout this section. It is interesting as an aside that Amanda spoke candidly about the warmth that she felt from Doctor Norris. She was caught off guard and stated that she was not aware that our group session had begun. To the therapist it was significant that Amanda was putting on her mask at the beginning of each session. Caught with her mask off, she related a sensitive interaction between she and her oncologist and communicated warmth in a fashion not acceptable during what she considered the "formal" group process, at least not at this exploration stage of the group's development.

Diana: You know, I think if he just showed you he cared. I get no feeling that he cares. I know that he must or he wouldn't be doing these. . . .

Amanda: Diana, I think that he does and the reason why . . . I'll tell you one brief experience I had. When we started on this thing, he knew that I had had a little altercation with Doctor Beam. I don't know if Doctor Beam was ever conscious of it, but I was, and I had passed it on to Doctor Maste. And so when he talked with me about getting into the group, he said, "Now I promise you I won't push you to do anything you don't really want to do." And then some months later I remember . . . or maybe it was when perhaps he questioned it. . . . And now many of you aren't going to believe this. *He put both hands on my shoulders!*

Diana: No! I don't believe it!

Amanda: . . . and said, "If this doesn't work out, remember I promised you . . . but I do want to talk to you about the other procedure. I want you to at least think about it." Well, as it happens, the medicine started working again; so we hadn't gotten back to that. But that was a real indication to me.

Diana: Well, you know, I've always had very strong doctors who would come in and say, "This is what we are going to do." And by his, what I consider nonchalant attitude, it's like he doesn't care! Or, it's like I said, "I don't want to take any medicine! And he said "That's up to you."

Jane: He's just not demonstrative.

Steve: You know we've had this conversation before. And I'm just going to get a little more directive because one of the things about the group is that it is good to vent. What I'm wondering is, we hear the different styles of the two doctors. And I'm sure we can talk about other doctors and nurses. . . . But the feeling I'm hearing has to do with the type of communication and warmth generated, and how you feel about or perceive that warmth.

Amanda: Oh! I thought this was just a preamble to starting. We were waiting for Carol. I didn't know this was a part. . . .

Steve: Oh, we're started. Really we start almost as soon as you walk in.

In a later session, also recorded on tape before the group's "official" convening, Carol, Jane and Diana discussed the "conspiracy of silence" that they perceived. Such a "conspiracy" may generate feelings of deprivation and dehumanization and incurs further anger and bitterness and feelings of impotence in the face of cancer.

Carol: Well, I had an appointment at the GYN at 11:30, and he gave me a pelvic exam, and that's it. I said, "That's it?" And I told the nurse, "You mean he can tell me where all my problems are with just that?" And she said, "Well, he'll get with Doctor Norris." I've been miserable these past two weeks. I've had such terrific pains in my stomach. I had it yesterday. And two weeks ago it got so bad; so I called Cindy, and she made an appointment at GYN. So, I had it today.

Jane: But you don't know anything?

Carol: I don't know anything. He just did a pelvic exam and that's it — took down some information.

Jane: Well, maybe he has to do some tests.

Carol: He didn't do any tests. He didn't do anything.

Jane: He didn't take a Pap smear or anything?

Carol: Just gave me a quick pelvic. It didn't take one minute.

Diana: I've been neutered. I should never have to go there.

Carol:	These doctors that keep silent, I don't like them. I like to know what's going on.

Again, Doctor Norris was the subject of discussion in session 4. Carol discussed her pain. Barbara asked whether or not she had discussed her pain with Doctor Norris. Jane offered that Doctor Norris never seemed to talk and that, through her indirect discovery, she had found his suspicion of a new cancerous mass in her body. Depression, hurt, and lack of self-worth are all feelings engendered by such treatment. A loss of control is reiterated in the often child-like treatment of the paternalistic interaction between physician and patient.

Carol:	I'm just concerned why I have all these pains. There has to be something wrong.
Barbara:	Did you ask Doctor Norris?
Carol:	Yes, and he said nothing.
Jane:	He doesn't talk.
Barbara:	"Everybody has aches and pains." That's what he told me.
Steve:	This old thing's happening again where we have too. . . .
Jane:	I was getting all these scans. Doctor Norris was sending me down to Bartlett Hall for a body scan and all that, but doesn't tell me why. And I thought it was just routine because I was always getting scans and X-rays etc. And finally he says to me one day, "I'm very glad to report that the mass was a cyst, not a tumor." I said, "What mass?" I didn't know what he was talking about. He never told me that he was suspicious of a mass on my kidney; you know, that one of my kidneys had this mass. Because he never talks! He never told me! And that was the first that I learned that there was suspicion of a mass.

In a later session, Sally alluded briefly to a situation in which she had difficulty in getting through to discuss the matter with her oncologist, also Doctor Norris. Again, all of us encounter such situations and feel like we are getting the runaround, and while all can be sensitive to the problems of time, commitments, and priorities by professionals, especially medical personnel, all also can identify with the unsaid feelings and frustrations of having to go through an intermediary to be able to have direct, intimate contact with the doctor. In the case of these cancer patients, Doctor Norris represented the link of hope and sanity.

Diana: What's his name?

Sally: Doctor Gates. I said, "Well, I want to see Doctor Gates!" "What do you want to see him for?"

Diana: What'd you say?

Amanda: And you bit your tongue and did not say, "It's none of your business."

Sally: No. I said, "Well it was something I particularly wanted to discuss with him." And Norris came on in. But I didn't see Doctor Norris other than that today. I understand he's here today.

Amanda: Yeah, I asked him, "Are you going to be one of those that passes through?" And he said, "No! "

Carol: Is he going to be Doctor Norris's assistant? That's good 'cause I like him.

TERMINOLOGY AND TREATMENT

In concluding this chapter, it is again important to note the cancer patient's opposition to the word *terminal*. During the course of the initial interviews, it was my responsibility to obtain consent by explicitly underlining the fact that each candidate for the group had an incurable prognosis and was, in effect, terminal. The opposition to the use of the word terminal is something that persons working with cancer patients should be aware of. They seem to prefer terms such as *incurable* or *metastatic*.

Jane: *See, I don't like that word terminal.*

Steve: Yeah, you don't, huh?

Jane: *No, I prefer to use the word incurable.*

Steve: OK, let's, well then. . . .

Jane: *You see, I think psychologically it's a better word.*

Steve: OK, fine, yeah, I guess it would be, and I don't. . . .

Jane: *See, because that leaves room for hope.*

Steve: OK.

Jane: *As soon as you say to a person, "you are terminal," get me my obituary. I'm going to die. I don't feel* *terminal*. And I know that I can hang on long enough until there's a breakthrough.

Steve: Well great, great, OK. So, you would prefer when I'm talking to you I use the word incurable. Fine. Well, anyway. . . .

Jane: See, I think it's a good word to use for any of those patients because, you see, a lot of these people are not advanced emotionally to the point that I am and have not accepted it. As soon as you say terminal to them, they're wasting away. They may as well get into bed and wait to die.

Steve: That's a good point.

Jane: When you say you're incurable, that leaves room for hope. "Well, gee, maybe tomorrow there's going to be a cure for me and I'm going to be living, and I can hang on." But with *terminal*, I can't hang on; I'm just waiting to die.

Steve: Well, you know this very subject. . . . I anticipate this very thing coming up in the group. The first couple of sessions you kind of get to know each other and stuff and then after that people start to come out and talk. And so, that gives me kind of an insight. Well, to get back to where I was. . . .

Jane: Well, Steve, don't forget that these are scared people; so you want to choose your words very carefully. You don't want to create more anxiety.

Simiarly, in her initial interview, Carol voiced the same concern. This may be perceived as a denial/coping mechanism. However perceived, it is significant for the informed and sensitive counselor. Persistence in the use of the word terminal in caring for cancer patients could destroy the rapport and have other deleterious effects. As in all other types of counseling, it is important to maintain rapport and, to the degree possible, operate within the client's belief and value system. Avoiding the use of this irritating word may facilitate meeting such a commitment to the patient.

Carol: You did mention one thing that bothered me about *terminal* patients. I have never considered myself as a terminal patient. I don't know how bad my condition is. Doctor Norris never said; he never told me. I was in the hospital in November of '75 for five days, then December, then January. After three months treatment I did very well. And I wasn't on any medication whatsoever until September when I started losing weight and my appetite just went kind of down. So we decided I had been too long without the medication; so he gave me a shot of chemotherapy, and I got better. Then he also put me on that horrible medicine that just set me back six months. I had a terrible reaction from it, and I'm getting better. But I'm still not feeling like me. But hopefully by the time all that gets out of my system I'll be good as new again. But really I've never considered myself as a terminal patient. I do know that in January of '75 I was very very ill and they didn't give me much hope at the time, and I was under the care of Doctor Moriarity. And he put me in the hospital here for a twenty-one-day treatment. And they put a tube through an artery which drained into my lung. And that did better than any. I think that sort of put me back on my feet again.

Steve: So the word terminal itself is. . . .

Carol: I never use it!

Steve: You never use it. Well, I'll try not to use it too.

Carol: Maybe some people do. Maybe they consider themselves terminal.

Steve: Yeah. The study is geared around severely, critically, or terminally ill persons, and so when I use that word, it's open to any interpretation that you want to use.

SECTION II

THE GROUP: COLLECTED
PERSONS—FALLING LEAVES

But I look at our group as a pie. And our whole life is a pie. It is a little bit-ty one-sixteenth of an inch. Here's the group and there's the whole rest of this big pie that no one in this group, you included [Steve], is even remote-ly aware of in my life. So there's no way you can take a sixteenth of my life and try to solve all my problems.

Diana

Diana has summarized the expectations of all of the group members regarding the impact of the group on their lives. That is to say, it was never intended for the group to solve all of its individual member's problems. Rather, it was intended to provide a vehicle by which these persons could share common concerns and feelings in an atmosphere of safety, trust, and acceptance. Likewise, by the end of the group, all expectations had been fulfilled in the spirit of the "con-tract."

Group process and group dynamics should be of significance to all professionals and lay persons interested in either structured or unstructured counseling groups. This interest should be even further heightened in the case of cancer patients. In light of ongoing developments in our society regarding care of the terminally ill in programs such as Hospice and in light of the proliferation of self-help groups, many persons will have opportunities to lead groups of cancer patients.

Groups move through exploration, transition, action, and ter-mination. The group facilitator must constantly be aware of nonver-bal cues and must strive to facilitate unexpressed affect. Clarification of thoughts and direction of interactions is important. Other tech-niques used to facilitate the group's movement through stages pro-vide the opportunity for the therapeutic effect.

In the course of working with cancer patients, the counselor is taxed even more because of the intimacy and awesome implications of the feelings, attitudes, and experiences being shared. As in other kinds of group counseling and psychotherapy activities, the counselor must be aware of needs and anxieties relating to subjects such as death, loneliness, fear, and hopelessness so as not to become part of the problem.

The human mind is extremely intricate. Thus, that which is stated or which is offered is often not what it appears to be. True meaning must be extricated and amplified in an artistic and sensitive fashion. As in any other therapeutic dynamic, the counselor must always be on guard for the possibility that what is being said is not what is actually meant. Furthermore, it is up to the counselor to create an atmosphere in which people are afforded the opportunity to clarify and express what it is they are actually trying to say.

In an effort to help the reader comprehend such dynamics at a deeper level, this section will examine each session for group process, counseling techniques, and sociometry. This will be accomplished by analysis of the unsaid, unstated dynamics occurring within the group during each session; commentary on the techniques employed; and the use of my personal journal, in which impressions of the sessions as well as group seating were recorded. Chapters are divided in accordance with group dynamics. For each of the four phases of group development, there are corresponding chapters: Chapter 6, exploration; Chapter 7, transition; Chapter 8, action; and Chapter 9, termination.

Chapter 6

EXPLORATION: "CHECKING EACH OTHER OUT"

COMMENTS ON THE INITIAL INTERVIEWS

THE first place to start in any discussion of group process is with the expectations of prospective members. During actual recruiting, it was interesting to find that while many of the interviewees seemed to have a genuine interest, they had much resistance to becoming a group member and discussing their problems. As will be seen in a later chapter, many of the candidates never joined the group due to fears of self-disclosure, intimacy, and the possibility of accepting the incurable prognosis. It was also interesting to note that many of the candidates camouflaged their own needs for such an experience under the guise of serving others. That is, it was acceptable to some interviewees to be in the group but only if they were there as a service to the other members. In my experience, this seems to be a dynamic peculiar to cancer patients. It appears that they will not "take for themselves" nor will they clearly express their own needs in terms of affect. There is always the concept of doing for others because "I can take care of myself."

Dave was a 47-year-old male Caucasian who was one of these persons who chose not to join the group. He had a number of physical difficulties including chronic heart disease as well as lung cancer. Early in our initial interview, Dave manifested some denial and offered as a rationale for his participation the need to help others.

> **Dave:** I should tell you that from the beginning I've had no apprehensions about my condition at all. I think I mentioned this over the phone to you. *But rather than them helping me, perhaps I could help them.* At least that's the way I view it at this point.

Later in the initial interview, Dave shared a fear of being in a group with people who had a terminal illness. This fear was common to other interviewees. It seems a curious composite of coping and denial and suggests anxiety when dealing with the reality of incurable, metastatic disease.

Dave: Tell me one thing if you can, or if you are permitted to. Do any of the people that will be in these sessions . . . do any of them have terminal illness?

Steve: Well, most of the group members have cancers that are under control. I don't know how the staff looks at them, but they are considered seriously ill. In a lot of cases they are under control but they are still progressing. So I guess . . . one of the members told me. . . . She prefers to think of it as incurable 'cause that kind of doesn't take away . . . you know with the present technology . . . they can't really cure it. So the members are in different stages. Some are under control, but all have cancers. I have been told they are incurable at this point in time with all we know. That's about all I can tell you.

Dave: That is the only part that is going to disturb me, I think. When those particular individuals open up. I know I had some adverse reactions to one death a couple of doors down the hall from me last trip into the hospital. And this is very unsettling to me. I still haven't really recovered from it in my own mind. It's justified I suppose. But for about two weeks therafter I was dismissed from the hospital, I was having some pretty bad nightmares concerning that. When you are that close to it, it sort of shakes you.

Steve: Yeah, I can see that it's a little frightening just talking about it right now. You are a little anxious. I can't promise you that somebody's not going to come out and just spill it right out there for you to work through. I can assure you that I'll try to ease the members through those kinds of crises as they come up in the group and try to help everyone in the group, including yourself, so you don't have that kind of bad experience again where you have the nightmares and those kinds of feelings.

Dave: I'm not squeamish as far as myself is concerned. But when it's somebody else, this disturbs me.

Two expectations from a candidate's point of view can be seen in view of the description of what the expectations would be of the group: (a) Being a member of this group implied that one was there to help others and in so doing, one might gain something for him or herself, and, (b) the persons in the group were dying. If, as Dave asserted, he was coping with his terminal prognosis and was denying that he was dying, then he was a poor candidate for the group. He would have used the rationale that "they" were dying and he was not for maintaining his distance.

Finally, Dave reiterated his fear of death and his difficulty with the emotions of others in response to deaths of loved ones.

Dave: No, not that part. As I said, the only thing that disturbs me at all during this whole process has been that one death. And that was very unsettling to me. And I think it was mostly because of the family's emotional outburst, which is quite understandable. But the fact is they waited until the wife and daughter got to the hospital right outside the room where the man had died when someone told them right then that it had happened. Of course, both of them just broke down completely.

Faye was another person screened for the group. With some difficulty, she decided not to become a group member. The following excerpt illustrates her problem with group discussions as well as her own interpretation of the stages of cancer.

Faye: Well, I guess you talked to several people; so you probably don't remember, but I told you at the time that right now I don't know how I feel about group discussion. You go through different stages and you go through fear. And you go through depression, and you go through adjusting to, "I've got something that the whole world is scared to death of." Then I have reached the point now to where I feel like it's time. . . . "OK! You've had this! You've gotten through it! Start putting it behind you!" Because I went through. . . . When I first found out I had it and got through the cobalt and all that it was like weird. I was thinking of that other Faye, that other person that didn't have cancer, that was completely healthy. And it was this other person. . . . It was like I was two different people, but now I'm getting back to, "I'm my old self again now," and it was the other person that had this cancer that had nearly choked to death and nearly died and all that. Of course, maybe next week I'll be right back down on the very bottom again and scared to death. And it gets easier though. I mean you put some time between you and the end.

Similar to circumstances in Dave's case, Faye had some concerns about the homogeneity of the group with respect to terminal illness. On inquiry as to whether or not Faye had any questions about group procedures, and following response was given.

Faye: I was wondering. What do you think? I mean, there are going to be people in the group who still have cancer. Are they going to be terminal patients?

Steve: Yeah, that's true. I don't think that would be any problem.

Faye: That scares me.

Steve: It scares you?

Faye: Yes, it scares me.

Steve: It scares you to be in a group with other people who are terminal and have the cancer.

Faye: Right. Because when you've had it. . . . You know, that could be me and you think I'm so fortunate that mine's gone now. Of course, you don't know if it's going to come back or not. It's just like I said. They can't guarantee it. But it scares me to think about it and I don't need to be scared. How do people deal with it when it's terminal?

Steve: I don't really know. I don't have an answer.

Faye: I wouldn't want to know it. No way. I don't think the

	Lord intended us to know when we are going to die. I mean, we are all terminal; we know that! But to have an idea of when it's going to be. No, I wouldn't want to know that!
Steve:	Well, one of the criteria for the group. . . . The persons in this group all have cancer, except for me, as far as I know. And now you're saying that yours is arrested, and so that might be a problem for you, you know. You'd have to think about that coming into the group. Now most of the people in the group, theirs is under control. A lot of them, a couple of them are without symptoms at the present time. But everybody in the group is considered severely ill . . . terminally ill . . . critically ill.
Faye:	Really?
Steve:	Yeah. . . . Yeah. So, that will be a subject that will be coming up, you know, talking about death and dying. And it could be kind of a scary thing, you know. I mean I don't want to. . . . I can see you are a little frightened now, and I think you should . . . we need to talk about that and think about that before you come into the group.
Faye:	Because, you see, I'm getting better! I'm learning to cope now and I don't want to do anything that's going to set me back!
Steve:	Well, there's going to be some times when the stuff that comes down in the group is going to be very heavy. I would say probably the first couple of sessions it'll be pretty easy. It'll be just getting to know each other and trust each other and that kind of thing.
Faye:	And then people are going to get into how they really think?
Steve:	People are going to get into how they feel about cancer and how they feel about their sex lives and their families and life in general and death in general. These are the kinds of things that come up in any group, but they'll be particularly pertinent right now. And that's, you know if you have fears. . . . I

can say you can drop out at any time in the group. But often once you get into a group like this, you develop a relationship with the other people and you don't want to really drop out because you'd be helping them so much. You know, each of you would be helping each other. And now, to the best of my knowledge . . . there's another factor you might want to think about. To the best of my knowledge I'm healthy. You know, I have headaches and colds and things like that. . . . So that's another factor that will have to be worked through in the group. How they feel about having a leader that's . . . who's healthy for all intents and purposes.

Faye: Well, that's me! I wouldn't know how to sit and talk with people and say, "Mine's gone!" As far as they know, mine's gone and you know I feel like really I have had it pretty easy compared to what some people have had. Because . . . well . . . it was bronchial cancer. And I take the mildest form of chemotherapy. And I mean this is encouraging to me. And some other people might say, "Well, I'd like to kill her because of that!" Because I'm sure if I was in their shoes, I'd feel that way.

Steve: They might say that about you, they might say that about me. There's another possibility. They might say, "Thank God for you and thank God for me!" You know, there's kind of two ways to look at it. The other thing is you'll never be forced to talk in the group; but you would be very helpful to them and think they could be helpful to you. I think it's always scary going into something like this. I'm a little scared myself.

Faye: Are you?

Steve: Sure, I don't know. . . .

Faye: You can't imagine!

Steve: I can't imagine. Right, that's No. 1, and No. 2, I have no idea where the group is going. I have an idea. . . . You know I have a little idea. So this is a kind of thing I'm responsible for. There's seven, as far as I know. If you'll be willing to join us and if I agree to accept you into the group, there'll be seven women and two men. And all the people in the group, to the best of my knowledge. . . . I've been told all the people in the group are cancer patients. Or, you know, they may be without symptoms at the present time. And most of the people are kind of like you; you know, walking around and doing reasonably well under the circumstances and with the shock and the anger and all these kinds of things. So I guess it comes down to; it's your decision whether you want to be here or not. I'm not trying to sell it one way or the other.

Faye: I know.

Steve: You may want to give it a try for a couple of sessions and then decide that you would like to join us.

Faye: Well, the thing about it is I wouldn't mind it at all except for the fact that right now . . . like I say . . . I'm learning to cope and I'm feeling better, which I need to do. And somebody can say something to me now. . . . Like when I can be feeling good, somebody can say something to me like . . . well . . . they had something that had reoccurred. That can send me off for two or three days, you know. Then I'm all depressed again.

Steve: Yeah, depressed and down.

Faye: Right! And so I'm scared to deliberately put myself in a situation where I'm going to get scared to death again. I've had that and it's miserable! And I've had not to rely on anything! The tranquilizers I took for some years got to where they depressed me again and I haven't had anything really to help me.

Steve: Well, I don't know. I get the feeling. . . . You know, I can see that you are anxious right now. I get the feeling that you would like me to say something whether you should or shouldn't join. . . .

Faye: Right.

Steve: . . . Put the decision on me. I'm not a medical doctor. I'm working on my Ph.D. I can see your fear and anxiety, and I can say to you that you know there may be risks that you will get depressed, that you'll feel rotten, and tranquilizers won't help. There are also the possibilities that you might be able to deal with your feelings better. Kind of like "misery likes company" . . . and building a new set of friends who understand how you are feeling . . . who are going through the same kinds of feelings you're going through. And so you wouldn't be forced to face your depression and anxiety alone. You'd be with other people facing the same kinds of fears and anxieties. So, of course, my opinion is that there's much more to be gained than there is to be lost; but that decision has to be yours. What I'm hearing is you're not sure whether or not you want to make that decision.

Faye: I don't know what to do! I can't make a decision!

Steve: That's a decision.

Faye: That's a decision that I can't make a decision? You know, sometimes you wish you were a child so somebody would tell you to do this and do that and you don't have to make your own decisions.

Steve: Yeah, yeah, that would be nice.

It should be reiterated that all of the persons interviewed had been informed of their incurable prognosis by their oncologist. Faye's method of coping with that prognosis could be interpreted as pathological. Life was difficult for those who cared for and loved her. It put the burden of knowledge and fear of disclosure on those who were closest to the patient and perpetuated guilt and anger in those persons as they went through the elaborate charade and masquerade of helping Faye deny reality. Certainly, eliminating that reality with brutal confrontation of the facts would not be in order. The removal of such denial could cause the development of psychosis, compounding an already complicated and tragic series of circumstances.

By example, Faye represented the kind of cancer patient that causes grief at many levels for those around her. She was not aware of the burden imposed on others as a result of her denial. Her death was even more cruel and tragic than it need have been because of these dynamics. Her's was the type of death that would be "wel-

comed" by those around her for their own relief. The subsequent
guilt that arises out of such "eager" anticipation of a patient's demise
(in some cases) could produce psychological and emotional problems
in survivors that might not manifest themselves for ten to twenty
years postmortem when the survivors, who were young at the time
of the patient's death, would be forced to confront their own demise.

In another initial interview for screening, Carl, a man in his early
twenties suffering from testicular carcinoma and its complications,
shared the theme alluded to earlier and common to almost all of the
persons considered for the group membership.

> **Carl:**   You know, a long time ago. . . . Well, when I found
> out that I was first sick and all that, I thought about
> meeting with other people to see how they reacted
> and sort of bolster myself. And right now there's not
> a whole lot I feel I can get out of the group because I
> consider myself very stable and in a fine mental
> sense. And like, possibly, if there is somebody in the
> group that's weaker, maybe I can bolster them. But I
> can't see myself getting any better out of it because
> I'm just great.

Here again, Carl *knew* that there was not much he could get from
the group but that he would have a lot to contribute to others.

A woman named Susan was also interviewed for the group but
could not participate because of apparent transportation difficulties.
However, closer inquiry revealed that Susan was unwilling to invest
the energy to participate in the group. In fact there were family
members who were willing to provide her transportation to and from
the group sessions.

In spite of her resistance, Susan did feel that such a group could
be of benefit to her and other cancer patients as evidenced by the
following excerpt.

> **Susan:**   I sometimes think that something like this might be
> helpful to all of us because you have times when,
> even though you think you have adjusted to it, you
> haven't. And sometimes if we get together, at least
> we will realize that other people have the same
> problem and then your problems don't seem quite as
> big. But it seems like a tremendous problem at times.

Steve: So what I'm hearing is that from time to time, it just gets overwhelming and maybe you wish you did have a group to talk with.

Susan: Well, you've got to have a sounding board somewhere and you don't like to use your family for that. Although your family is sometimes too close and they are too sympathetic towards you and sometimes sympathy is not exactly what we need. We need kind of a boot in the backside sometimes and the family doesn't give you that.

Steve: So it would be helpful to you to have a kind of a session or a place where a group could meet and act as a sounding board and see if they are feeling the same kind of things.

Susan: That's right! That's right!

Later in the interview, Susan, too, acknowledged that on the one hand, she, ". . . thinks it will be beneficial to me." On the other hand, she expressed her interest in helping others stating, "I hope I can be of help to somebody else."

Of the members interested in being in the group and eventually joining, Barbara was one who shared honestly that she was the most important person in terms of benefit from the group. When asked as to what she would like to see the group do and what she would be able to find of benefit in the group, Barbara stated the following:

Barbara: Well, I think the main thing is to see. . . . Well, most of the things I would be interested in would be the different types of malignancy and how the other people are responding.

Steve: How they are handling it?

Barbara: . . . Accepting it. If they are doing some things that I could do that could change my way of thinking or my attitude or something, it would be helpful to me. Is that what we do? We discuss the different problems they are having and you tell them your problems?

Steve: Well, something like that.

Similarly, Louise shared a need to be able to talk in a more open environment when she stated the following.

Louise: Well, maybe where I can talk more openly I guess.
My family and I, we talk pretty openly but sometimes, I don't know . . . I feel like I can't. I don't want
them to worry and I know they are worried. My husband tries to act like a big strong "he-man" and says
he doesn't worry. But I think deep down, he does.
And I try to seem happy because of that. And I feel
like maybe people in the same condition . . .
maybe we could talk to one another.

It becomes more and more apparent that cancer patients both
need and fear the opportunity to discuss their problems with those in
similar circumstances. Sally echoed what Louise and Barbara had
earlier affirmed.

Sally: I tell you, sometimes I get awfully depressed, and it's
not. . . . I thought maybe I might get something to
help me with that. And, well, I've never had anyone
close to discuss the problem with. I have a little
niece who has gone through lung cancer, and she's
much, much younger than I am. But she's fighting a
battle. We talk by telephone about every two or
three weeks. She's had to take cobalt and she's on
chemotherapy. And we have problems about how
we feel or what we can do. But I've never had anyone that I could discuss this with. I'm not used to discussing problems, and I mean to sit down and talk to
people about it and "yaw-yaw" about it. But I feel
that sometimes I would like to have somebody
maybe that's had a similar operation to this. You
know some things about it we could discuss the matter with.

Two key persons responsible for the organization and evolution
of the group were Carol and Diana. They, along with Jane, re-
quested the opportunity for a group to be conducted through the oncology unit. It was significant that in both of their initial interviews
they suggested their desire to help others. Here is one example.

Carol: Well, I think this will be quite interesting. It'll make it
something if I can help someone else. Perhaps that is
why God has left me here. I don't know.

Note that in her search for purpose in the time that she had left in life, Carol tried to define what God might have her do with this time. The link with her spiritual roots seemed to give Carol the energy to continue her life and to have almost mini purposes and goals in order that each hour, day, week, or month might be full. The importance of a strong religious belief and its relationship to the ability of one to accept death has been well documented in the literature. Carol seemed to personify an attitude of acceptance with grace apparent in those persons who have deep-seated and inner-directed feelings of relationship with their personalized concept of God.

Finally Diana is seen looking forward to the group with an optimism seldom witnessed during the ten-session life of the group. She also summarized the most common vocalization of all of the members when she stated the following.

Diana: And I guess the thing I'm looking forward to is being with people that have something really in common because most people don't really understand.

SESSION 1: EXPLORATION

Session 1 exemplified the exploratory phase of group process. During this phase members had difficulty discussing specific issues involving their treatment and chose instead to discuss "safe" subjects. There were many safe types of disclosures, with members putting their best foot forward. Much anxiety was manifested.

Much time had to be spent in terms of instruction regarding the instruments developed for the group. Group process consisted of people meeting for the first time, introducing themselves to one another, and telling something significant about their lives that they wished to share during this first session. An interesting dynamic of this early session occurred when Diana verbalized some of her frustration, indirectly, at being so young and wished out loud that she was fifty-one. In a very natural and caring fashion, both Carol and Amanda attempted to facilitate Diana's verbalization and help her to clarify it. Incidently, this native ability to facilitate by other members made the job of group leader easier. Much less time was needed to teach and model good communication skills for the members.

Diana: I wish I was fifty-one. My children would be grown, married, established.

Carol: You know Diana, the older they get, they just have bigger problems. When they are little, they have little problems.

Amanda: Don't you wish you were fifty-one because that would suggest a certain length of survival.

Diana: Yes, Yes, or even my husband going up in his company and the benefits. I have a pang of jealousy that he's going to do all this without me and, you know, I want it all because. . . .

Carol: . . . You want to be there to share it with him.

Diana: Because my life has been in cycles. I ran . . . literally ran the first three years. I tried to live a lifetime. They said I had six months to live and I began to buy everything in sight. We began to go everywhere.

Carol: I did the same thing.

Diana: . . . Do everything because I was not going to live, and I looked at each day saying, I wasn't going to live. And I think that's such an empty feeling to never have tomorrow. People say, well, "I can walk out of here." Terrific, but you don't have something in your body eating it away.

Carol: That's right.

Another interesting phenomena that appeared early was the supportive nature of the group as typified by an interaction between Amanda and Carol. After Carol had expressed a fear of growing old alone, Amanda stated the following.

Amanda: It's not so bad as it was twenty years ago.

Steve: So you're saying that you can share some of your feelings with Carol that you've kind of been where she is.

Amanda: Well, no. No, I can't honestly say that because I didn't have any threatening disease and I didn't have four children. I had one. . . . But there's a big difference between one and four when you start buying shoes. No, I think you have far greater things to contend with than I ever did. But you just mentioned growing old alone. It can happen. It's amazing how you can fill your life with other things.

Technique

In terms of technique, the counselor was concerned with organizational "housekeeping" dynamics. It is extremely important to begin to establish a rapport in any group at this stage, and it is even more significant with a group of cancer patients. If one is physically healthy and is facilitating a group of people who have terminal disease, one must be aware of anxieties within himself regarding terminal disease, death, and dying. As the only healthy person in the group, one is in a sense the group isolate. During the course of the group there were occasions where anger and hostility about relative good health could be sensed. It was as though they wore a badge as members of a special club and ". . . You're not! How the hell do you think you can help us?"

The counselor must be able to facilitate the expression of affect. For instance, during the first session anger at the medical establishment was suggested, but not directly verbalized, for being lackadaisical in the diagnosis of Jane's cancer. Much of the literature has shown that the expression of anger is difficult for the cancer-prone personality. Thus, it is the responsibility of the counselor to verbalize the unspoken affect in a way in which the group can deal with it. Of course, this does not necessarily mean that the group will deal with it as evidenced by the closing quote at the end of the following excerpt.

Steve: You're trying to give Diana some support because she's young and all that. But what I'm hearing is that everyone in here to some degree is angry at the injustice of the situation regardless of what your age is or what spectrum of life you are. I was hearing that maybe the group might be saying to Diana, "Hey! You're alone in this because you're the youngest member in here." But now I'm hearing something different. The group is saying, "You're not alone in this. You're just seeing it at a different point in your life. We're all angry."

Amanda: Well, Steve, intellectually we all know that there's nothing fair about life. If it was, everybody would have enough to eat; everybody would be warm; everybody would have a good house. So we know this intellectually. But emotionally we just don't accept it. It hits you. You just say it's not fair. Well, what right do you have to expect everything to be so fair?

Incidentally, it is very typical for counselors to feel anxious when starting any new group. Anxiety is even more acute in a situation as tense as one dealing with the dynamic of imminent death just below the surface of conversation. It would be of some concern if counselors were not experiencing some anxiety out of empathy with the initial meeting of such a group, especially if it was the counselor's first experience with a group of persons who were dying.

Sociometry

Figure 6-1 and 6-2 illustrate the seating arrangements and primary patterns of communication during this session. In the first figure, members of the group are listed by names. The second figure shows circles indicating the therapist with each member being represented by a subsequent circle with the first letter of their name inserted in the circle. Arrows represent the primary directions of communications. For instance, the communication pattern between Amanda and Diana was one in which Amanda was doing a lot of advice-giving. Thus, such communication is illustrated by an arrow going from Amanda toward Diana. Similarly, Amanda did some advice-giving to Carol as indicated by the directional thrust of the communication. Much of the communication during this session was directed between individual members and the leader or with the leader as a go-between in facilitating communication. This is indicated by lines with double-ended arrows. In the case of Amanda and Barbara as well as Diana and Jane, there was some cross communication as indicated by arrows going in two directions. (Future figures in this section will be illustrated using the first initial of each member's name only.)

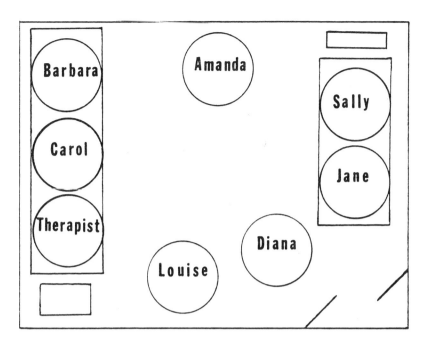

Figure 6-1. Session 1: Seating of group members and therapist.

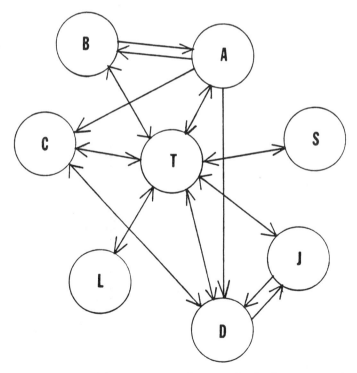

Figure 6-2. Session 1: Primary patterns of communication between members and members and therapist.

Journal

As stated earlier, during the course of our group, a journal was kept of personal recollections of each session. Those recollections for the first session will be shared at this time. In subsequent reviews of technique and dynamics during each session, journal recollections will immediately follow the brief explanation of the figures.

Joy! Yesterday seven people showed for my group! Louise, Carol, Diana, Jane, Amanda, Sally, and Barbara were present. Carl lacerated his liver in three places trying to see if he could hit a car on his motorcycle at 40 mph and survive. He was in serious condition and had emergency surgery; but, thank God, he's alive and will be OK. He'll be worked with individually. He may make a good paraprofessional cancer counselor. Behind his confident personality, Carl has to have many concerns, such as testicular carcinoma.

Jane was disappointed that there were no men in the group ("What about me?" I wondered aloud. "You don't count.") Amanda and Diana were glad that no other men would be there as they felt free and open with me and felt freer to talk in more intimate terms about their disease with other women.

Louise is on a treatment called hyperalimentation. They give her 3,000 calories a day through a nasogastric tube. They'll keep this up for three or four weeks to try to get her weight up so they can try to administer chemotherapy, for she will lose weight. Anyway, she brought all of the paraphernalia with her to the group (tubes, meters, etc.) Of course, the humorous one that I am, I asked her who her plumber was. These women are so courageous outside and so scared inside.

The group spent most of this session comparing symptoms: hair loss, muscle control loss, limbs, aches, drugs, pain, pain killers, weight loss, weight gain, deep voices, hormones, neutering by removal of ovaries, and breasts. But feelings are already beginning to show. We spent some time in processing, trying to get them to listen to one another and reflect feelings in the first person *I* or *me* and to look into each others eyes as they talk to one another, addressing each other by name.

I noticed touching (physical) between Sally and Jane and cross talk between Barbara and Amanda. Carol has found God and relates to joy, peace, and love; each day is extra time. She was at one time in 1974 given forty-eight hours to live. Her complaint (shared by other members) was the following: "Don't tell me how long. Just tell me my condition. Treat me like a human being, not as an organism growing a cancer culture for 'boy wonders' to experiment on." Diana is angry. Her cancer is accelerating and involves both lungs. She's had trouble breathing lately and has had pain in her chest. Amanda tried to claim that it seemed most unfair that one as young as Diana (33) should be faced with cancer (Diana's had it for 7 years), and that Diana had a right to be angry. It seems that Amanda has lived her life and has no resentment. I doubted this, of course, and felt that Diana, unwittingly, was being isolated with her feelings of anger and resentment and wondered out loud if this was what she was alluding to. The other group members chimed in to the effect that they were resentful and angry, especially Jane. Jane said that she had really, at sixty-eight, just begun to find meaning to life as a mental health volunteer at Georgia Mental Health Institute and is not that concerned with cancer or fairness. Barbara said that she was really open with her family about cancer. She has metastatic breast cancer and still has *the breast* (notice "the breast" not "my breast"). Sally is a widow and is lonely. Louise remained quiet throughout. I must keep in my mind that many statements made could be sophisticated defenses.

The group decided to meet at 12.30 P.M. instead of 1:30 P.M. the next time so that Amanda wouldn't miss a group due to physical therapy. They're all so interested in having each other's names, addresses and telephone numbers. They are also keeping their journals; however, there is one mechanical problem: The damn tape recorder ate one of my tapes. If there is anything mechanical within 5 feet of me it will eventually destroy itself or generally screw up. God has endowed me with an ineffable streak of mixed luck with machines. I'll save $2 on labor doing it myself and spend $60 on the part I broke fixing the other broken part. However, He has also endowed me with an awareness of this limitation. I had two tape recorders going and only missed a few minutes of the group.

SESSION 2: EXPLORATION

Session 2 also was exemplary of the exploratory phase of group development. Early in this session some avoidance was apparent. Attention was given to developing trust and rapport. The members seemed to be concerned with more discussions of the treatment as opposed to emotional effects of the treatment. This seemed to reinforce an hypothesis of avoidance: avoidance that did not seem unusual considering the group's developmental stage. Jane and Carol seemed to have ease with self-disclosure. However, as in any other group, subjects of self-disclosure were subjects with which Jane and Carol had felt comfortable and had apparently discussed in other similar situations. Toward the latter third of the session, there seemed to be transition toward action.

As the session unfolded, various members verbalized feelings of hope and manifested denial (coping) in their reactions to changes in medications. There was optimism regarding the beneficial potential of the new drugs they were trying. There was some verbalization of suicidal ideation by Diana and an avoidance of addressing the problems that Jane shared regarding her relationship with her son. The dynamic was one of offering advice to Jane about managing her relationship with her son as opposed to trying to help her clarify her feelings and solve the problems for herself. Support by other members for one another was very apparent and it was a dynamic throughout the entire course of the group that, in and of itself, was enough reason to justify such groups in outpatient settings in oncology/hematology clinics.

Techniques

Following the review of the previous session, humor was used to try to relieve some of the tension and anxiety in both the therapist and the group. For instance, in a discussion about urine collection, some of the following comments were made by the therapist.

Steve: Are you girls ready for this? Now you're going to have to pay close attention to this. That's a real "pisser" [laughter].

* * *

Jane: I said, "Why do you want this special stuff of mine?"
Steve: They are probably selling it on the black market.

* * *

Steve: You ought to collect a vial and frame it.

During a particular segment when Jane was self-disclosing

regarding her problems with her son, in an unconscious move to avoid addressing the conflict, Amanda tried to distract Jane into discussing her symptoms as well as Jane's feelings about being a guinea pig for experimental chemotherapy. At that point, as a therapist, it was important for me to structure the group and bring into their awareness the importance of sharing affect in dealing with the personal problems in their lives that were being compounded by cancer.

Steve: There's a lot of stuff going on here and you're really sharing a lot of things, but I think we all may be missing some subtle points . . . some things that aren't being said. And that's what I'd like to point out right now. I heard Jane say a number of things. Her son's driving her up the wall, and Carol's sharing the same thing. Especially right now it's a very pressing thing for you [to Carol].

The structuring had to be repeated a number of times throughout the sessions. One of the characteristics apparent in this group was extreme difficulty with conflict and affect, particularly during the early sessions. As the group progressed, structuring and facilitation continued. Summary, interpretation, and reflection were all utilized. In the middle of this session a small example of transition toward the action phase of the group became apparent as evidenced by the following confrontation and subsequent avoidance.

At this point, the group had been discussing the purpose of life and the reality of cancer. The reality of living a normal middle-class existence with a so-called idyllic death doesn't seem possible. The therapist confronted Jane and Carol. Louise offered a "pat" solution in an apparent attempt to avoid the particular reality that cancer patients must face. The technique to be observed is the facilitating nature of the confrontation by the therapist.

Steve: Yeah, and the reality is it doesn't seem to be possible. But what Jane is saying and what I hear Carol saying is "So what? OK, maybe the reality is it isn't possible. What can we do about it? What can we do to make the best of the situation?" And what you [Jane] are saying is that "yeah, if I let the emotional stuff get to me that's going to get me before the disease." That'll drive you up the wall. And I'm hearing some of that from you [Jane] even though you're not really saying it.

Louise: I think Diana should live each day. That's what I'm trying to do to the best. Let tomorrow take care of itself. Get through today. Enjoy your children; enjoy your husband.

The session proceeded along these lines with very low-level (psychologically speaking) verbalization regarding suffering, depression, and anger. As the session ended, Louise offered indirect positive feedback about the nature of the group by sharing efforts to continue attendance following discharge from the hospital. It was interesting that none of the group members would acknowledge that they were in group *therapy*. Rather, they were participating in group *discussions*. Of course, a facilitative group discussion should be therapeutic, and perhaps it is an issue of semantics. On the other hand, it could be an issue of avoidance and an attempt to deny that persons suffering with the emotional impact of cancer need professional help.

Louise: After I leave the hospital, which I guess I'll be here a couple of more weeks, I feel sure. . . . Now I have a friend who has a mastectomy, and I have talked with her about coming with me. I know my husband is not going to want me to drive or come by myself, and I don't see no need for him to come and hang around somewhere else. And I have talked with her and she said she felt she would enjoy coming with me. Would that be all right if she came here and sat in on the meetings? I need to know.

Steve: How does the group feel?

Jane: It's all right with me.

Steve: The only reservation I have is, and it's a selfish one. . . .It's in terms of my studies . . . in terms of biasing the results. And if we. . . .

Carol: Well, if she can drive Louise, just let her come in and. . . .

Amanda: . . . Just sit.

Steve: OK, but just let me share this with you. Barbara sat with us today and she was for the most part quiet, but don't you believe for a minute that she wasn't involved in everything that was going on and that's the thing.

Notice how one of the group members deals with the possibility of having an observer present who would be providing transportation for another member, Louise, once she was discharged from the hospital. While none of the group members had the sophistication to appreciate the intricacies of biasing research, Carol's primary concern was for Louise being able to continue as a member of the group regardless of whether or not another member would have to be present in the group: a member who would be more or less an observer since that person was not being treated for metastatic disease. It is as if to say that "our needs are more important than your need to have unbiased results." Such an assertion was taken as a sign of rapport between myself and Carol as she had the courage, at least at an unconscious level, to confront me with the group's needs as being above the therapist's needs.

Sociometry

In Figure 6-3, the seating arrangement for session 2 is illustrated. In comparision with session 1, Diana and Carol had moved closer. Amanda and Jane were together. Sally moved over to the sofa. I, Barbara, and Louise were sitting in individual seats. Not much in the way of significance should be made of the seating, at least at this stage.

Figure 6-4 is an illustration of the communication patterns between therapist and group members during session 2. Note that the communication was not two-way as it was in the first session in which group members were looking for direction. In an effort to avoid addressing thorny issues, the communication patterns were more of persons talking through me to one another, as well as not responding directly to the open-ended statements by the therapist with appropriate interactions. This type of one-way communication is represented by two parallel lines with arrows indicating the primary direction of communication. Notice that Sally, Barbara, and Louise offered only random comments throughout the session. This is represented by broken lines with no directional thrust indicated.

In Figure 6-5, one will notice that the primary focus of the interaction during this session was Jane. She shared much information about her problem to the whole group. Pointed comments were directed from Jane toward Carol, Amanda, and

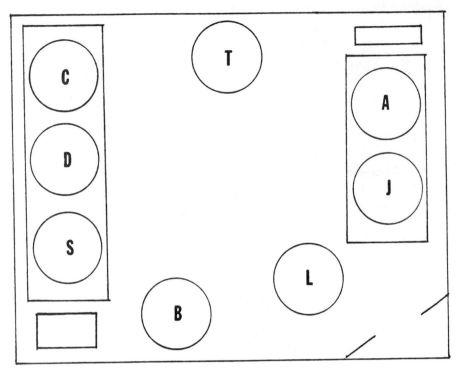

Figure 6-3. Session 2: Seating

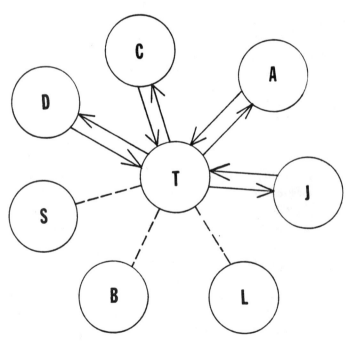

Figure 6-4. Session 2: Primary patterns of communication between members and therapist.

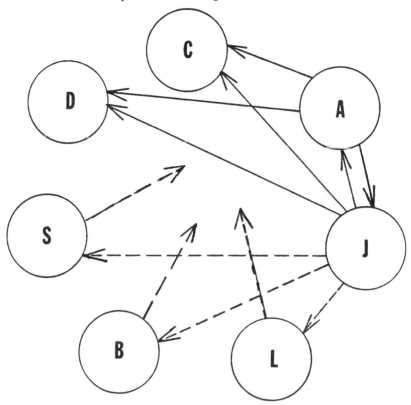

Figure 6-5. Session 2: Primary patterns of communication between members.

Diana, respectively. Generalizations and random comments about her plight were directed at other members of the group as evidenced by the broken lines. As stated, Sally, Barbara, and Louise offered random comments not directed at anyone in particular. Again, the emphasis is on the fact that at this point in the development of the group, members were talking *at* each other as opposed to communicating *with* one another.

Journal

Our session today was nothing short of tremendous. Everyone showed up even though Louise and Jane were late. Jane might have had a few drinks prior to coming to the group, but I'm not sure. She seemed somewhat relaxed but sober. The group was very verbal, and I expect that some of the action dimensions will be slower in therapeutic emergence because each member seems to be venting and each one wants to talk. We discussed chemotherapy, widowhood, children, death, suicide, life expectancy, day-to-day living, and the future and past. There was more personal sharing than last session, but it was at a cognitive level and not a deep feeling level. However, it moved quite well. Frankly, I expected more problems in facilitating interaction due to resistance and denial, especially in light of the literature. But with my ladies, I can hardly get a word in edgewise and find myself raising my voice to be heard. I'm trying to make it a therapeutic group versus a discussion group. Loneliness and depression seem to be the main concern, not the cancer per se. Some of the members felt loneliness, and other emotional problems were worse than the cancer.

The women seem to love the group. Cohesion was evidenced by touching and by the members contacting each other by telephone between sessions. Also, Cindy said that a few persons I had previously interviewed had wished that they had joined the group. One woman goes to a "Christian" psychiatrist. Doctor Norris seems pleased with my work.

Chapter 7

TRANSITION: TRUSTING AND DISCLOSING

SESSION 3: TRANSITION PHASE

S ESSION 3 was one of transition. It was an important and significant session in that more emphasis was given to the here-and-now dimension of the group as opposed to the previously, safe discussion involving the dynamics of treatment. Feelings about the therapist were expressed by Amanda early in the session. Of course as therapist, one has the choice of accepting that feedback or viewing it as part of the resistance in terms of therapeutic dynamics. That is to say, many persons will offer good feedback early in the process of therapy as an ingratiating (seductive) gesture of submission in order to protect themselves from penetration of their ego defense system by the therapist.

Amanda: Yes, but I think he has that kind of personality. He's attracted to it. I hope Steve will forgive me. Psychology and psychiatry in my view attracts two kinds of people: one, really very warm, outgoing, caring kinds of people, and others are just nutty as fruitcakes. It's the position of a "heal thyself" proposition. We'll leave you in the first category for the time being.

Another indication that the group was in transition was suggested by Jane's confrontation occurring briefly after Amanda's previous verbalization regarding the therapist's expectation.

Jane: I'm a little confused. This is the question I wanted to ask. You said before that you were concerned about my feelings of depression and somebody else is concerned about their children, etc., etc. I thought that our feelings were supposed to concern themselves with our reaction to cancer and chemotherapy. Now how does the other relate to this? Because I would

249

	have the other problems . . . my inability to cope, whether I had cancer or whether I didn't have cancer.
Steve:	OK, I agree with that. But I'm not sure what you are asking. Are you asking. . . ?
Jane:	What I'm asking is, how does my inability to handle my situation with my son relate to what we are supposed to be doing here?
Steve:	You see, I'm not sure if you are saying there's no relationship between you and your son. The way I see it, that's all a part of your life space.

Transition was further exemplified in the session by persistent attempts to redirect the focus of the group from *out there* to *in here.* Techniques of clarification, facilitation, and low-level confrontation by the therapist were similar bench marks of movement from exploration toward action; movement typical of the transition stage. In the following exemplary excerpt Amanda was sharing her resistance to the expression of affect in the group. One will notice the subtle confrontation by the therapist of Amanda's reluctance to express affect; one will also notice that in her assertion she was not willing to express affect; Amanda's cynicism, satirical vocalizations, and anger were evident in the context of the expression of the resistance.

Amanda:	You see, Steve, that's where I disagree with you. It is impossible, in my view, for me to separate your cognitive attitude and abilities from your feelings. I simply cannot be governed by feelings! I think that's undisciplined, and I think it leads to nothing but chaos!
Steve:	We'll talk a little bit more about the force. I mean. . . .
Amanda:	What do you mean? You say I may be misinterpreting what Steve is saying, but it seems to me that you are emphasizing very strongly, almost exclusively, what we are to do here is to discuss how we feel. Well, I think feelings need to be controlled. And of course I might wind up in a mental institution because I control them too much, but that's the way I feel about it! Perhaps I am misinterpreting. And I'm willing to be corrected. But do I detect an attitude on

your part? Unless we just get burst into tears or something of that sort, then we are not expressing our feelings!

Steve: Do you feel like bursting into tears right now?

Amanda: Heavens to Betsy, no!

Steve: *Are* you expressing some feeling now?

Amanda: Yes, I'm expressing. . . . Well, true, I'm expressing some feelings, some reactions to what I think you are saying.

Steve: OK. And what I'm hearing is a little . . . not really anger, just frustration in trying to clarify what you think I am saying.

Amanda: It's just a difference in attitudes and opinions. And I think you are basically an emotional person, perhaps, and I'm not! And somehow we have got to get a balance in here.

Steve: So when you hear me talking about feelings, you think I'm talking about just people who come out and break down and cry about all the problems they are having. Is that how you are picking it up?

Amanda: The way I'm picking it up is that my impression is you feel that people should be governed by their feelings without reference to anything else. And I cannot agree with that.

Steve: I guess the response I would have to that would be that I think you have part of what I am saying. I think we are governed by our feelings, and I think one way. . . . For instance, in your case that you've chosen to compensate for that . . . is rather than to be governed by your feelings . . . is to control those feelings to the point where you feel comfortable in your interactions. Because you shared that you do believe in a cognitive control of feelings. And I think, what I am hearing, is that that's the way you have chosen to adjust to. . . .

Amanda: Not just to this!

Steve: No, right, but in the real world. . . .

Amanda: I think you should make allowances for people who operate that way.

Steve: OK. Now let me see if I am hearing you correctly. Are you saying that you are feeling some pressure that I might not be making allowances for you to feel the way you want to feel?

Amanda: I think I may disappoint you. Because I just simply am not going to overflow with tears.

Steve: So now you are saying that I might be expecting you . . . everyone in the group . . . to overflow with feelings. And I might be disappointed because you won't perform.

Amanda: Yes! That's exactly what I think!

Steve: OK. Well, can you talk a little bit more about the frustration that I'm feeling or that you are feeling or that we are both feeling. . . . Is it possible we are missing each other because of *your* expectations? Because you don't feel you can meet my expectations. You know I get the feeling that you might feel that you are letting me down a little.

Amanda: What would we do without that word *feeling*?

Steve: We wouldn't be anywhere.

Amanda: We'd be absolutely paralyzed.

The reader will notice that there seemed to be a playful banter between Amanda and me. Such banter was evidence of the transference occurring between therapist and "patient." More significantly, such banter clearly facilitated the establishment of rapport and trust. It is a dynamic as well as a technique that has been found to be very useful in facilitating any group's movement to action. Such banter tends to humanize the therapist and develop a family dynamic within the group; a dynamic vital to cohesiveness and progress.

Immediately following the previously excerpted interaction, the therapist confronted Amanda regarding her feelings in the here-and-now. Such a confrontation was seen to be very vital during the transition stage of the group, especially in the existential theoretical model. In the existential model of group psychotherapy, the emphasis is on what is happening in the session at any given point in time regarding any member's life space. Ideally, generalizations of self-awareness into everyday life and relationships produces healthier life-styles. Notice Amanda's assertion that she was perfectly relaxed following a rather lengthy interaction in an early session with the therapist. Also, notice that she immediately took the focus off of herself and attempted to manipulate the situation to focus on the therapist/researcher's needs as opposed to the importance of her own therapeutic experience.

Steve: Let me ask you this question. How do you feel right now?

Amanda: I'm perfectly relaxed. I'm afraid you may wind up. . . . Well, let me say this. If the object of this study is to get the people in this group really to literally bear their souls, then you may be disappointed.

Rather than confront Amanda's denial and resistance, the technique of choice was to interject a little humor and sarcasm in a subtle attempt to call into the group's awareness the dynamic occurring.

Steve: OK, the object of this study, to clear it up for you, is for me to graduate [laughter].

Throughout this particular session the group seemed to continue checking out their ability to trust the therapist balanced against their need for acceptance by the therapist. They looked for clarification of the ground rules and for safety in the ability to express feelings. Subsequently, as these dynamics unfolded, there was more significant self-disclosure. Members discussed loneliness and purpose in life as well as family. Other themes of major importance were also discussed. Toward the last quarter of the group session, there was more action. As often occurs toward the end, there was a winding down of the intensity of the group and more discussion about the mundane issues connected with every day life. Significantly, positive feedback was given at the close of the session.

Carol: Well, last week, Steve, Diana, and I were talking to Cindy, and we were. . . . Diana and I were telling Cindy how interesting this was, and we recommend it for every hospital to go through this. And she said when our group is finished, we all should write a letter to Doctor Norris and tell him what we got out of

it and whether or not we feel this should continue
on, you know, with other people.

Amanda: Well, I was probably the most skeptical one of all because. . . .

Steve: Yes, you were.

Amanda: Well, I admit it! As I told Doctor Norris, I said,
"When you spend twenty years hearing people recommend counseling when the faucets leak, you just
kind of get a bad feeling about it."

Steve: No, I recommend a plumber when the faucet leaks.
Counseling when you get your bill.

Carol: . . . But if I found this thing too depressing, I wasn't
going to come anymore. But I thoroughly enjoy it.

Amanda: Well, I think we all. . . .

Jane: I was very enthusiastic about it.

Diana: How do you feel now?

Amanda: Well, the way I feel now, there have been some very
interesting sessions. I like to talk for one thing. I can
see a real danger, though unless it's a carefully
screened group, which they admitted. They took
great caution, although I think Steve would have
taken somebody in off the street just to get the right
number [laughter].

Notice the therapist's persistent use of humor in otherwise confrontive and possibly antagonistic situations generated by a
member's verbalizations. The therapist also shared some of his own
anxieties about this particular group through the use of humor. It
was a way to maintain a certain degree of distance so as not to become a part of the problem by entering into a combative style of interaction with other group members.

Techniques

Following a rather lengthy interlude (also cited earlier) regarding
expectations in the group, one technique used by the therapist was
role clarification.

Amanda: What you really need is to pick up a two-by-four and
let go with it.

Steve: Well, I don't know if I'm going to endorse that kind of thing. But what I'm saying . . . I guess where I am with the group right now. . . . I'm going to take a little more of an active role this week. This is our third official session as a group, now since we started meeting with Sally, Barbara, and Louise joining us.

It is not clear whether the long interchanges between verbalizations by the therapist and patient are positive or negative. As the sessions began to unfold and move into the action phase, therapist interaction and instruction became less lengthy and more poignant.

It was necessary to redirect and clarify regarding group expectations versus therapist expectations on numerous occasions. An example of such redirection and clarification can be seen in the following excerpt.

Steve: This is our third session and what we've done to this point; we have been talking and trying to give each other support and advice and build some cohesiveness in the group. And Diana was asking, "Well, how is this going to be different from a discussion group?"

Carol: This is our fourth session isn't it?

Steve: Well, we are calling it our third therapy session because the first session, we only had four people. So for some of you, I guess it is a fourth session, but for the group that we have now, it's our third. And I was trying to talk about the difference between talking about our concerns up here [pointing to head], you know, at a cognitive level and talking about our concerns at a gut level. And we should try to help each other with how we feel. Where we are headed now is to talk a little more about the feelings. And I was trying to answer Jane's question about, "What does my problem, my depression, and loneliness, and problems with my son have to do with my cancer and chemotherapy?" And I was trying to remember one of our earlier sessions where we talked about the fact about how resentful you all get when the doctors just treat you as a body and as a subject and that you'd like to have the whole person treated.

Well, that's the way I am about the mind. You can't
separate just. . . . We can't. . . . You know, if Jane
brought up a problem about her son, we said, "Jane,
what does that have to do with your feelings about
chemotherapy?" Well, probably nothing directly.
But yet you all know that there's nothing that goes on
in your life space that doesn't affect you. And I try to
provide. . . . We are building a kind of a caring atmosphere where I'm treated as just another member
of the group. And you are all calling each other from
time to time during the week, and so we are building
a unit here. And that's what we have to try to do
more of. And so I guess I'll take an increasing role in
trying to help you verbalize your feelings and we'll
see how it goes in that way. So if I cut you off at any
time or say something and try to get you to make a
statement in a feeling kind of sense, I'm not correct-
ing you as a teacher; I'm trying to facilitate as a
therapist.

Later in the session there seemed to be a manifestation of
Amanda's resistance as evidenced by the verbalization of motherly
feelings toward the therapist. Rather than confront Amanda with
her resistance, the therapist chose to utilize the opportunity to
facilitate cohesive bonding with Amanda in order to develop feelings
of trust and security.

Amanda: This is a question of semantics. You use the word
feelings very freely. You use the words *caring* and
love very freely. I don't! And that's the basic
difference between us. But maybe we both have the
same attitudes, but we just give them different labels.

Steve: You seem to be very sensitive to me . . . like right
now . . . because you are worried about how I might
be feeling. Are you wondering if you might be a
source of my anxiety? I used the word feeling again.
But I'm just trying to clarify. . . .

Carol: Maybe it's a motherly feeling?

Steve: OK! That's a feeling. A motherly feeling is a feeling.

Amanda: You see that's what I'm talking about. I think it's truly a question of semantics. When I say feelings . . . I mean when I hear you say feelings, I think you mean some deep emotional thing that's way buried deep and nobody's going to be happy until it comes out.

Steve: Well, that might be the case, but it doesn't have to be.

Amanda: Doesn't have to be? But you see I think, that's it!

Steve: Can I ask you something? What kinds of feelings go along with feeling motherly toward me?

Carol: You *are* old enough to be his mother.

Amanda: I think you are working very hard to graduate, and I want you to graduate, and I want you to get an *A +* !

Steve: So, you are kind of proud of me, in a sense.

Amanda: We all have a vested interest in you.

Steve: You have a vested interest in me. You all have "shares" in me, in a sense. Right? So there's a caring.

Sally: We want a big dividend!

Steve: A big dividend, right? So you are saying you are kind of proud.

Jane and Amanda began to engage in a rather direct confrontation regarding the group norm and the idea of expressing feelings. Notice the technique involved in *facilitating* the discussion *between* Jane and Amanda as opposed to *directing* a discussion between Jane and Amanda *through* the therapist.

Jane: You know what's confusing me is you have a certain idea in your mind. . . .

Steve: Who are you talking to? 'Cause you are pointing at the wall.

Jane: I'm sorry. I'm talking to Amanda and I'm looking you straight in the eye. I'm saying that you feel you can discipline your feelings, that you can control how you feel. How do you know where to separate this? How do you know what consists of your feelings? And how do you know you're controlling this? And how much of this is an honest expression?

Steve: What are you trying to say? Wait a second. What are you trying to say about yourself to Amanda?

Jane: Well, actually, I'm trying to say to Amanda that many times I will say things which I think the public or a person wants me to say and will present a certain image of me which I think is desirable. But it isn't the way I really feel. I could be very polite and all that and think to myself, "I wish you'd go to hell!"

Amanda: We've all done a lot of that.

Jane: And so I want to know where I'm being honest with myself, where I am trying to present an image, or where I'm really feeling a certain way and would like to say, "I wish you'd go to hell!"

Steve: So, are you saying, you would like some of the members of the group to help you to identify when you are really being up front versus when you are camouflaging?

Jane: Yeah! I would like to be able to say, "I'm not being fought about how I feel." I really feel a certain way, but I'm not presenting it honestly because I don't think it would be popular. I don't think it would place me in the best light with people. And that's what I wondered where we separate. Is it really a discipline? Are we really disciplining ourselves or are we trying to create a certain impression which shows strength?

Amanda: Don't you feel the way one can express themselves varies with the situation?

Jane: Yes!

Steve: Are you saying that for anyone or are you talking for Amanda?

Amanda: I'm just trying to be correct, Steve. I feel it depends entirely on the situation. There are some. . . . In all the years that I was an administrator, there's been many times that I just wanted to say, "Just get out of my office and stay out!" But I had to keep in mind what I was after — my goal. And if it involved placating someone, OK. I just gritted my teeth and placated them. Because what I was trying to achieve was more important than venting my feelings.

Jane: Yes, there was a difference. There were feelings.

Amanda: Oh, sure! They were there. But the point I'm trying to make with Steve. . . . There are times when they are inappropriate.

Jane: Yes, I agree with you. But you were disciplining yourself so that you could present it.

Amanda: You're darn right!

Jane: But actually you were not expressing your feelings or else there is a distinction when you think about it. I don't say go ahead and manifest to everybody how you feel, you know, with a disrespect. I don't say that. But I think to myself I like to separate how I really feel from what I'm thinking. Maybe sometimes I have come to the conclusion that thinking a certain way will perhaps eventually change my feeling so that I will have feelings that I am actually more comfortable with. But I have to separate them.

Another important facet of the therapeutic interaction was the therapist's ability to verbalize awareness of nonverbal process. In the following passage, it was evident that the therapist had accurately observed and verbalized (interpreted) Jane's shaking voice.

Steve: You know I can't help notice that your voice is so laden with emotion right now. And I felt your hand and it was warm. And I noticed that while you were talking your hands were just kind of like this [clutching hands together over breastbone]. Like, "This is right coming from my heart."

Jane: It is! It is! It's the way I feel!

As with any other group, the therapist maintains a repertoire of techniques to be utilized in building group trust and cohesiveness as well as developing acceptance by the group members of the therapist as a human being. One such technique is self-disclosure as exemplified in the following passage.

Steve: I can speak for myself. If I'm really angry with somebody, I don't want to tell them to go to hell, and yet I might be feeling that inside. I guess on the other hand, there have been times when it has been really important for me to tell somebody how I felt, and I blew the chance where I could have really helped them; where I could have really helped myself by just saying, "Hey! I don't need this aggravation!" You

	know, "This is how I feel!"
Carol:	I never get so aggravated that I tell someone to go to hell!

Notice Carol's strong verbalization following the therapist's self-disclosure. If there was ever any doubt in a professional's mind of the positive effects of self-disclosure in helping to bring out other members, this distinct excerpt should satisfy that doubt and illustrate the power of the use of appropriate self-disclosure in facilitating group process and the intensity of the therapeutic experience for group members.

In the following, rather lengthy passage, one can see the beginning of confrontation of group resistance to the expression of feelings by the therapist. Diana kept quiet during the entire interaction until the very end where her sarcasm and anger became very apparent. It was the intense discussion and confrontation of that affect that prompted the spontaneous and telling remarks by Diana.

Amanda:	Yes, well, I'll try. I'll have to go back to my work experience. I've had people come charging into my office just mad as wet hens, and if I cannot get involved emotionally but maintain my objectivity, I can handle the situation every single time. And that's the whole object of being an administrator. You've got to keep things going. Now, if I react on a feeling basis, then we are just going to wind up in a knock-down drag-out and we won't accomplish a thing.
Steve:	What I'm starting to hear you say is that the expression of feelings or control of feelings is an all or nothing proposition. And I've heard you talk about the two extremes like, "Hmmmm, I can't do this."; where you are saying, "I must. The show must go on . . . This is going to go on," you know, "We are going to get through this." And on the other hand you are saying that if you really express your feelings, you'll be pounding the table and jumping up and down.
Amanda:	Yes. See that's what I think!
Steve:	Is there a middle ground where you could still express your feelings? And I'm asking the whole

group. . . . Have you been in situations where there is middle ground? Where you could still tell somebody how you feel and not necessarily hurt them and feel like you've expressed your own feelings in such a way as to get them out?

Amanda: And you see that's what I call maintaining rational control of your feelings. You have them. You don't deny that you have them, but you don't let feelings control.

Steve: What is rational control? I don't understand that term.

Amanda: Well, just doing. . . . You think you just want to throw something at them. That's how you feel. But your head tells you this is not the way to handle the situation.

Steve: Do you ever feel. . . . Have you ever felt like that type of a rational kind of control has taken itself out somewhere else on your person? In your mind or your body?

Amanda: Maybe! I just know I always thought I wish I could slam a plate against that wall! But I'd have to clean it up!

Carol: I have never been in Amanda's situation. I have never been in charge of an office. The only thing I'm in charge of is being a mother and a housewife. So I have never gone through all that you have. I work for someone else, and I live by his rules, and when I leave the office, I live by somebody else's rules.

Amanda: That's the end of it!

Steve: Sally, you were starting to say that you've been in that situation.

Sally: I say I understand what she is talking about.

Steve: Can you talk about it a little?

Sally: Well, I worked in the courts for thirty-one years. I was an executive secretary for the judge. And in that capacity, well, he ran the office. He did the framework. I mean he sat in there and listened to the cases, but you did all the rest of it. All the details and this and that. And you fought to keep all the people out of it who were not supposed to be in there. You had to decide who was to get in there. Really! I mean, whether it was legitimate or not. You'd be surprised in a judge's office what you'd have to come in contact with all the time. But you've always got to keep one thing in mind, you know. You are paid by the taxpayers. And if you don't remember anything and you can't do anything else, you've got to place that smile on your face and be just as nice as you can.

Steve: I can't help feeling the resentment in having to play that kind of a role. I heard it from Amanda too. When you are in that kind of a role, "This is a reality and I know it up here" [pointing to head], but there's a little resentment.

Sally: You can get just as mad as hornets, and you just go around and around and carry on. But you couldn't get angry. You couldn't say to them get out, blah, blah, blah. You have to sit back.

Amanda: Well, maybe we are! I'm speaking for myself. Maybe I'm simply overreacting to a misinterpretation of what Steve means by feelings. Obviously, you don't mean an either/or proposition, but that's apparently the way I had interpreted it.

Steve: What I want to help you all to do is to be in touch that first of all, you do have feelings. And secondly, be in touch with what those feelings are and maybe learn ways to help each other. Learn to express these in constructive ways; in productive ways; helpful ways.

Amanda: I don't like cold-blooded people. I'm scared of them, people who are unable to feel. I just don't know what to do with them, but also I don't know what to do with people who have no control over them.

Steve: Has there ever been a time in your life where you wished you knew how somebody else felt about you?

Amanda: Well, I have to. . . .

Steve: Have there been times in your lives? I guess, and I'm asking the whole group; I'm not just talking to

	Amanda. . . . I feel like she's getting a lot of pressure today.
Amanda:	I'm not getting a lot of pressure.
Steve:	But have there been times when you wish that you could hear how someone felt about you? I mean to really know that they care or if they hate you, or whatever it is. I mean to just know because it's important.
Amanda:	Steve, I think that depends so much on your family situation, on how secure you feel, and that kind of thing. I remember a friend telling me one time, "When you meet somebody, do you ever think they don't like you?" I said, "Well, it never occurs to me that they don't think I'm the cutest thing around." So that goes back so far. And you don't even know how it occurs or how it developed that you felt totally secure. I hope people think well of me, but if they don't, well, I'm sorry.
Steve:	But I guess I felt like you kind of sidestepped my question a little bit. What I was really asking you personally . . . and anyone else in the group to share. . . . This is a time for sharing. . . . Have you been in a situation where you really . . . somebody important to you . . . maybe somebody you really cared about . . . it was important to you to know that friend maybe . . . or that you would really like to know, "How do you feel about me? What are your feelings when you are around me? How do you feel about life in general?"
Sally:	I'm afraid I'm not that analytical.
Carol:	Well, I can sense when someone likes me, or whether they like me a whole lot or whether they don't care to be. . . .
Steve:	Would you like to hear them say that? Or would you like to be able to say that to them?
Carol:	No, I can see it. I can feel it.
Steve:	So, what you are saying is that it is not important to you to have them verbalize . . . like to say, "I love you," "I hate you," or "I'd like to know you better," or

something like that.

Carol: Well, those that I'm very close to, even women, tell me many times when I'm in the office that "I love you." And when they say, "I love you," like when one woman tells it to another woman, it doesn't necessarily mean that we are both lesbians. But we just have this feeling that we care about one another.

Amanda: Nowadays you can't even express honest affection without getting a label.

Carol: There are some people when you first meet them you love them right away and you feel as though you've known them for a long time. And that's how I feel about Diana. The first day I met her I thought, "Well, I really care for her," and I feel as though I've known her for a long time. And not just four sessions. And would it make you smile if I told you I felt the same way about you?

Steve: Well, of course it would. But that's not what. . . . I'm not fishing for anything like that. But yes, it does make me feel good.

Carol: And then there are some that it takes me awhile to care for them. And then there are very very few that I don't ever care about.

Steve: How are you feeling right now?

Carol: Well, I feel better today than I did yesterday, but I'm still kind of weak.

Steve: OK. That's physical. But how do you feel right now as you are sharing this with us. You know, "I am glad. . . ."

Carol: My heart is bubbling with happiness.

Steve: It's a feeling of joy that you are experiencing.

Carol: Right.

Diana: And I'm thinking, "How does this make any difference?" This seems so irrelevant to me. Big deal who likes you and who doesn't like you. We're in a life and death situation, gang! Don't you see? What difference does it make? I don't care!

The movement from exploration toward action is more apparent in the interaction between Jane and the therapist later in the session. After Jane had gone on at some length about her loneliness and the fact that people didn't seem to seek her out and develop relationships with her, the therapist confronted her. The accuracy of the confrontation was indicated by Jane's immediate verbalization. The awareness brought to light by the confrontation was translated into insights regarding her relationships with others.

Steve: I wonder if it's possible because you don't expect it. I don't know if that's the case. Could it be that you might be *pushing* it away?

Jane: It could be. It could be the fact that I'm so unaccustomed to it and it's such a strange feeling for me, it's hard for me to grab so that I cannot very closely and intimately respond. I feel it, but I feel strange about it.

Later in the session, following a rather intense confrontation of Jane's loneliness, the therapist facilitated a group discussion of alternative ways for Jane to solve her problems. Again, this suggests a significant point in the transition where the focus turned from oneself to someone else in terms of concerns. It illustrates the constant development of cohesion and involvement between these members: a process so vital to the evolution and effectiveness of this type of group.

Steve: You can't see a way that you could interact any differently with those you care about than you are. Is that *your* problem or is it *their* problem? Because we were just talking about Jane pushing people away. It's as much her pushing them away as it is them pushing her away, and you all kind of shook your heads at that up and down. I guess I'm saying, whose problem is it? Is it yours?

Carol: Well, yes! I can see it in Jane's problem but I don't see it in me.

Steve: Isn't that always the way it is?

Carol: I don't push people away; they gather; they come to me. Yesterday . . . not yesterday, but the day before yesterday . . . I went to work for the first time after two weeks and the whole office stopped to welcome me back home. And I got several gifts when I went back to work, which I don't expect. But I know they are happy that I am well again and back to work. And I don't like it when they give me gifts because I know it costs them money to buy.

Amanda: Yet, you appreciate the expression.

Carol: Right! I appreciate it and I know that they care for me.

Steve: And are you able to communicate that back to them that you care?

Carol: Oh, yes!

Steve: And I think . . . I'm not sure, but I think Carol might have some of the secrets to the question you are asking, Diana.

Diana: But you know people do come to me. People just love to pour their problems out to me.

Amanda: See, that's just the penalty you pay for being a strong person, but you can't deny it.

Diana: · But I guess I don't have any. . . . You know, I can't show weakness. I can't. People come to me.

Steve: It's not that you are so strong as it is that you feel that any show of a crack in that strength is a weakness. Does any one in the group agree with that?

Diana: I mean, the people who come to me with their problems, they don't really have problems. They don't know what a problem is.

Steve: But you would like to tell them that sometime.

Amanda: But Diana, the fact that they come. . . .

Diana: Well, it's the worst thing that's ever happened to them, yes. But you *know* it's not!

Amanda: It can't compare to what's happened to you. But the fact that they come at all shows how receptive you are to relationships with people.

Carol: Diana, my problem's bigger than yours. I lost my husband, and then on top of all that, I get cancer. You still have your husband and you still have your children. So I feel that my problem is bigger than yours.

Steve: Wait! Wait! I'm lost! What are you trying to say to her?

Carol: Well, she's saying that people are always coming to her with problems and their problems are not as big as hers. And she's saying that no one has any problems bigger than Diana. And I'm saying that in my situation, my problem is bigger than hers. But I don't let it bother me to accept people and . . . .

Steve: You know what I found for me? That my problems always look worse than yours.

Amanda: Diana, I truly feel that it's a testimony to the warmth of your personality that people come to you. They don't expect you to solve it for them, but they feel like you are listening.

Carol: That you are listening. Right!

Group cohesiveness was further suggested by the following excerpt. Notice that Jane attempted to support Diana.

Diana: I feel like I'm coming across as a very weak . . . .

Jane: No, I think there is something very warm and very compassionate about Diana. That's why it was very easy for me to talk to her. And the strange part . . . . Even though I revealed the fact that I did have this need when I was ill for somebody to talk to me, nevertheless, the impression that I give is one of self-sufficiency. People will say, "Oh! She doesn't need any help. She's so self-sufficient."

Steve: But isn't that responding to their expectations? Isn't that what people expect you to be so you respond to it?

Jane: Yeah, and I could be dying. I don't know how to cope with that situation.

Steve: So who are you being fair to? I guess the question I'm asking all of you . . . , "Who am I being fair to when I get into that kind of a *strong* world?" Because the expectation in our society is to be "strong," and I'll put that in quotes because I don't agree with that definition; to be strong in the face of adversity. I'm not advocating coming apart and coming unglued and just falling apart.

Sally: Sometimes I wish I could have that opportunity.

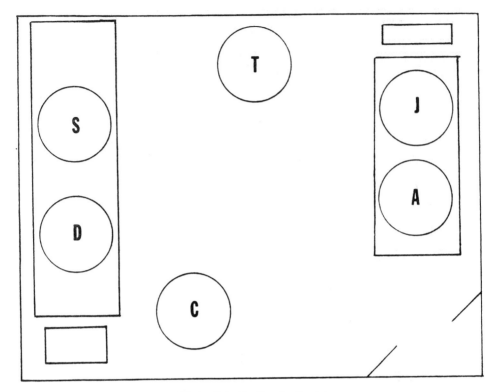

Figure 7-1. Session 3: Seating

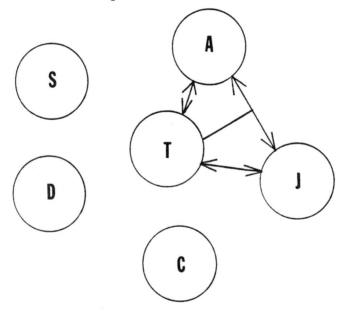

Figure 7-2. Session 3: Primary patterns of communication between two members (Amanda and Jane) and the members and therapist.

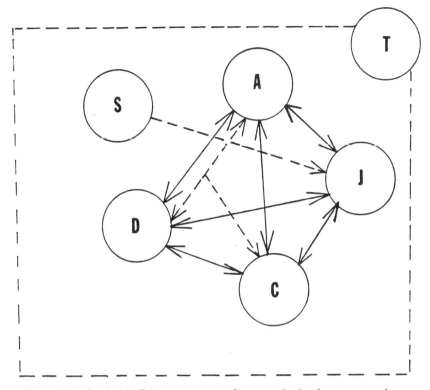

Figure 7-3. Session 3: Primary patterns of communication between members

Sociometry

The evolution of communication in this session went from mono-
logue to soliloquy to person-to-person, two-way communication.
Figure 7-1 indicates the seating arrangement for session 3. Figure
7-2 illustrates the primary mode of communication early in the session as one of two-way communication between Amanda and the
therapist, Jane and the therapist, and Amanda and Jane. One will
see that the line intersecting the two-way communication symbol
[between Jane and Amanda] represents facilitation of their interaction by the therapist. In Figure 7-3, it can be seen that the communication patterns during session 3 became less random and more
two-way in nature. This dynamic was particularly true in the cases
of Diana, Amanda, Carol, and Jane. At this point in the development of the group, Sally made random verbalizations of support for

different members without becoming part of the direct communication/interaction patterns. Therapeutic presence envelopes the group and became more significant as the group progressed toward action. Verbalizations other than significant facilitation of communication decreased. The group members became their own facilitators. The therapeutic process had begun.

Journal

Session 3 begins today! Louise is very sick from chemotherapy and was unable to attend. Barbara's daughter couldn't stay; so Barbara had to go. Amanda, Carol, Jane, Diana, and Sally were there. Themes today centered around the relationship between disease and the real feelings involved in others. Loneliness and what to do about it was also a theme. It was interesting to hear the older members talk about their inabilities to change their personalities at this late date in their lives. I posed the question that if their bodies were changing as a result of cancer, why couldn't their attitudes about life and their relationships to others change as well? I was more active this session and this was possible because the group was becoming more cohesive. It was a good session!

We had a Christmas party afterwards and that went well too. The hospital staff is giving me great support. I wish I could say the same about Georgia; however yesterday I spent three hours defending my research (written) to the final committee (of all committees). It seems that they are concerned about the "great" psychological risk to my group members. It's really asinine since by the time they approve or disapprove of my research, my group will be almost finished. Most of the members of the committee are probably afraid of their own deaths and seem to be projecting onto my group members. Anyhow, the whole thing is absurd. I spent twelve to fifteen hours to get permission to help these people.

Chapter 8

ACTION: CONFRONTATION AND CARING

SESSION 4: ACTION PHASE

S ESSION 4 was action-oriented. Group members began to confront one another. There was cohesiveness of the group, strong affect expressed by various group members, self-disclosure at deeper levels, and the members began to confront the therapist. Modeling the therapist, the group members facilitated one another toward the expression of feelings. This was taken as a sign of progress since such facilitation was directed toward more than just problem solving. There seemed to be less dialogue about symptoms and treatment in the group and more discussion regarding members' respective personal problems. The expression of affect became more intense as the group progressed.

Session 4 commenced with the focus on Jane's birthday. There was an atmosphere of joy and warmth. There was concern for members who had the opportunity to join the group but avoided it. Along with Carol's assertion regarding commitment to the group, this dynamic coupled to suggest that some of the members of the group were seeing the process as beneficial.

Louise was very sick throughout most of the life of the group and could not attend after session 2. While she did not die during the course of the group, there was much concern voiced by all of the group members for her well-being, and, by innuendo, their own anxieties were expressed regarding the course of their cancers.

The therapist set the tone for action when he said, "I guess what I'm trying to say is that we can start to cut through some of the facade we all put on and kind of get into who you are and what it's all about."

Techniques

After Jane's party there was a brief discussion involving the group's interest in the therapist's welfare. This dynamic suggested that an excellent rapport and cohesiveness existed between the group and the therapist. There was also a deeper level of self-disclosure and good feedback to one another, as well as to the therapist.

A technique utilized in action is confrontation of what a given member is *not* saying through structuring. For instance, early in the session the therapist stopped the group interaction and tried to structure by taking time to teach the necessity of sharing feelings.

> **Steve:** Let me just stop it here. I don't think you are saying what you mean. I think it's important that the other members of the group know how you feel because I think you are asking "how-do-you" questions. Let them know where you are now and what you are feeling so they can have an idea whether or not they have ever been at a place that you are in and how they worked it through. I think that would be more helpful to the other members.

Structuring was indicated a few minutes later in the session when Jane tried to take away the anxiety created by the confronting situation. The therapist restructured the group toward focusing on Diana.

> **Steve:** Jane, I just want to interrupt here for a second because I want to keep the focus on Diana. I think there's something going on here that is very important for her to work out. And I think it's important for her to do it now. When you hear people telling you that you've got youth on your side, that you are young, and that hope is just around the corner. . . . How does that make you feel?
>
> **Diana:** Like I could throw my coffee up all over the floor.

Notice that anger was expressed by *suggestion*, and not by the actual *verbalization* of the feeling of anger. This dynamic remained a problem for all of the group members throughout this action-oriented session. Focusing on feelings and expressing those feelings directly was more threatening than showing feelings by example.

The following excerpt further exemplifies the technique of structuring to bring a group back to task. The object was to focus the group's attention on a particular aspect to make the session less chaotic and more action-oriented.

Diana: Well, it's just, you know, I get humored from Cindy and from Doctor Norris. I get humored from my husband and my parents. I get humored from my friends and all, and they pat me on the shoulder and tell me what a good girl I am and how strong I am. And I know, I told my Uncle when I was home, I was tired. . . . You know, "I'm tired of being told how gallant I am." Or I'm always told what an inspiration. . . .

Carol: I hear that all the time.

Jane: You know it would be great if they didn't talk to you at all about this.

Diana: But they do.

Jane: If she had a respite from this and didn't hear it. . . .

Steve: Well, I think that to be able to talk about these things is the purpose of the group. And I think that an example of what Diana is talking about happened when Cindy came in before the session today and opened the door and said, "You don't look fat at all. You look marvelous! You don't look like you've gained a pound!" She was really being very warm, very sincere, and friendly. And Diana instead of saying, "You know, Cindy, it makes me feel good to hear you say that, but that's not what I need right now. I need to be able to fall down and to lean once in a while." . . . Instead of saying that, she just smiled and said, "Thanks Cindy. Thanks a lot." But that's not what she wanted to say. Diana has shared with me that she's feeling some of this happening in the group too. That some of you are giving her that and meaning well. And she's sensitive enough that she doesn't want to blast anybody so to speak and just say, "Darn it, this is the one place I come where I can really just be myself and scream if I want to, and yet you are not allowing me to just let out my feelings so that I can get a handle on them." And I think, you know . . . correct me if I'm wrong . . . but I think that's what she's trying to say.

Diana: And I know you love me, I know you love me, and

it's like I love Cindy. If I hadn't had Cindy, I wouldn't
be able to make sense today.

After discussing her loss of self-control, the therapist tried to help
Diana clarify a pressure she felt in having to perform in order to satisfy others needs and expectations as opposed to being able to release
her own feelings. Clarification is another important action technique. One of the dynamics that occurred in the group was the
avoidance of dealing with intense affect that Diana was sharing at
this time.

Steve: And you get this from your husband; you get this
from your children; you get this from your family
and friends; and they mean well. And another thing
she [Diana] shared, is that she is not sure that this
happens with the rest of you all.

Barbara: Oh, it does!

Amanda: I think you are wrong about that! Excuse me, Barbara,
go ahead.

Barbara: I feel the same way. I can look in the mirror. I know
what I look like. And I'm not used to being this fat. I've
got a fat face, no hair hardly. And I'm ugly; I know
that. But you look so good; you just look so well.

Steve: But you know what I'm going to say something. I did
the same thing, didn't I? Because when I came in you
were saying about your wig, and I said. . . .

Carol: Is that a wig?

Barbara did it again. Carol then took the pressure from Diana by
focusing on some of the side effects of the chemotherapy as evidenced by her attention to Barbara's wig. It seemed so much easier
to retreat to the "safety" of symptoms.

Several members verbalized their difficulties in sharing their innermost feelings of anger with patronizing "healthier" people. The
therapist continued to use clarification to try to help the group members verbalize their feelings about such interactions.

Steve: I appreciate that sharing, but I think we are getting to
the core of something here. We are getting into an area
where I'm hearing that you would like to find ways to
communicate to people without hurting them.

The importance of knowing what the prognosis was in the case of one's cancer was also shared in this session. At one point in the session the therapist confronted the significance of prognosis in planning for life's events in the here-and-now. Such technique exemplifies an inherent principle involving existential types of group counseling and psychotherapy.

Jane: I'm still kicking around. How in the world can he tell me so I don't place him in that position. Whatever's going to happen is going to happen anyway regardless of what he said.

Steve: I'm kind of concerned about what's happening in the group right now.

Carol: I think we all want to retire.

Steve: No, I wasn't thinking about that, but I don't particularly want to retire.

Amanda: Well, I hope not.

Steve: I was just wondering what was happening in the group. There was kind of an interesting dynamic. There were two conversations. One had to do with retirement going on here, and the other had to do with not wanting to know or not being able to put a time limit on it. But the importance of knowing the prognosis. . . .

Barbara: The word *disability* is such. . . .

Steve: Is that the word that triggered the whole thing?

Carol: This is what decides. . . .

Steve: Is disability necessarily a state of body or a state of mind?

Amanda: Well, as far as the Social Security Administration is concerned, it's a state of body.

Jane: You know what seems to me happens, and not necessarily with the patient who is getting psychotherapy, but with any patient who would have an incurable illness? I think a hypersensitivity steps in so that if people say something where they have no ulterior motive at all, immediately the patient twists it around and gets a very cute little response that adds to depression.

Diana made an intense disclosure about having to live in a co-coon-like world where everything seems fine to persons on the outside and all of the pressures that such behavior puts on her own self-concept. The group began tangential discussion regarding the temperature of the room in which we were meeting. A technique that counselors in all groups must use is one of confronting avoidance. The ability to confront avoidance signifies the action-oriented stage at which the group is functioning.

Steve: It's really interesting. I noticed that we moved into an area that was pretty tough. It was interesting how you all backed away from it. Changing the subject . . . and a little humor and a little laughter. And I guess I think that's a safety valve for the group. And I don't know if it's good or bad, but the only thing I'm concerned about is when we are together, when we get an hour-and-a-half or two hours together, that this is the place to take a pretty hard look at some pretty hard things that aren't always the greatest to look at. What I was hearing from Diana and from everybody is that you are not allowed to do that out there. I think what Amanda said was very insightful and perceptive . . . that other people can't handle it. And so you have a choice as to whether or not to be selfish and deal with it in your own way so that you feel better out there, and hurt other people, or there might be more alternatives. It also seems that you're saying that rather than verbalizing feelings you keep silent. Kind of grin and bear it. And I think that one of the purposes of this group is to get together to look at those hard issues. There have been a number of things that have happened today that have happened in the past that interfere with discussion of hard issues, and I feel more of a need to call your attention to them . . . your awareness to them. There is cross talk: the small conversations and the levity. For instance, the little anecdote about the radiators and stuff like that is kind of a way of moving away from confrontation. It's a safety valve and it's been

	going on, but I think we really need to confront some of the harder issues and work them through.
Amanda:	And, if they exist?
Steve:	And if they exist?
Diana:	Well, there again, we go back to the beginning. It seems like I'm the only one who, you know. . . .
Barbara:	Well, I understand a little bit, Diana, because I really wish people would treat me now like they did before they ever knew I had cancer. Like when I go over to my stepdaughter's house; before I found out I had cancer, I just walked in there, picked up the broom, and swept up the floor or whatever I wanted to do. But now when I go there, the first thing they do is get me a pillow for my back, then they bring me a glass of coke and then a pain pill. And I'm not even hurting! You know, she's trying to be helpful and I don't want to hurt her feelings. You know.
Carol:	Well, I don't want anybody feeling sorry for me.

Following the confrontation, the group came back to task. Barbara shared that she too had experienced some of the difficulties of trying to maintain her composure with people who were somewhat solicitous and oversympathetic.

The latter part of the fourth session was concerned with Jane's loneliness. Also discussed were other imposed and self-imposed dynamics of loneliness/aloneness. Interestingly, there seemed to be a dyad between Jane and the therapist with the other members in more or less an observer's role. Thus, toward the end of the session the therapist confronted the other group members regarding their verbal inactivity in attending Jane's problems. Such a confrontation was an effort to not only offer Jane alternatives for coping with her problems, but also to facilitate cohesiveness that occurs through the sharing of similar feelings by other members.

Jane:	And even many times like recently; there's a woman at the church, a very intelligent person, who called me on a few occasions. And I could have seen her and gone to church with her. But she was attaching so much significance to me and what she thought I was capable of that I was scared to encourage this

relationship because I felt that I would be disappointing her, that I was not what she thought I was.

Steve: I heard that somewhere in this group before. I heard Diana saying the same thing.

Diana: You're [Jane] ending up with the same thing I am.

Steve: I heard her saying the same thing to you and to some of the others in the group. And you're saying right now about the woman who called you that you felt that there was an unrealistic encouragement there, that it wasn't an honest communication. And I think that's what Diana was trying to say earlier: that she needs a more honest communication.

Diana: Well, you know, I'm sitting here listening to her and I'm thinking that, you know, earlier in our conversation, that she was sitting over there saying, "You all have those problems," like she didn't, and she does; she has them. You have them just like the rest of us. I'm sorry I'm not looking at you. But, you know, you do, which makes you even more a part of us.

Steve: I was going to say, what were the feelings that were going on in you as she was saying . . . as you were identifying with that?

Diana: Well, that she's not so much. . . . Well, it seemed like earlier that she was saying, "Well, you know, everybody does have those problems and I don't."

Steve: So do you feel closer to her now?

Diana: Yeah, I feel like she's closer to us whether she counts us as her six most intimate friends or not.

Sociometry

Figure 8-1 illustrates the seating arrangement during session 4. Figure 8-2 illustrates the primary patterns of communication during session 4. Notice that the heavy arrows from the symbol for the therapist (T) to both Jane and Diana suggest confrontation. The double-arrowed line between Amanda and the therapist suggests the process of developing a rapport to facilitate the working through of defenses and resistances on Amanda's part. It symbolizes both direct and indirect confrontations between the therapist and Amanda. The

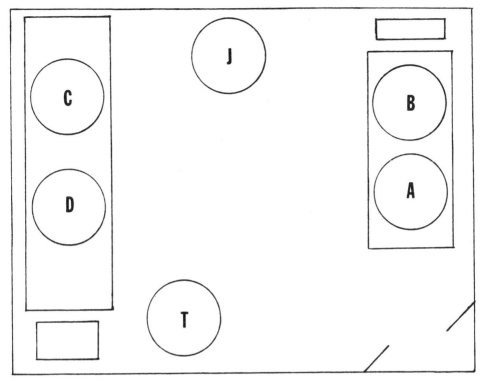

Figure 8-1. Session 4: Seating

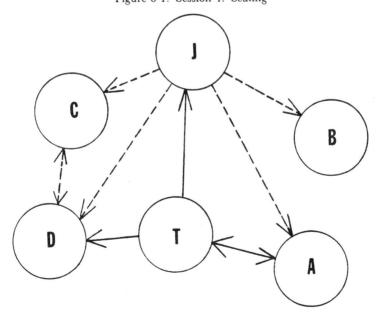

Figure 8-2. Session 4: Primary patterns of communication between members and members and therapist

dotted lines with arrows emanating from Jane suggests her reaching out to the other group members without reciprocity. The dotted line with double arrows between Carol and Diana suggests the unique rapport between the two as Diana searched for support from Carol during the more confrontive segments of this session.

Journal

I had a good group at Emory. Louise is very sick. All members have filled out their second semantic differential (an instrument used in the research). Depression was very evident in Jane, Carol, and Diana. Jane has been calling Diana and Carol too frequently to complain. We are getting away from symptomology and talking about feelings. The group members are confronting each other more also. Jane is starting to become more aware of what role she plays in her own loneliness. I'm beginning to feel more confident about the group, and my fears about working with my clients are abating. They are beautiful people and have so much courage.

SESSION 5: ACTION PHASE

Session 5 can be best characterized by stating that it was confrontive and action-oriented. Early in the session, Jane confronted the therapist with her irritation regarding something that she had heard said to her the week before. It seemed that some of the confrontation that Jane had been getting regarding her loneliness and her role in perpetuating that loneliness had hit home. In the following excerpt, she shared her irritation with the group. Her ability to verbalize such frustration suggested that the group was very cohesive. Otherwise, Jane would not have dared to take the risk of rejection.

> **Steve:** I also heard you say, besides just sounding disappointed. . . . I also heard a little anger. Not anger; but you were a little peeved with her for maybe suggesting that you might have a role in her [the friend's] life.
>
> **Jane:** You know I think that's true.
>
> **Steve:** And you are doing it a little more. Where is that irritation coming from?

Jane: Where is the irritation coming from? Of course, I think in my mind maybe I was forced to say that. Could some of it be true?

Steve: You were questioning it while we were doing it, and you also were questioning it over the last week.

Jane: I have been questioning it, and I have been wondering about a lot of it because of how certain things go. I might get angry about something that isn't making me happy and isn't desirable. And many times I was thinking, when you just said that, sometimes we become irritated when somebody tells the truth or a partial of the truth. So when you said that, I had been thinking about it. But as you said it, I thought, "Well, maybe it is."

Steve: Are you saying now that maybe you are a little irritated with me for seeing something that might be?

Jane: Yeah, that's what I just said. I wasn't really irritated. I wasn't aware of the fact that I was irritated. But when you mentioned it I thought, "Well that's like a mosquito bite. It's irritating."

The session was intense. The focus was Jane's relationship with her son: a relationship of a divorced woman and her only son with a somewhat sadomasochistic feature in which the son psychologically and physically abused the mother and the mother responded by becoming a rather shrewish martyr.

There were significant confrontations during this session. The group members communicated more directly and concretely with one another. For example, the following excerpt illustrates the group's confrontation of Jane's problem with minimal interaction on the therapist's part. One can see that Jane's best defense seemed to be acceptance of all confrontation as valid. It is difficult to argue with one who is always in agreement.

Steve: When Diana would start talking, you'd say, "You have youth on your side, and the worst thing for me is the loneliness and the pain my son gives me." And I don't think we . . . and I'm not saying. . . . I'm not trying to hurt you. . . . OK? This is all in an effort to help you become aware of some stuff. But a lot of times you would try to get into yourself and where you were coming from with John, which just gives me further information that this is so heavy on your mind. And it's also something that's interfering with your relationship with other people because you can't possibly. . . . If you've got that much energy churning into such a negative kind of relationship, then how much energy can you have left over for forming meaningful relationships with other people?

Jane: That's right. And I'm also aware of the fact that it doesn't make for the most interesting conversation because people can listen to it up to a certain point and be very sympathetic. . . . But I'm aware of the fact how much advice can they offer. I know pretty well much what I ought to do.

Amanda: You see, Jane, I think you may have put your finger on something right there. Because in twenty years at the speech school I used to listen to people pour it out. It just simply does not last too long because very soon you think you deserve it; you're asking for it. And I have no sympathy for you until you take some drastic action to change these circumstances. So if you are really trying to change them, I'm in there behind you and I'll help all I can; but just don't come crying to me about something you could change if you wanted to. I mean I've encountered that kind of situation many times.

Jane: I agree with you completely.

Steve: Can you [Amanda] say that to Jane? Are you saying that you are getting to that point in the group?

Amanda: No, I don't think so.

Steve: We're trying to be honest here.

Amanda: I'll try to be honest. . . . Yes! I think, Jane, it is of such paramount importance for you; it is so all consuming: your interest; your energy; your everything, that it's getting to be a bore for people who have to listen to it!

Steve: To you?

Amanda: That's right, it is. And that sounds so unkind, and I

	don't mean it to sound that way. But sometimes it takes blunt action to shock you into looking at something.
Steve:	Are you finding that your sympathy is almost turning, then it becomes anger? Then it almost becomes withdrawn because you almost shut your ears on it.
Amanda:	Yes, and you don't want to do that when somebody's obviously hurting. You don't feel that you should shut the door but you just can't help!
Steve:	You can feel the pain, but you can't help?
Amanda:	You could do something about this if you want!
Jane:	Yes, that's right! That's right! I agree with you! As a matter of fact you were merely confirming what I felt. You can listen to a person up to a certain point, then it's a broken record.
Amanda:	Well, and then it's cruel to say, "OK, I'm sick and tired of hearing that!" And yet you lay yourself wide open to that sort of statement.
Jane:	That's right! That's right! Anybody could say, "Well, maybe she's masochistic if she's putting up with it."
Steve:	OK, there's another one of those words.
Carol:	What does that mean?
Steve:	What does that mean?
Jane:	That I enjoy hurting myself, perpetuating a situation which I say is distasteful but which I continue. I know I'm playing some kind of neurotic game.
Steve:	While Amanda was talking. . . . I hate to cut off . . . I have to pull in the whole group. I noticed Diana was shaking her head too.
Diana:	Well, Friday, we were talking and I told her [Jane], "Until you take some positive steps I don't want to hear about it any more." And that's as positive as I could be with her until she takes some sort of a step to show us.
Amanda:	I think, Jane, it would be just as wrong and just as hampering and crippling of us if we were to do the same thing to you as you have been doing to this boy all these years: not to take any positive action about this. Anything you want we just listen to you.

Jane: I know you are absolutely right.

Carol: Jane, what do you want to do?

Jane: I've got to cut this relationship off. I've got to tell John. I've got to make John realize that he's got to stand on his own feet, that he's responsible for himself.

Amanda: My feeling would be I have no more responsibility. I cannot accept any more responsibility. Period. And of course, that's like Steve said: You wouldn't want to sever this relationship permanently. But the one that's caused you so much pain, I don't know if that's any great loss.

Jane: I don't see him that often. Even when he picks up his check. . . .

Steve: You are still making excuses; you are doing it again.

Jane: No, I didn't mean that. I mean that if I stopped seeing him, it wouldn't be a great loss.

Steve: But you didn't say that. You started by saying, "I don't see him that often." You were defending him.

Jane: No! No! This was not an appropriate. . . .

Steve: Can I bounce something off you? I just want you . . . what I'm feeling. . . . The group's with you, OK?

Jane: I know that.

Steve: Let me bounce something off you. A while ago you said if you severed this relationship, you may have hell to pay, and my feeling is you are having hell to pay right now. Of course, you can't know about physical abuse because of John's past history, and I'm not willing to take that responsibility to say, "Here go ahead and do that." That's kind of what Amanda was saying; but here's another thing to throw into the pot. Are you aware of what's happening to you in the group, here?

Jane: I'm aware of this; that I perhaps dwelled on the subject and have been unwilling to employ effective measures to terminate the relationship.

In an action session, group cohesiveness is paramount. Group cohesiveness was evidenced by the abilities of the group members to confront each other while maintaining a good rapport. For instance, in the following excerpt, Carol and Amanda offered concrete verbalizations to help support Jane and to help her clarify her feelings. In this excerpt there were only two verbalizations by the therapist. One was an opening to Jane to facilitate the expression of her feelings. Later, the therapist made a verbalization to try to help the group appreciate the nonverbal dynamics of Jane's tears during the confrontation.

Steve: Let me ask you this. I just laid a lot of heavy stuff on you. How do you feel?

Jane: How do I feel?

Carol: She looks like she has the whole world on her shoulders.

Jane: No, I really don't feel that way. I feel that what you have told me. . . . I really appreciate it. I think it's better for you to tell me. . . . Actually how giving me this feedback of how I'm coming across, and I think this is very valuable to me, and I'm very grateful for it. [crying]

Amanda: Jane, it's frequently shocking when you find out, "Gosh, do I sound like that? Or do I look like that?"

Jane: I know I must sound like a broken record. I know my weakness. I know that I'm not functioning like the adult I should be.

Amanda: Let me ask you this. Do you indulge in this sort of conversation outside of this group? Is this the only place you really talk about it?

Jane: No.

Amanda: Well, then, honey, I'm not surprised at all that you have difficulty maintaining relationships. I thought maybe you just kind of unloaded in here because you felt it was private and confidential.

Jane: No! No! I do, but not always. But with certain friends I do talk about it, and I think they are pretty disgusted with me.

Amanda: And see, you don't want that to continue. You are punishing yourself.

Jane:	That's right. That's right.
Carol:	And you are going to find, Jane, that all your friends are going to cut you off if you don't do something.
Jane:	And you know the strange thing is I'm very grateful to all of you for telling me this.
Amanda:	You are very generous to say that because you could say, "I don't like any of you because you all don't like me. Goodbye!"
Jane:	No, no!
Steve:	I think she's genuinely grateful, but I feel there's a lot of pressure. And this is very loaded. This has been the most pressure that I've felt in this group. Right now.
Jane:	Because you know what it's going to do? It's going to. . . . It's given me an awareness. It's going to make me . . . it's got to make me act. What it's done, it's going to make me act.

In addition to developing interpersonal skills towards facilitating communication in the group, some members developed the ability to verbalize awareness of nonverbal behavior by other group members. For instance, in the course of the excerpt above, note that Carol made a verbalization, which led to Jane's tears. Notice that Carol said, "She looks like she has the whole world on her shoulders." Such attention to nonverbal behavior during the course of deep confrontation suggested sensitivity. Sensitivity served as the foundation for this action-oriented session.

Toward the end of this session the group began to interact on a more intense and intimate basis with minimal interference from the therapist. The members were helping themselves.

Techniques

As therapist, one must remember not to fall into the role of advice giver but must remember to be a mirror for the group; a mirror that attempts to reflect at deeper levels the psychological processes that are involved in human experience and relationships.

Along with continued redirecting and occasional structuring toward facilitation of deeper levels of communication, a new technique utilized in this particular session was verbalizing the illustration of the group being a microcosm of reality. As such, the group offered each member the opportunity to confront current behavior, to develop insights, to integrate such insights into possible behavioral changes, and to reenter the larger reality of the world with alternatives for new behavior previously not considered.

> **Steve:** And you can see what's happening here. I think the group is a microcosm. Group interaction is an example of what's happening with the real world. You [Jane] are turning the group off. You are isolating yourself from the group or being isolated from them because week after week, you come back with the same thing and you aren't willing to explore alternatives for taking action. You keep making excuses for John, and you are turning off some of the other group members, and in effect you are causing your own loneliness.

Because of the group's cohesiveness at this point, it was much easier for the therapist to confront Jane regarding her denial.

> **Steve:** It's not helping you, you are just churning it over and over again, and you give the picture of everything is rosiness with the cancer and the disease, and the world is hunkey-dorey, when we know it's not. And so I guess another feeling that comes along is that you are not being honest.
>
> **Jane:** No, I'm not being honest.
>
> **Steve:** Upfront.
>
> **Jane:** When you say that I give the feeling that everything is hunkey-dorey with the cancer and everything like that, I don't know where you get that impression.
>
> **Steve:** I guess what I was trying to point out is the inconsistency that everything is pretty fine with you considering all the things that are going on in your life. But on the other hand, we all know that the problem of John is there, and that's a pretty big thing. And so that presents an inconsistency to me as to how can everything be pretty OK when this is happening? When I'm hearing it in the group every week. When

you are talking to the group members outside of
group about it. When you share it with me.

Because of the intensity of the confrontation during this session
the therapist took time at the end of the session for summation and
closure. Particular attention was given to Jane's feelings as the result
of this session. Whether she was encouraged or not did not seem to
be as important as the opportunity for her to verbalize her feelings.
One might suspect that she was still being defensive even at the end
of the session. At least several alternatives had been provided for examination during the interlude between sessions. It was interesting
that persons in all groups, and particularly this unique group, seem
to have a reflexive defense mechanism that allows them to tell others
that they are feeling alright while genuinely experiencing discomfort. During the interim period between sessions, members often
had the opportunity to reexamine what happened during the session
and bring fresh insights to the group at the next session. Thus, it is a
good idea to ask persons who emerged as principals during confrontation to reflect on their thoughts regarding the previous session at
the session immediately following.

Steve: I'm going to do a couple of things here, then we'll
stop. One is I want to ask how you [Jane] are feeling?

Carol: I think she looks better.

Jane: How am I feeling? I'm feeling very encouraged. As I
say, I've learned a great deal through everyone here
and I'm glad. But to tell me precisely how you felt, I
think that's very valuable.

Steve: I think that this is a sign that everyone in the group is
concerned or we wouldn't bother. And I want to
make sure you are still a member of this group.

Jane: I am.

Carol: And I want you to join the Retired Persons Association. It's the best thing for you.

Jane: I've been there twice, and they couldn't take any new
members in the evening. It was an evening session. I
guess, you know, there are some chapters that cannot
take any new people because of fire regulations.

Could it be that Carol was trying to take care of Jane between
sessions?

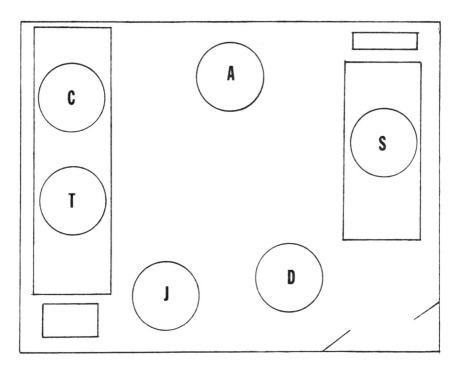

Figure 8-3. Session 5: Seating

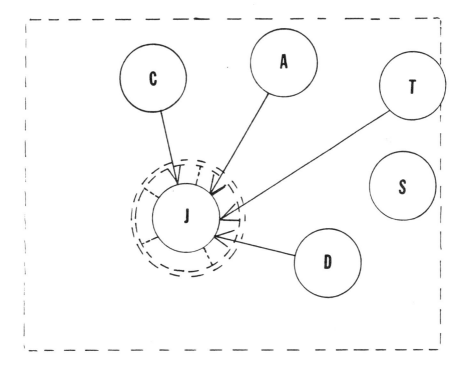

Figure 8-4. Session 5: Primary patterns of communication. Therapist and most members communicate to a member (Jane)

Sociometry

The seating pattern of session 5 is illustrated in Figure 8-3. Notice that Amanda has begun to occupy a different seat.

Figure 8-4 illustrates the primary patterns of communication during session 5. The therapist is peripheral, enveloping the group with facilitation as indicated by the dotted square pattern. The other members confront Jane, and she defends herself (indicated by the random dotted lines and the two congruent dotted circles). Sally had much difficulty handling the intensity of the confrontation and remained isolated, by choice, from the group interaction during this session.

Journal

We had our fifth meeting yesterday and focused mostly on Jane's problems with her son, John. In essence, the group said that they wanted her to do something about it or to stop talking about it. It was a very confrontive session and the deepest of all those we have had.

I also called the group's awareness to the fact that they seemed to become anxious in therapy and to begin to talk about extraneous "out-there" concerns. Anyway, I'm glad that Jane was in the hot seat today, for it was necessary for her to come out in order to help the group move on. She was becoming an isolate in the group. She was calling the members in between sessions and trying to continue therapy over the phone. She just kept playing the same "tapes" about her son. This had a tendency to push other members away.

I know that we are getting more cohesive as a group for another reason. At the end of the session we were just chit-chatting and someone suggested that we should stop. I said, "Good, 'cause I have to pee." Amanda said, "I wish you would stop your vulgarisms. . . ." The rest of the group seemed to agree. I will respect their requests, of course, though I don't agree that I was vulgar. However, that's the first real negative feedback that they have given me. It is a good sign.

SESSION 6: ACTION PHASE

One of the important dynamics hoped for was the appearance of deeper level discussions of death and dying. Session 6 had death and dying as its theme. The session centered on the very moving recollection of Sally's experience with her mother's death. The ability to discuss her recollections in such emotional detail signified the action-oriented nature of this session.

The session opened with Carol discussing a very painful episode that she was having with the course of her cancer. Amanda reflected her anxiety about discussions of members dying as she tried to reassure Carol. Immediately Sally began to recall the story of her mother's death in an indirect, emphatic fashion in response to feelings generated as Carol was sharing the imminence of her own death. As she began to recall her mother's death, Amanda's anxiety became more apparent. Sally recounted how her mother did not wish for the children and other family members to see her pain. Her mother would just go off into the bathroom so no one would be able to observe her. Amanda replied as follows.

Amanda: Well, I think that's good. That's considerate of other people. And, you know, I feel strongly that you should be. . . . I mean being considerate of other people is far more important than expressing your own feelings. I know we [to Steve] don't agree on that, but I feel that way.

Amanda continued to support Sally in an effort to avoid the intensity of Sally's sharing regarding her own cancer. It seemed that Sally's mother died of breast cancer. Sally was experiencing déjà vu.

Amanda: Well, they can do so much more now. I really think that they can allay some of that suffering that other people had to experience. But I remember my mother was very different. Mother had an extremely low pain threshold. And she didn't have cancer; but she had some surgery once. And the night nurse with her gave her as much medication as she wanted. And the nurse said, "You will be a drug addict!" And mother said, "You let *me* worry about that! I'm not going to suffer!" And I sort of feel that way. I don't want to be a vegetable. I don't want to lose control. But I see no great power in just suffering.

Steve: There are a lot of strong feelings that I'm feeling here

	as you were recounting your mother's experience. I could see that this is still very vivid in your mind.
Sally:	Still? I know when I found out what I had to go through ... had the same thing in the same place. . . . I just went into six tailspins, you know.
Amanda:	I'll bet you did! I'll bet you went into shock.
Steve:	It's almost like a replay of the same events.
Amanda:	That's the thing about it. You have to be governed by your . . . by the knowledge you gain from your own experience.
Sally:	And I know the doctor that sent me out here to have the examination. . . . And he knew all this because my father was in bed with pneumonia when my mother passed on, and he couldn't even get up. So anyway, afterward, after he got out of bed and he had at least started to go to this Doctor Williams, who just started practicing. . . . So Doctor Williams had known me through all those years, and he knew all about my mother, and he twitched too when he told me.
Amanda:	You know, sometimes I think these doctors have the lousiest jobs.
Sally:	He said, "Sally, you are going out there and let Maste do that biopsy." And he says, "There's nothing else. You've got to do it! You've just got to do it!" But he tried to encourage me.
Amanda:	Well, I think it was not false encouragement, Sally. I really think not.

While Amanda continued this somewhat hypocritical position of offering the same false support and denial that she had accused friends of offering her, the group demonstrated its maturity and evolution by confrontation of core issues. One sign of group maturity was that there were very few references to treatment. Also, it was evident that Amanda began to unmask and share some of her feelings. The ability to confront death and dying as a theme in the group was also a manifestation of its intensity. Significantly, the group seemed to function almost autonomously with the therapist interacting only to structure, facilitate, and confront. The suggestion here is that group process was self-sustaining with member trust, confidence, and other attributes being exhibited.

Interestingly, at approximately halfway through the session, Amanda seemed to show further anxiety about the subject of death in both attempting to manipulate the group away from the subject and by an unconscious double entendre with the use of the word *death*.

Amanda: Carol, do you feel you've said everything you wanted to say? I hate to feel that you've been cut off, but you can't just keep beating your subject to *death*!

Techniques

Responsible, facilitative behaviors that had been suggested earlier were continuously employed. Additionally, and relative to this session, the leader facilitated discussion of the subject of death and pain without communicating his own anxiety. This reflected the therapist's trust in the ability of the group to be facilitative with one another as well as the leader's growing confidence in the group as a unit.

There was a continuation by the therapist of the use of confrontation regarding denial and an inability to deal with affect. However, a somewhat gentle approach was manifested in confronting Amanda's resistance.

Amanda: And maybe if there was just some super person who could give me all the answers. . . . But I don't know anybody that can give me all the answers.

Steve: Are you looking for answers or are you just looking? I don't hear you asking for answers, I hear. . . .

Amanda: I'm really not.

Steve: I hear you just wanting a place or some situation that would enable you to explore your. . . . I don't like to use the word feelings with you because we are having a semantic problem. I think we are saying very close to the same thing.

Amanda: Well, I guess one advantage that I have is that I live alone. And if I want to talk something out to myself, there's not a soul to listen to me. I can talk all I want to out loud. And I think sometimes it helps to vocalize.

Amanda began unmasking, finally sharing, in an indirect fashion, that there may be some benefit to verbalizing feelings regarding cancer as well as those concerning death and dying.

There is a technique manifest in existential-type group psychotherapy and involves an effort to focus on the here-and-now dynamics of the group in an attempt to minimize vague anxieties that might inhibit personal growth and improved satisfaction with the world. The following excerpt illustrates facilitation of that dynamic as well as mild confrontation in helping Carol focus on her feelings about her own death.

Steve: Carol, I hear a lot of anxiety, particularly this week, and I know that there's been. . . .

Carol: Right! These last two weeks have really been sitting on my mind.

Steve: It's just been an awful time, like sitting on pins and needles. And I, in a way, I kind of hear you asking the group, "Where am I?" You know, "Give me some feedback as to where am I." And I'm wondering to help us know where you are. Where do you see yourself right now?

Carol: Well, I think I'll see tomorrow but whether I'll be here in six months, I don't know.

Steve: OK. You are thinking about that right now. And when you think about whether "I'll be here six months from now," you say that in a very matter-of-fact way. But I'm sure that that's very emotionally ladened.

Amanda: Well, it has to be Steve. Nobody can talk about dying casually. And if they do, then it's just put on. I don't think that's a genuine attitude.

Following the disclosure that perhaps her life was coming to an end, that she had achieved her purpose in life, a technique was employed by which the therapist shared unstated feelings and summarized those feelings, reflecting them to the initiator of the disclosure. In this case, Carol was the initiator.

Steve: Carol, I'm hearing a feeling of uselessness.

Carol: Yes, I really do. I really feel useless.

During the action phase, the leader used his knowledge regarding the dynamics of cancer and incorporated such knowledge with sensitive confrontation. This was an example of the technique of integration. Also, there was a continuous effort to keep the group's focus on the here-and-now particularly in helping the emotional aspects of death and dying. The here-and-now dynamic cannot be emphasized enough, particularly if the counselor is focusing on the existential dynamic as his theoretical orientation. In the case of this group, it sometimes meant confrontation when drifting away from present centeredness, as exemplified in the following excerpt.

Steve: Another thing that goes along with that, and it's happening here too, is that when somebody is sharing or talking about their other problems, that forces you [the members] into committing some kind of a feeling or becoming involved in that problem. And if you've already got a lot of stuff going on in yourself, it's hard to get over to where someone else is and hear that too. It's a lot easier to talk about how you are feeling than to hear about how someone else is feeling. I mean, whether it's physical or whether we are talking about feelings. . . . It produces a lot of discomfort. It's evident right in here in the group.

Sometimes the counselor must offer suggestions, verbalizing alternatives not thought of by the other group members. Such verbalization is often in the form of teaching where, after all, much of the therapeutic effect of counseling and psychotherapy is to be found. The following excerpt illustrates the technique of offering an alternative in a teaching mode.

Steve: But I guess what I'm feeling is that you [Carol] have a right to live for yourself. You are not being responsible to yourself. I'm wondering if this is a case where you should be a little more selfish.

Sociometry

Figures 8-5 and 8-6, respectively, illustrate the seating arrangement and the primary patterns of communication for session 6. It is noteworthy that Diana and Jane were both absent during this session.

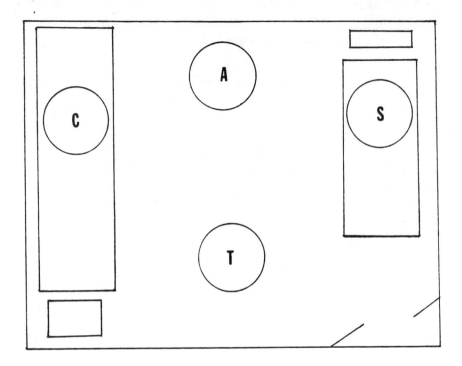

Figure 8-5. Session 6: Seating

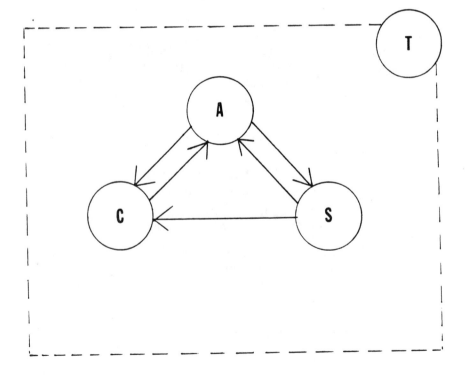

Figure 8-6. Session 6: Primary patterns of communication between members

Perhaps the absence of Diana's anger and Jane's depression, which had preoccupied the group, allowed the remaining members to vent their own concerns about death and dying. At any rate, Amanda seemed to take on the role of the facilitator with the therapist's presence being a secondary factor. Sally seemed to be preoccupied with venting and sharing the grief from her mother's death. Carol similarly seemed to be interested in sharing her feelings about pain as well as death and dying. She also shared some of her concerns about her children's irresponsibility. There was little two-way communication.

Journal

Last week Jane's fixed bridge fell out and she had to go to the dentist. Diana's kids were ill and she was not present either. Barbara didn't show, and Louise is very sick. I doubt that Louise will be with us anymore. I was disappointed that there were only three present, but we had a very significant session. We dealt with the feelings of uselessness and the occasional desire for death that Carol was experiencing. Also, I confronted Amanda about her inability to let Carol experience her feelings in the group. As I said, it was pretty heavy, and I expect it to be more so the next session. It was a good session.

Like in Jane's case, we also discussed problems that Carol was having with her adult children. Sally shared a very moving account of her mother's death from breast cancer. Her mother died in Sally's arms. In short, we were really into action, and the group seems to be less anxious; so do I.

SESSION 7: ACTION PHASE

Early in session 7 Jane indicated that she had taken steps toward solving problems regarding her son. Significantly, there was spontaneous interaction with positive feedback in terms of the group experience.

Jane: I felt it was a very significant development. You see, that's why I like group therapy, particularly if you are in a group where you respect the people, and they tell you, and they tell you how you are coming across.

Amanda:	Well, I think you have reacted admirably.
Jane:	Thank you.
Amanda:	Not only did you take it, but you did something about it.
Jane:	I did! I did!
Sally:	That's the important thing: to do something. You may want to do it, but when you get right down to doing it, then that's something else.
Amanda:	We all need a little starch in our backbone from time to time.
Sally:	Absolutely.
Jane:	I could see this little weakling, this crybaby.
Amanda:	Not any more. Are we going to flip a coin to see who breaks the silence? [Looking at Steve]
Diana:	You know, I have a lot of reservations. I see the good that it's done, and if we had to do it over again, I think it would go the same way; but I still have a lot of reservations about, you know. I think we see each other once a week, and we know just a little bit about each other; only a little bit. Not even. . . . We haven't even gotten down to basics, other than perhaps, we all know Jane better than we know each other because we all have talked with Jane. She's talked with us more than we talk with each other. And you know, there's a lot of things we don't know about each other. So sometimes I think as I'm looking back . . . and I thought on the things we said to Jane. . . . I can see where for her, it's good. I can see where we might take the bull by the horns and look over here at you and say, "This is what I think." But we don't know what it's like at home. We don't know what's really in Amanda's mind. You know, I have a lot of reservations. I have a lot of reservations about even. . . .
Amanda:	You mean the effectiveness of this kind of thing?
Diana:	Yeah. Yeah. And maybe it's because. . . . Maybe I'm afraid now we are going to go around the circle and it's going to get here on Diana.
Amanda:	Somebody's turn now.

Diana: And I'm not ready, you know. I don't know if I could handle it because I would keep saying. . . .

Jane: I really feel not everybody fits immediately into a group situation. Some people never fit into a group situation. I have. On the other hand, if the group is of the quality that this group is, I find it very easy to talk and I solicit and I welcome the reactions.

Diana: I think it's super that we can definitely see a change but I still have reservations.

It became apparent that the group members were very anxious about confronting one another. The therapist verbalized awareness of this anxiety. Diana elaborated on this verbalization and seemed to suggest her desire to enter into more depth while expressing her fear of doing so.

Steve: I think what I'm hearing is that you are verbalizing the group's anxiety about confronting each other. It seems like we are going around. It was Jane's turn. And like last week, the focus happened to be on Carol. And you are wondering, could you handle that? Could Amanda handle that? Could Sally handle that? And is that the way it has to go? I guess the way that I feel is that anxiety is present in a group. You know, there's a group anxiety. And if it happens that a person seems to take a turn, that's the person's choice. And if it doesn't happen that way, that's OK too.

Diana: But I think what I'm saying is you're not going to hear too much how I feel because I'm . . . you know . . . I've lived on top of it for seven years. I experienced a breaking down in the group, and here I preached I want to get down to basics. I want us to get down to the problem instead of talking about how to make instant coffee. Now I'm sitting here and I'm saying I experienced it with Jane. And maybe what happened with Jane just kind of brought my mind to it. But I'm saying I feel like I've been on a charade. I've been on it continually because there's so much you don't know about me, you couldn't possibly know about me. But you wouldn't want to know, and I put on my smile, and I'll be set.

The action-oriented aspects of the session were further underlined by the tendency of this session to focus on Diana's story. The group turned its attention to Diana and her anger as well as Diana's job hunting difficulties. Significantly, Diana verbalized her thoughts and fantasies regarding suicide. In any therapeutic group, it is significant when action occurs. Each member seems to be in the so-called hot-seat at alternate sessions. For instance, at an earlier session Jane had been the focus, followed by Carol and Sally at subsequent sessions.

Other characteristics of this session included group problem-solving activities, often with suggestions to Diana regarding the pursuit of career opportunities. Also, there were discussions of self-worth. During the course of the session, there was very little discussion about treatment or symptoms. It was critical that a group of this type go beyond symptomatology into inner feelings in order to demonstrate the therapeutic effect of this medium. The absence of the discussion of treatment and symptoms, therefore, was clearly an indicator of group progress. Also, deeper levels of sharing were evidenced.

Techniques

Without belaboring the point, the techniques utilized in the action sessions can be summarized by listing those techniques that seemed most effective:

1. Confrontation
2. Structuring
3. Offering alternatives for problem solving
4. Facilitation
5. Empathic response

The effective group therapist minimizes intervention and allows the group to take the course of discussion to the ends it desires. The chief function of the therapist is to verbalize what is not being said and to keep the group to task. Other group members, such as Amanda, seemed to have modeled the therapist by taking over the role of facilitation. Cohesiveness and trust allowed the group members to share spontaneously at much deeper levels. This was a

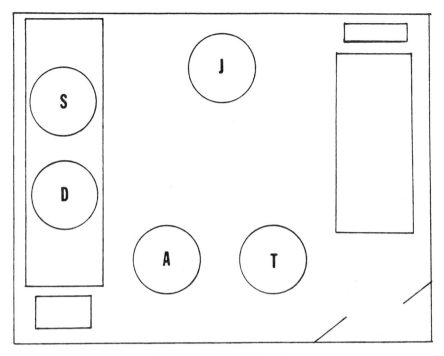

Figure 8-7. Session 7: Seating

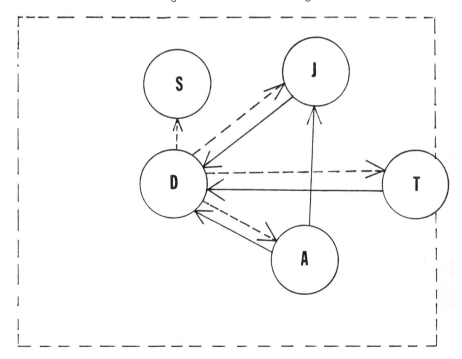

Figure 8-8. Session 7: Primary patterns of communication between members and a member (Diana) and therapist

manifestation of the therapeutic dynamic that had been established by the presence of the therapist and was maintained by that presence. Technique at this point was less important than the warmth, genuineness, and caring of the counselor.

Sociometry

Figure 8-7 represents seating arrangement, and 8-8 represents primary patterns of communication for session 7. While there seemed to be no significance to the random seating pattern of the group, there was significance in the fact that Amanda had a more facilitative role, which directly contributed to dialogue between Diana, Jane, and Sally. The therapist's presence as a facilitator is symbolized by the dotted square around the group in Figure 8-8. Also, the therapist was more direct with Diana regarding problem-solving behaviors and verbalization of feelings than with the other members of the group. The dotted lines emanating from the symbol *D* represent Diana's random dialogue to the entire group.

Journal

Session 7 was a good one. Lots and lots of action occurred. The action centered primarily on confrontation of Diana's bitterness and anger. We confronted her martyr role with her husband. I also administered the third semantic differential. Carol couldn't make it because the radiator in her car broke. Amanda's disease has progressed. She knows it, but she is still putting up the brave front.

Chapter 9

TERMINATION: ENDING/BEGINNING

SESSION 8: ACTION-TERMINATION

S ESSION 8 could be described as one of action-termination. In other words, while many of the dynamics that were present during the action-oriented sessions described earlier still existed, various comments by group members suggested their awareness that the group was coming to an end. For instance, there was demonstration on Diana's part to begin to try to solve some of the problems she was having regarding her family, particularly in relation to her husband.

Several examples exist to further demonstrate the group's movement toward termination. All of these examples have something to do with feedback regarding the group experience. For instance, Diana described a situation in which she had just received new medication. She could not tell whether her feeling better had to do as much with the new medication as it did with her attitude.

Diana: Yeah, but I can tell a complete and total change. But I don't know. . . . I know it has something to do. . . .

Amanda: Does it make any difference where it is?

Diana: . . . Whether it's psychological or what. But it's fantastic!

Amanda: I really don't think it makes a nickle's worth of difference whether it's physical or mental. You feel better. Just say, "Thank you Lord," and go on.

Carol: That's right! I feel great!

Another example of the possible effects of the group was the verbalization of the willingness to attempt new behavior by Jane regarding her relationship with her son. As the reader will recall, Jane and her only son had a history of a tumultous relationship. Immediately following a discussion on death and dying, Jane shared the action step that she had decided to take regarding her son.

303

Jane: Well, I accept the fact that people are not here for-ever, and I also was very grateful and always will be grateful to the fact that you people conked me over the head because now I am making every day count. And every day is meaningful, and I'm having. . . . Wait until my son gets my masterpiece of a letter.

Carol: You going to write him a letter?

Jane: Oh, I've written most of it. It's a masterpiece.

As mentioned earlier, positive feedback was evident throughout this session. The following excerpt offers an example.

Carol: Well, I feel since we have had these sessions, we all feel as though we have a new lease on life. I know Diana doesn't feel as frightened of her problem.

Diana: Well, I think. . . . Yes.

A little later Diana shared positive feedback regarding the group.

Diana: But anyhow I think what I said a minute ago. . . . I am just as afraid of cancer as I was when we began this, and I probably have just as many hang-ups. To-day I feel like I'm in more control. And I've been able to come here and I've been able to say, "I'm scared." And I've been able to, you know, to hear it. And I've been encouraged; even though sometimes I say I don't want to be, I have been. So I'm on top of it. But I still feel like I'm just as afraid. I don't want to die anymore today than I did. . . .

Carol: . . . *Yesterday!*

Diana: Yeah!

Some of the most significant feedback regarding the group therapy and its benefits was suggested by Diana's comments to the group members near the end of the session. She discussed how she had felt growth over the past few months as a result of the group. She now had renewed hope in her life as a result of the experience.

Diana: But, you know, I've been there and it's got thrown in my face like a pie. So, you know, I'm saying, maybe there's hope for me! I don't know; but I can see where I've grown in a few months.

Amanda: That's marvelous!

Diana:	So maybe from now until summer . . . maybe there will be another growing process. Maybe I'll come in here six months, eight months from now, and I'll be a totally. . . .
Amanda:	Maybe you'll be the leader! We'll fire Steve!
Diana:	But . . . but, you know, we've kind of grown with our problems. They've started out here, and we've grown, and I don't feel like now. . . . I'm getting back into my reasons why I don't want to get back in another group. I don't want to have to regress. I want to keep going forward, and I don't want to hear anybody elses' problems.
Amanda:	You don't feel strong enough at this point to help anybody else.
Diana:	We really get involved with each other. We've gotten involved with each other. We care, and I care. And, I just right now don't feel like I can add any more people!

The above excerpt was taken from that segment of the group in which the topic of discussion was the possibility of continuing the group beyond ten sessions. While Diana and Amanda both suggested growth and positive aspects of the group experience, they were unwilling to regroup and invest more energy.

During this session there were minimal discussions of physicians and treatment. Attention was given to problem solving. Cohesiveness allowed autonomous behavior regarding facilitation and confrontation by the group members of one another.

One other significant dynamic occurred during this session. Since much support from within was available to the group members, a very pertinent excerpt follows regarding accepting the reality of cancer. Certainly, such a discussion would not have been possible without the process and dynamics of the group being at a level significant enough to engender confidence, trust, and caring for this very personalized unmasking.

Amanda:	But you are just stiff when the day is coming when you won't be. . . .
Diana:	Well, there again I'm going to put it this way. I'm not going to kid myself into believing it's not going

to come.

Jane: Well, I think you are right. I think you are exactly right about that.

Diana: And I don't go around with a long mopy face. And I will leave this room, and I'll be just like I was when I came in.

Steve: I wanted to. . . . Amanda I think what I feel you are trying to do here is say to Diana, "Maybe there is a way you can deal with the reality and accept it and still free yourself up to be relatively happy today."

Amanda: I hope I can get that across. As I say, I'm the original realist." My husband used to say, "She'll make you lie because she just pins you down." So I can quite understand that part of your feeling. I just hate to see you make yourself unhappy by. . . . I mean, you know it's coming. I know it's coming. But I just can't live today thinking what's going to happen tomorrow. I just can't do that.

Carol: Enjoy today!

Steve: Amanda, is that what you feel some of the writers mean by acceptance of the reality — that is frees you up to . . . ?

Amanda: I think it does. I really think it's quite liberating to be accepting of reality . . . not pessimistic . . . not stupidly optimistic. Just say, "OK, this is the way it is!" And I always hate to bring the Church into it. But I remember our minister making a statement . . . , and I have quoted him a thousand times. He was talking about somebody losing a relative. "Every experience can be redempting." Now it's not going to be if you don't let it be. But it can be, and I'm not saying that you should develop any marvelous beautiful saintly character because of this. I'm just saying you can use this experience not to deprive yourself of every drop of happiness to which you are entitled. But just say, "OK! That's the way it is. Accept that." But I'm going to accept the other part of it too. I'm still here, and I'm going to enjoy it.

Diana: I guess I'm stupidly optimistic. I hang on to those two words. I was stupidly optimistic.

Amanda: I think we can be! I think we can be! We fool ourselves, the worst person in the world to fool.

Steve: I wonder if your reaction to that and the anger and the bitterness you carry around with you and that you are gracious enough to share with us here isn't defeating your enjoyment of the things. . . .

Diana: But maybe I need more time. Maybe. . . .

Amanda: You may need more time. You may need more time!

Diana: Maybe this will come about. Right now maybe it's coming about and I'm not even aware of it right now. Like I say, I know things are better but . . . like I say . . . everything I believed in was totally . . . well, thrown back in my face. My face was just literally. . . .

Steve: Like somebody stuck a boot right in your face.

Diana: Yeah! Yeah! Everything I believed in . . . everything I preached and shared and everything . . . all of a sudden was just thrown back at me. Everything! It's like everything I said was lies, but I believed it.

Steve: Almost like you wanted to scream out, "You liars!"

Diana: And so now I'm a. . . .

Amanda: You may really have hit upon it. You just need more time.

Diana: And, you know, definitely, [with] this new turn of events with the new medication, things are better.

Amanda: You know something, Diana? This just occurred to me. This was borrowed from a psychologist friend. . . . Not you [to Steve]!

Steve: I heard that "Not you!" I'll remember that.

Amanda: Well, I mean I'm not accusing you. But actually I felt at the time, "Oh Lord!" But I really think it's true. When very bad things happen to us as that certainly was to you, you have to go through a period of mourning, and maybe you are just coming out of that period of mourning. And it's very wrong for people to try to suppress it. You do that a lot when there's been a death in the family. You try to cheer them up and just let them cry. Let them be. Just get it out and let them mourn. And maybe that's what's happening to you: that you really are coming out of it. And it's good that you had that. It kind of cleanses your whole system.

Steve: I guess my concern now, like today, is that the longer the process of coming out of this takes, that you don't really mourn. I think that's an accurate analogy too. My concern is that as you mourn, that even now with the anger and the bitterness [and you accept the reality of the time limitation], you don't know how long. My concern is that you keep putting off finishing that kind of mourning and accepting the reality as Amanda says without overoptimism or without overpessimism, but just, "This is the way it is!" The longer you put that off, the shorter time span you have to enjoy the things that you and your husband seem to be working so hard for.

Amanda: Diana, we are going to save you if it kills us all.

Even in the face of the ultimate reality, there is hope. It must be reiterated that the art of counseling with the cancer patient is one of helping each one to accept the reality of their condition and the finality of the prognosis when the condition is incurable. While helping them to maintain hope at whatever level.

Techniques

Techniques used in this session did not differ significantly from those of other action-oriented sessions. Pressure was maintained on the group to focus on the here-and-now. The therapist's function was to be a guidepost and to be as inobtrusive as possible. In any group, the leader's presence and caring is much more significant than any techniques used during the course of treatment. Confrontation was used regarding dynamics such as resistance and denial. Confrontation was also used in an effort to help persons clarify meaning and priorities in life.

Sociometry

Figure 9-1 indicates the seating arrangement during session 8.

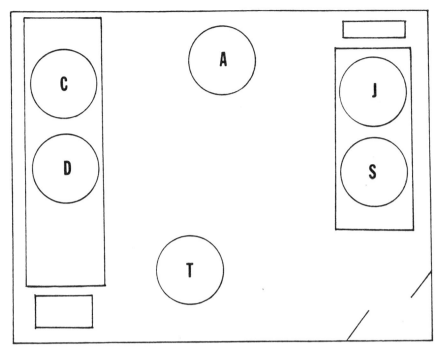

Figure 9-1. Session 8: Seating

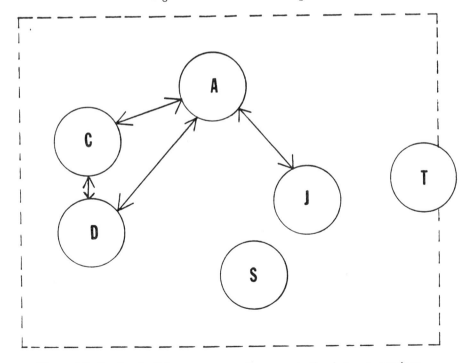

Figure 9-2. Session 8: Primary patterns of communication between members

Figure 9-2 represents the primary patterns of communication. Amanda's roles were to act as facilitator and group leader. The therapist's presence is indicated by the dotted line bordering the sociogram. Primary patterns of communication involved Amanda, Carol, and Diana. There was some two-way communication between Jane and Amanda as well. Sally interacted minimally with the group during the session. Two-way communication is indicated by double-ended arrows between members of the group.

Journal

Another heavy session went on today. I feel like the group is beginning to work through some things. Amanda is doing volunteer work with the deaf, and Diana is seeking the opportunity to do volunteer work toward solving her problem of feeling as though she is not doing meaningful work. Carol got more hours in at her job but is still having considerable pain. Jane and her son are still having problems, and the group is really turning off to Jane. Jane's son came into the clinic and complained that it is Jane who throws things and has tantrums and claimed to be concerned about her. I think that the way to resolve this is to get them both together after the research. Diana has torn up her journal and thrown it away in anger. She says that what she wrote in there no longer applies because she has grown during the group. I think she's really working, but her anger and bitterness upset me. Jane told me after the session that she was trying to be accepted by the group and that she was not afraid of death because it would be almost a welcome relief after the kind of life she's had, whereas the other members wanted to hold on to life for as long as possible. This seems to be particularly true in Diana's case, for she and her husband struggle for material things and go into debt trying to get them; they in a sense rush life. I don't know if I believe Jane.

SESSION 9: ACTION-TERMINATION

After unmasking and confrontation regarding one another's feelings and a brief discussion on symptoms, some housekeeping chores were done in preparation for termination. Specifically, the early part of the session centered on issues regarding the use of the research instruments.

Early in the session Diana shared some animosity and sarcasm. As it turned out, her sarcasm was really an attempt to redirect her anger with Jane. Jane and Diana confronted each other on several occasions during the session at rather intense levels.

Approximately one-third of the way through the session, it became apparent that Jane was also angry, but her anger was projected away from its source onto Diana. The source of her anger was a meeting that she and the therapist had following the last group session. There were two significant processes occurring. One was that group members were dealing with honest feelings such as anger. This is significant because the literature suggests that cancer patients typically have difficulty verbalizing strong emotions. Secondly, group members were having the courage to confront the leader much more directly. In this case, the leader switched roles with Amanda and became a group member while Amanda became the group facilitator.

Jane: I was upset about many things. It was not. . . . It wasn't you [to Diana] who really. . . . It wasn't you, because if I said I didn't feel. . . . You're not a trained person! You're not a psychiatrist! You're not a therapist of any sort! You are a human being with certain feelings! And you have a right, just as I had. . . . And I did express my feeling for a long time in the group. This was your prerogative as well. I couldn't be angry at you! But I was angry at the way Steve handled certain situations because I didn't meet your [to Steve] expectations . . . .

Steve: So are you angry with me because I didn't meet your expectations?

Jane: . . . Because you said certain things to me which did not indicate that you understood that I had certain needs . . . that I was expressing it a certain way. Maybe I wasn't expressing it the right way! If I knew exactly how to express it, I wouldn't have many emotional problems. And I've got some emotional problems!

Amanda: I think you are very honest about that 'cause I'm inclined to agree with you. But may I repeat some of the conversation you had with me about the reasons for your disturbance? You said that . . . I believe . . . that it disturbed you that Steve felt you were not telling the absolute truth about your lack of fear of dying. He didn't really believe that, and I don't know how you [to Steve] can resolve that. If that's what she really feels, Steve, whether it's an honest. . . . Don't you think she has to determine whether that's an honest feeling or not?

Steve: Yeah, I guess I wasn't saying that. I wasn't questioning that part. But I was saying she shares the same frustration about the disease and the uncertainty of dying that all the members of the group share but from a different perspective. So I wasn't questioning that the lack of fear was genuine. And I agree. I tend to agree with you. I can't question that.

Jane: When you say I shared but from a different perspective, what do you mean?

Steve: Well, I think I was trying to reflect what you were saying to me, which I thought. . . . It was your words, but apparently there was some miscommunication there.

Amanda: The English language is the poorest vehicle for communication known to man.

Steve: Feelings are difficult to communicate too. But what I was hearing was that you were telling me that you had had a pretty bad childhood . . . that you lost both your parents when you were six. . . .

Jane: No, when I was twelve!

Steve: . . . When you were twelve . . . you had lost both of your parents . . . you had had a bad marriage with your husband and had all this hassle with John for whatever reason and the guilt associated with that. And at sixty-nine years old . . . you had lived a fairly rich life, but . . . death at some times would almost seem like a relief.

Jane: I never said that! You said that! You said that death to me would be acceptable only because [of] the life I had lived! I hadn't said it was a rich life! Those are your words! You said that [compared to] the kind of life that I lived, death would be preferable to that! That was the reason I was being dishonest when I said I wasn't afraid of it, but I'm not afraid! For instance, they give me injections . . . they gave me all kinds of surgery that you can imagine, and I had never really been scared, and I have a high pain threshold. This is my peculiarity! It's hard for people to understand!

Steve: I guess I feel like we are miscommunicating because I don't think I ever said that you were afraid. I don't know where you are picking that up. I don't think I said that either in the group or at our meeting afterward. And perhaps I overstated what I was seeing with not enough sensitivity at the time. It's possible. Perhaps I wasn't being sensitive to what you were communicating to me. I do make mistakes.

Diana: Don't you [to Jane] realize that there are some of us here who have, as far as the surgery goes, have had just as much surgery as you've got. And whose to say that your particular disease is even further along than mine or than Amanda's or Carol's? But this is important for you to think it is!

Jane: No it isn't!

Diana: But you are always telling us this!

Steve: You are talking about something different now.

Diana: No! No! It just seems like. . . .

Jane: I have only once, that I can recall, said to you . . . and that was last time. I was told, when we were talking, about how many times you were disappointed because you were given hope and then they didn't materialize. And I said, "But I have had extensive metastasis and I was given a short time to live." But things change. I feel always that the hope of other medication. . . .

Diana: I'm sorry! I must not! I'd do better not being here! I guess I don't understand what's being said.

Steve: Well, OK. Let's stop it here for a second because I feel like there are barriers being built up. We were communicating even though. . . .

Diana: *I'm sorry I said anything!* I don't think I understand what's going on!

Steve: No. What I think you are responding to, Diana, is the situation in the group last week where Jane started talking about her surgery and stopped. . . .

Diana: Jane talks about her surgery. I've heard this story a million times! And on the telephone! Here! And we are hearing all this for many, many, many times. So I don't understand what's going on.

Steve: So what you are saying is that it makes you angry.

Diana: I don't understand her anger today. I don't understand what's going on. I don't understand why she's upset with you. A lot of times I don't understand the words she uses; so maybe that has something. . . . She has a better vocabulary than I do; so sometimes I don't understand what she's saying. So maybe I don't even know what's being said.

Steve: So that produces frustration between what she seems to be saying and what you think she is saying.

Diana: I guess I don't even know what she's saying!

Jane: Well, how can you be resentful toward me if you don't know what I'm talking about?

Diana: I don't think I'm resentful. I just don't think I even know what's going on. *I'm sorry!*

Amanda: I do think you all are talking in cross purposes. I'm not sure you really are talking about the same thing at all.

Diana: But I don't understand what. . . .

Amanda: And I'm not sure it can be resolved.

Steve: That's not a reason *not* to discuss it though. That's my feeling. I mean, I think it's important to work it through here. What you are saying to me, Jane, is that I'm a professional and that you had an expectation of how I would respond to you in the scene after the group last week. And you felt I let Diana talk about things to you in a way that was not acceptable to you. And in that way, I did not fulfill your expectation of what a professional therapist should be.

Jane: See, I just can't figure out one thing. How I had the

	time. . . . I'd really like to time this. . . . How I had the time to talk so much about my physical ailments and about my son and how many sessions . . . ?
Steve:	This is our ninth.
Jane:	. . . Our ninth session. I didn't know how I had so much time to talk about all my physical ailments, and I don't remember spending too much time talking about my physical ailments.
Amanda:	It's very difficult, don't you think, to reconstruct conversations because so often we remember what we wish we had said rather than what we did say, and it just revolves until you did and you didn't. And that's why I don't see too much to be gained by continuing. For instance Jane's given me permission to repeat the conversation she had with me. Diana's name did not enter into it. All her antagonism was directed at you (to Steve) for the very reasons that you had said that you had not lived up to her expectations. I think that's something between you and Jane. . . . It's unfortunate to pull Diana into it and become an accessory when my only impression is Diana didn't have anything to do with it; but maybe I'm wrong.
Steve:	That's fine.
Jane:	No, she didn't. . . .
Diana:	OK! When this whole thing started today, she was lashing out at me, not Steve.
Amanda:	She was getting around to it.
Diana:	She was looking at me and lashing out at me and saying, "Are my problems not as important as yours?"
Jane:	I want to tell you something. Sometimes when you are upset about a situation. . . . I could have looked at Amanda the same way.
Diana:	No one asked if they wanted to listen to my problems; but it was asked if we wanted to listen to you. . . .
Jane:	And it wasn't that. Not only your problems. . . .
Diana:	. . . And you couldn't have looked at Amanda and said that because it was me.

Jane: . . . Not only your problems but anybody's problems here. Not only yours, and I haven't singled you out. And I understand your situation very well, and I'm not the villain that you think I am. I think I'm a friend, and I would like to think so. But sometimes well-meaning people don't always express themselves quite the right way. But if their intentions are good, sometimes I think there are certain things that can be overlooked.

Diana: I thought honesty was part of our makeup in this group. I thought we could say things here that we couldn't say elsewhere!

Amanda: I think we are getting an overdose of honesty today.

Jane: I think we have! I think I say a lot of things that I wouldn't elsewhere! So I think that has been accomplished. I don't think that that's an issue.

Amanda: Maybe what we are really saying, Jane, is that if honesty is a part of it, then we have to simply steel ourselves to accept what that person who has made the statement thinks is honest, even though it may hurt a little bit. It may even be offensive. For instance, when I spoke to Steve about some of the language he was using, it was very offensive to me, and he could have said, "Well, if that's the way you feel about it, go on and get out of here." And we could have gotten into a real fight about it. But he apparently was sensitive after the fact. [I think some day he's going to have to be sensitive before the fact!] And so he accepted it. But it was quite critical . . . quite derogatory really. . . . But it was quite honest and he accepted it. Now I'm sure he didn't think, "My she's a fine upstanding person!" He may have had some moments of resentment; but he accepted it, and I think maybe that's what we are saying. When things are said in here that really kind of get your back up, you just have to say, "Wait a minute! We all have the right to be honest in here and nobody is deliberately trying to be hurtful!" And it may be kind of hard to hold onto sometimes. But isn't that essentially what we are saying?

Jane: Hey, you know! I'll tell you one thing I can honestly say this is a step ahead for me. And this is really constructive for me because in the past I would not have had the nerve to be honest with the group and to say exactly how I feel. I would have kept quiet. And this, I think, is a step ahead because I have been able to feel, and I really feel this is a loving group. I don't take offense . . . actually . . . honestly . . . at what is being said. . . . I know that people here aren't malicious with their words. I think they are kind; but sometimes, just as I don't say. . . . Well, I feel and mean any words that should convey my emotion and my interest. Other people have the same feelings and don't say it properly. I think basically there should be no malice, and for me I've already forgotten about it.

Amanda: Now you see you have worked through it. You've come full circle!

Jane: But I felt that I wanted to show you all I wasn't sissy, and as some of you said, "Tell the group!" I was going to tell the group. In the past, do you know what I would have done?

Amanda: Just not come back?

Jane: I would not have appeared!

Amanda: Well, that's good!

Resolution was brought about by the confrontation and the growth that Jane shared regarding her inability to confront persons. She verbalized that in the past she would have avoided such a situation. The intense confrontation seemed a positive indicator of group progress and personal growth in each of the members.

The above excerpt was interesting also in that there was an intense confrontation by Diana of Jane regarding Jane's persistence in making her scars and "war" stories sound more dramatic than those of anyone else in the group. However, Diana then began to "waffle" (to avoid confrontation) and feigned inferiority when she apologized for saying anything. In so many words Diana seemed to say that she was not as bright as Jane and was not as facile in terms of vocabulary. She claimed to not even be understanding about what it was that Jane was saying. However, as the group moved toward resolution with Amanda facilitating, it was noted that what had occurred here in this session was honest and open communication, even though it might have been an overdose.

It was also during the ninth session that Carol told us that the current condition causing her acute distress was diabetes. The group cheered! Diabetes was treatable; metastatic disease is incurable. Again, there was the maintenance of hope with the possibility that Carol might be able to live for a longer period of time. After all, maybe Carol's whole problem was metastatic *diabetes*, which could be miraculously cured by insulin and other drugs instead of metastatic *cancer*!

Another significant dynamic of this session was the termination anxiety shared by Diana. She had a fear that she might not resolve many of the conflicting feelings that she had regarding her cancer and the prospect of death.

Steve: And you kind of look . . . kind of down. . . .

Diana: *Down* is definitely not the word. *Definitely!*

Steve: Not strong enough?

Diana: Uh huh!

Steve: In the pits?

Diana: [sarcastically] Oh, no! I don't feel like I'm that way at all!

Carol: I think Diana has come a long way since we had our first session. She was concerned about her weight, her face, and she had this great fear of dying. And I can see a big change in her. I can see a bigger change in her than all of us put together.

Steve: And she needs that feedback.

Carol: And I think it's for the best.

Steve: I know what you are trying to say to Diana. [to Diana] She's [Carol] giving you some support. Do you hear the support? I think we worked this thing through from Jane's point of view but we haven't from your point of view. And I think it's important that we do this before this session is over today, seeing that we are going to meet only one more time in this particular group.

Diana: And if we don't work it out, what do you think is going to happen to me?

Shortly after verbalizing her anxiety Diana exhibited feelings of anger and resentment that she was having regarding the here-and-now dynamics of the group. Significantly, she was able to confront Jane with the intensity of her feelings. The confrontation of Jane also led into a confrontation of the role Amanda had played regarding her intimidation of some of the other members.

Diana: I think right now everything's OK. I just put this. . . . I don't . . . . I didn't really understand everything that was going on. I've listened to you. I understand what you said last Wednesday out in the waiting room and what she said and all that. I understand that.

Steve: I hear what you are saying, but I feel like you are repressing your feelings . . . that you are just not saying how you feel right at this moment in the group.

Diana: My feelings?

Steve: You can look at her [Jane] like that if you want. . . .

Diana: Well, I just. . . . It blows my mind to think that somebody can say something and not remember it when it happened right now, within the last hour. . . .

Steve: So you are still hurt. You are still a little angry.

Diana: You nearly said it. You nearly came out with the right word ["pissed"].

Steve: I almost said the right word?

Diana: You would have offended Amanda.

Amanda: Please don't! I'm not accustomed to that kind of language!

Steve: So, I won't say the word, but it has the same first letters as *post office*. I'm feeling that you are feeling that way.

Diana: Well, you know we've listened to each other. We've listened to each other a whole lot. And I. . . . Like sometimes Amanda can come out and explain what we just said. But it really bothers me for all that to get thrown back in our faces as it was earlier to me. . . . Thrown back in my face! 'Cause we've listened to each other a whole lot. More than we wanted to at times. Then to get . . . sometimes you deliberately focused on us. Sometimes we've not really had. . . . Like you are doing to me right now. You know. I don't really have a choice in this. Then to have it thrown back in your face when you've listened to people tolerantly. It really is a whole lot more than I can. . . .

Steve: Are you saying that at times you've listened when . . . ?

Diana: No! Don't say that!

Steve: . . . That you've listened to people in the group. And when you hear from another group member that you haven't been listening, that makes you the way you are feeling?

Amanda: You just want credit for being tolerant. You've listened tolerantly and, by golly, you want the same privilege as everybody else!

Diana: Right! That's what I'm saying!

Steve: Without feeling like you've monopolized . . . without feeling guilty?

Diana: Yes!

Steve: That the people in the group have been where you are. . . .

Diana: No! I don't think you are understanding what I'm saying! But that's OK! That's OK!

Steve: No, that's not OK. I'll shut up this time.

Diana: No! Amanda understands. Then it's OK. And Carol hasn't been here the whole time so she doesn't know what's going on.

Carol: No, I'm lost in this.

Amanda: Diana, I think what you are saying is pretty clear. You are saying, "Listen, I've listened to all of you all, and I listened tolerantly. And sometimes I was bored to death and sometimes I wondered why in the devil do you put up with that kind of thing? Or, why don't you do something so I don't agree with you? But I've listened and you owe me the same privilege. OK, if I seem to have dominated the conversation, I really haven't 'cause I haven't talked any more than you have." That's really what you are saying. It's as simple as that!

Diana: And remember, I got that thrown in my face earlier today! And *that's* what I'm referring to!

Steve: But you are not talking to me when you say that.

Diana: No, because I don't want to hurt anyone's feelings.

Amanda: We're already done with that! You aren't going to hurt anybody. Don't you know that?

Steve: I guess what I'm feeling is that sarcasm shows your feelings indirectly and it's not being honest. Your feelings are showing whether or not you say you don't want to hurt anyone's feelings. The sarcastic way that they come out could be more hurtful than just saying what you are thinking.

Jane: I think she said it.

Diana: Jane, I have listened to you almost every week since we've met and I've listened to you call me. I've enjoyed our telephone conversations, and I've listened to you again. And I've heard about your sickness and about John. And it upset me tremendously at the beginning of this meeting when you looked at me with daggers in your eyes and you compared the situation that everyone listened to *me* and wasn't given a choice. And yet when we all listened to you we simply didn't want to hear from you anymore.

Jane: See you interpreted it that way! I didn't say that it was you specifically that we didn't want to listen to.

Diana: Yes you did!

Jane: No, I did not mention your name!

Diana: You mentioned my name! You looked at me and you mentioned my name!

Jane: Did I mention her name? Do you [Amanda] remember?

Amanda: When you talked to me, Diana's name never entered into the conversation.

Diana: But earlier today you looked at me and you said last week. . . .

Jane: When I came in today you were talking to Amanda.

Now I couldn't stick my nose right in there and start talking about me.

Diana: I'm saying after you were telling about your situation with Steve, that's when you looked at me and said. . . .

Amanda: Let me ask you this, Diana. Did you have a little prior notice of this type of conversation?

Diana: No! No! Maybe that's why I was so confused.

Amanda: I mean it wasn't that you had a little preconditioning.

Steve: Now wait a minute. I feel like that's directed at me.

Amanda: No! I didn't know whether you had seen her or not.

Steve: Yeah, but it was directed at me. I mean you were saying. . . .

Amanda: Well, you would have been the only person it could have come from.

Steve: See, I think that was kind of an oblique remark, and it kind of hurt me.

Amanda: I'm sorry.

Diana: Well, I knew last Wednesday. I thought that she was upset because Steve came through the office, and Carol and I were there, and he said that Jane was upset or Jane was crying.

Steve: I said I needed to to talk to Jane, that I couldn't stay and talk to you two right now . . . that she was in the waiting room.

Diana: OK. And somehow it got back to something that I had said to her, because of something that I said to her, or the fact that Jane couldn't help me. . . . And she was upset about it. OK! That's all I had been aware of and all this. . . .

Amanda: I didn't know about that. Well, is it sufficient to say that you . . . ?

Diana: It's all said, "The way I feel. . . ."

Amanda: And Jane said, "I'm sorry I didn't really mean you specifically." Does that take care of it? Or do we still have some more feelings to express?

Steve: [to Amanda] You give me the funniest looks when you say that!

Amanda: I'm just a neat person. I want to tie up all loose ends.

Steve:	Everybody's looking at me. I'm feeling a lot of pressure.
Amanda:	Good! Maybe this is our way of getting even with you!
Steve:	I can see by looking at you that you feel better just by having said it.
Diana:	OK . . . if you can see that.
Steve:	I mean that's what I feel.
Diana:	Apparently it's written all over my face!
Steve:	You don't like me reading your face?
Diana:	Does it matter?
Amanda:	I have no illusions that they'll [the Clinic] be ready for me on time, but I allegedly have an appointment.
Diana:	They usually are not busy. There we go again. You are doing it again.
Amanda:	I know it, and I intend to keep on doing it. I just honestly feel this way, Steve. I know there are sometimes when it's a mistake to break the mood because you are sort of moving in and you want to take advantage of it. But sometimes the situation, the tension gets intolerable, and you need to sort of back off and start again.
Steve:	Yeah. It gets intolerable for you.
Amanda:	That's because you thrive on it and I don't!
Steve:	Well, I think we've touched on it before.
Sally:	I don't either!
Steve:	And I hear Sally saying it now. But I'm feeling that a lot of times you are taking the responsibility for how much pressure the other members can stand. I don't feel they've given you that consent. . . .
Amanda:	Well, you are right about that!
Steve:	. . . Consent to do that. And on the other hand, I feel that because there is a lot of caring in the group, and because the group members trust me, that there's an implied consent to use those techniques that I'm skilled with to do what it is I'm about. I guess I'm teaching now, and I'll shut up in a minute, but when you are getting into things that personally produce turmoil, either in the group or outside of the group, you are going to touch on feelings and emotions that

are sensitized and there's always a risk in looking at those things. And so when you are feeling that pressure for the other people, I think that shows a remarkable amount of sensitivity and caring for the other members. . . .

Amanda: . . . But quit it!

Steve: And you are saying to me, "Quit it!"

Amanda: No. You are saying to me, "Quit it!

Steve: Yeah, I guess I am because I feel that it takes the responsibility away from the other members of the group. I know they haven't said it, but you are an intimidating woman at times, and it's hard to confront you.

Diana: I feel like I can say things, and she can interpret what I'm saying.

Steve: I guess I was speaking for myself.

Amanda: I'll be very careful now. I'll just let them sit there and sweat!

Steve: Well, I think you are a very sensitive woman with a lot of experience. And I think you've held a leadership role in the group, and it helped a lot of the members.

Amanda: Well, there's a difference. You *can* talk too much!

Steve: Yeah, I know I can.

Amanda: No, I don't mean you! I mean me! I'm using the wrong pronoun. I can talk . . . *anybody* can talk too much!

Amanda had insight about some of the problems that she had been causing in the group.

Technique

This session was particularly intense. It featured many dynamics including confrontation of subject material as well as confrontation of the leader. The session was laden with anxiety about the termination for the group as well as possible "termination" of one of its members, Carol; *termination* at two levels caused fear.

Early in the session irritation with the therapist was evident, particularly on the part of both Diana and Jane. As the therapist confronted the group's avoidance, Jane's anger with the therapist became more intense as exemplified by the following excerpt.

Jane: Then I tried to tell him [Steve] that I appreciated what he did and, I don't know, some other thing. . . . And I put my hand on his hand, and he said to me, "You don't have to tell me who I am. I know who I am." And then he whispered, "I'm pretty good!"

Amanda: Do you beg to differ with him?

Jane: What? Yes, on the basis. . . .

Steve: I feel that you are leaving some things out.

Amanda: Well, I wish you would add them! I wish you would add them!

Steve: Well, it's more important to hear them from your [Jane's] perspective because you are angry. You are angry with me.

Jane: Yes, for you asked me upstairs. . . .

Steve: You feel like I've left you vulnerable somehow.

Jane: You made me feel that what I said was foolish, was utterly superfluous! Now, as I said, you said something that did not make sense. You said that I could not show to a human being a feeling of gratitude, and I didn't like it!

Steve: So what you are referring to at this point is the part of our conversation when you first told me that you . . . that this was really a terrific experience for you, and how good you felt about it, and how good you thought I was. And I think I said thank you in my own way. And I said, "I don't need that. . . ."

Jane: No! You didn't say thank you because if you would have said thank you or anything else — anything subsequent would have been great because I would have forgotten this!

Steve: Well, maybe I didn't say thank you.

Amanda: It sounds like you both got a little emotional.

Steve: Let's presume that I didn't say the thank you and let's just presume. . . .

Jane: No! As a matter of fact you pushed my hand away.

Steve: I don't remember doing that.

Jane: I remember it!

Steve: I think I held on to your hand and I said, "Jane, I don't need that. I don't need those kinds of strokes because I feel confident in who I am, and I feel confident about what I'm doing." And a number of times you have told me thank you in the group and how wonderful you thought the group is. You've called me on the phone to tell me how wonderful it was. You've called all the members in the group to tell them how wonderful it was and how good it was going and all that. And I guess what I was thinking at the time is, if it's going so well, why do you need to tell me all the time? . . . I guess if I'm honest, I was beginning to feel a little bit manipulated.

Jane: I'll tell you some people are effusive in their expressions! Some people are very demonstrative! I'm a demonstrative person! If I had said something offensive to you, I could understand it becoming annoying because it was excessive. It was and it wasn't a pleasant thing. But there are different ways. . . . You are a skilled person! There are different ways of dealing with it! You don't have to conk me over the head! *I'm not stupid*! I don't have to be conked on the head! You don't have to *tell* me! You could have said it in another way so that I would not have felt demeaned, and I felt very bad. I felt so badly that I cried that whole night!

Amanda: Well, that is *bad*!

Jane: And you know what I finally did? There's an organization that you call during the night. I called them because I couldn't sleep. I was so disturbed.

Diana: Because of what you [Steve] said to her?

Jane: Because of the whole picture.

Diana: Because of what happened in here and up in the waiting room?

Jane: Yes! Right! And the fact that I was singled out to have the group query about whether they still wanted to listen to me or anybody else. Anybody can talk about what they wanted to talk about eternally. And nobody was asked . . . the group wasn't asked, "Do you want to listen to this person? How do you feel about it?"

In terms of technique the therapist attempted to verbalize what was occurring outside of the group during the course of the group session. It was very important that Jane's manipulation of the therapist as well as her possible manipulation of some other group members be exposed and interpreted verbally in the group. Jane reacted somewhat defensively near the end of the excerpt where she felt persecuted and singled out in the group.

Diana immediately, and probably justifiably, personalized Jane's remarks and confronted her.

Diana:	So you're against me too!
Jane:	I'm not against you! I'm not even talking about you!
Diana:	Yes, you were! Yes, you did! You mentioned. . . .
Jane:	No! Because. . . .
Amanda:	I really think all this is. . . .
Steve:	I think you [Jane] are talking to me, and I think you are talking through Diana to me.
Jane:	No! Didn't Carol talk about herself and about how she felt in her office and how great it was and the jewelry and all these things? She talked about that many times! It doesn't have to be a derogatory thing that may be distasteful. Even too many cream pies can give you a belly ache too!
Steve:	Let me just say that I can feel your hurt, and I can see that you are hurt and that you are angry with me. And I want to say that I think I cut Carol off a couple of times the last time because the group was not helping you, and Carol knows this too 'cause I talked to her after the group. I said I cut you [Jane] off, but I felt that we needed to focus on Diana, and while we were dealing with Diana's thing, you started talking about John again. And I think what I may have said . . . "I'm not sure the group wants to hear that right now."
Jane:	I don't remember that! No, I don't remember that, so I can't. . . .

Steve: What I felt was happening was that. . . . I felt this happened before in the group; that a couple of the members specifically you, since you are the only one here right now, . . . You will sidetrack from whoever is talking at the time to get back into your relationship with John. And what I was feeling . . . what I was picking up, I thought, was the frustration of some of the other group members. And you're taking away from their time to deal with their concerns in the group.

Jane: You know I wish you could replay some of the tapes and find out exacly how many times I did actually talk about John. How many sessions were actually devoted. . . .

Steve: I would say that you talked about John probably every session that we had.

Amanda: May I suggest this! We are all grown, and we all have tongues, and if we found it intolerable and suffered it, then it's nobody's fault but ours.

Steve: I think you are speaking for yourself. But some of the other members have come to me and talked to me about the problem, and they brought it up in the group . . . specifically Diana and Carol. And they brought it up in the group that they did want to see Jane commit herself to some action with John. And I had felt that it had gone real well.

Amanda: I think she has, don't you?

Steve: Well, I had thought so until we talked at lunch. Now I'm not sure.

Jane: Why? When you suggested that maybe you could talk to John and talk to both of us at the same time. . . . First of all, I happen to know John. I happen to know his reaction. For me to reveal to somebody else . . . particularly someone who is specialized in your field, that would indicate to John that I don't think that he recognizes that he's got emotional problems, which he would resent.

One can recognize the techniques utilized here in which the

therapist brings the group into a confrontation of the here-and-now dynamic. What was happening in the real world and what was happening in the group at this point were congruent.

Again, Amanda became the facilitator and the therapist took on the role of just another group member. Such a reversal of roles was conclusive evidence that the group had proceeded to a point at which it was no longer stilted and inhibited. Rather, it was now free flowing and spontaneous.

Amanda: Well, don't you feel, Jane, that you are sort of getting that under control now?

Jane: Oh, yes!

Amanda: Well, I think that's grand, and hang on to that positive aspect!

Jane: That's right. I have! I have! John was supposed to come to see me Friday or Saturday, and he never showed up. And I had given myself . . . I had told myself. "Now I'm giving him this opportunity. If he doesn't do it, I have a letter written which I mailed, and that's it." It was as simple as that.

Amanda: But you know it's. . . . When something's been so omnipresent for so long, it's awfully hard to just dismiss it, and the tendency sometimes is to sort of hash and rehash. I've run into that over at the cerebral palsy school. They've had some very unpleasant experiences over there; some changes in personnel at the administrative level which were not clean cut. A question of firing or forced to resign. And they just kept bringing up, "Well, so and so said". . . . And I finally said, "Now look, this is a new day. I never want to hear that woman's name repeated in my presence again because it's always a preface to something unpleasant. Forget it!" I know it's hard to forget things that have just colored your thinking for so long, but you just *have* to! And it seems to have worked. So maybe that's what we are saying. Try to put the bad part out of your mind and try to focus on the good things that are going to come out of it.

Jane: Yes. As a matter of fact, it was a relief to me, and it was very. . . . I was glad.

Amanda: Well, I think you've made that very clear. . . .

Jane: . . . that the group did say this to me and I think I expressed to everybody in the group because it brought
to a head what I must do. It activated me. It made me
realize many things. It made me realize that I couldn't
do this . . . keep dragging this thing interminably –
that there had to come a time when this had to be
concluded right away.

Diana: So what have you got to be upset about? I guess I
don't understand what you are upset about.

This series of excerpts represents a unique type of confrontation
that occurred in the group. It was both a confrontation of member
and member; confrontation of member and therapist; and a confrontation of dynamics in the group. As the dialogue progressed between Diana and Jane, the "waffling" of Diana (alluded to earlier)
came to represent avoidance of being more direct with Jane. Finally,
Diana verbalized that Jane was not *just* angry with the therapist, but
she was angry with Diana as well.

Diana: OK! When this whole thing started today, she [Jane]
was lashing out at me, not Steve.

Amanda: She was getting around to it.

Diana: She was looking at me and lashing out at me and saying, ". . . Are my problems not as important as yours?"

Jane: Do you know, I want to tell you something. Sometimes when you are upset about a situation. . . . I
could have looked at Amanda the same way.

Diana: No one asked if they wanted to listen to my problems; but it was asked if we wanted to listen to you.

Jane: And it wasn't that not only your problems. . . .

Diana: . . . And you couldn't have looked at Amanda and
said that because it was me!

Jane: . . . Not only your problems but anybody's problems
here. Not *only* yours! And I haven't singled you out.
And I understand your situation very well. And I'm
not the person that you think I am. I think I'm a
friend. And I would like to think so. But sometimes
well-meaning people don't always express them-

selves quite the right way. But if their intentions are good, sometimes I think there are certain things that can be overlooked.

Diana: I thought honesty was part of our makeup in this group. I thought we could say things here that we couldn't say elsewhere.

Amanda: I think we are getting an *overdose* of honesty today!

Jane: I think we have. I think I say a lot of things that I wouldn't elsewhere; so I think that has been accomplished. I don't think that that's an issue.

In what may have been one of the most important dialogues in the life of the group with regard to implications for technique, Amanda facilitated the confrontation between Diana and Jane. She discussed the subject of honesty and offered a critique of the use of honesty by the therapist. In what appeared to be a resolution of the confrontation, Jane responded to Amanda's efforts. Amanda shared that Jane had appeared to "work it through." It appeared that Jane, Diana, and the therapist had worked through a particularly natty issue. It was as though the textbook use of the focusing on the here-and-now in an existential approach to group psychotherapy had become manifest in reality.

Amanda: Maybe what we are really saying, Jane, is that if honesty is a part of it, then we have to simply steel ourselves to accept what that person who has made the statement thinks is honest, even though it may hurt a little bit. It may even be offensive. For instance, when I spoke to Steve about some of the language he was using, it was very offensive to me. And he could have said, "Well, if that's the way you feel about it, go on and get out of here." And we could have gotten into a real fight about it; but he apparently was sensitive *after* the fact. I think some day he's going to have to be sensitive *before* the fact. And so he accepted it. But it was quite critical. Quite derogatory really. But it was quite honest, and he accepted it. Now I'm sure he didn't think, "My she's a fine upstanding person." He may have had some moments of resentment; but he accepted it. And I think maybe that's what we are saying. When things are said in here that really kind of get your back up, you just have to say, "Wait a minute. We all have the right to be honest in here, and nobody is deliberately trying to be hurtful." And it may be kind of hard to hold onto sometimes. But isn't that essentially what we are saying?

Carol arrived late, shortly after this intense emotional confrontation. After bringing Carol up to date, the therapist redirected the group toward coping with Diana's feelings. It seemed that Diana was feeling as though she were being targeted as the focus of Jane's anger. The most interesting feature of this exchange, from a point of technique and group dynamics, was the fact that cancer patients have notoriously difficult times verbalizing and coping with anger.

Steve: I'm not going to try to bring you up on what's happened. It will just suffice to say that we have had a very emotional session this far, and it's been very confrontive. We are just trying to tie up and end. . . . So I feel a lot better about what's happened here today. I feel the group . . . particularly Diana and Jane . . . has had some angry expressions. But, we said how we felt. I'm a little concerned about how Diana's feeling.

Diana: I feel like I'd like to walk out and not ever come back.

Steve: That's what I thought.

Diana: You know this whole thing has just been tense!

Steve: Is that so bad?

Diana: No, we're not. . . . The one thing we are not going to do is focus on me!

Steve: Well, I don't think we are focusing on you. I think we are focusing on a group feeling because this is a feeling you have and you are part of the group. This does not necessarily have to do with anything outside. It has to do with what's happening in here. And frankly, I would hate to see you feel that way by the time we finish.

Amanda: Well, how much longer do we have? I hate to put a

	time limit on it.
Diana:	One more meeting!
Amanda:	No, I'm talking about today.
Steve:	Well, I mean today. I don't want you to go away feeling that way. I think Amanda senses Jane's pressure and is trying to get some kind of closure on working this thing through. I feel a concern for that too; but I still feel it's not completely finished because I don't think Diana's said everything she feels.
Diana:	Well, I just don't understand a lot of it. I don't understand. And I don't! It's fine!
Steve:	Could you share the confusion a little?
Diana:	No! . . . Well, I said from the beginning, I don't understand, or I can't comprehend Jane's problem even though I've listened to her. Maybe when she lashed out at me, I quit listening to her.
Steve:	She turned you off?
Diana:	Right! Maybe that's why I didn't understand what she said.
Jane:	When did I lash out at you?
Diana:	Oh! . . . Ohhhh . . . !
Steve:	Just in the last. . . . I'm being serious now. I'm not trying to be hurtful. In the last . . . even though you [Jane] may have been directing what you were saying to me, you were talking to Diana for the first fifteen minutes.
Jane:	Well, I didn't mean it, you see.
Diana:	Well, to not mean something, it sure seemed. . . .
Steve:	This is the confusing message that she's [Diana's] getting, I think. . . . I'm not sure. . . . Is that possible?
Jane:	. . . You see, when actually I didn't feel that way. See, I'm amazed! That's why I said to you! When did I lash out at you? Because I wasn't aware of it.
Diana:	OK!
Steve:	No! It's not OK!
Diana:	No, that's OK! Please don't!
Amanda:	*I'm OK, you're OK!*
Steve:	[to Diana] OK, I'll take the pressure off of you. But I'm feeling like some of your feelings. . . . I'm going

to try to verbalize. . . . And if they are wrong, you stop me. OK? There is one remark that is particularly triggering some of this confusion for Diana while the focus has been on her for the last two sessions . . . and I think it's a heck of a lot of pressure for her. It happened last week when Diana was dealing with how she's trying to meet her needs about her fear of death. At some point, with good intentions, you [Jane] entered into the discussion and said, "But Diana, there's hope! Look at me! You know, at my age." . . . And you started to compare. . . ." "And I had all these operations." . . . I think that was said in a helpful tone and with interest. And I feel what's happened is that Diana is turned off from that, because, first of all, it came across as motherly to her. Secondly, you weren't really listening to what she was saying. You were missing her feelings about it. And I think sometimes when that happens to me, I get turned off because I feel like the person is more preoccupied with what's going on with themselves than what's going on in me. And it makes me feel like they are trying to say that their values and how they cope is better. Like, if I were Diana I would begin to wonder, you know, if you were trying to teach me your values and how you cope instead of accepting her values and how she copes. And I think this is where part of the barrier's coming from.

Jane: Well, I'm very sorry if I'm giving that impression. I really am. Because this was not my intention.

Steve: . . . And I think what's difficult for her is to believe you when you say you are sorry. Because. . . .

Jane: I am! I'm genuinely sorry, because I would not have wanted to provoke this kind of situation. But when I said what I said, I sincerely meant it. I guess I am not as sensitive. . . .

Diana: Well, why did it upset you that the last two meetings have been focused on me? . . . which if I had to do it over again, I wish it hadn't been during the time. But let me finish. Why? You said that we didn't go around the room and ask, "Do you want to discuss Diana's problem again?" Yet, when this thing with John. . . . Somehow we said we don't want to hear any more until you do something positive about it. And you were saying to me . . . "Everybody listened to my problems!" And we didn't ask, "Does anyone want to?" But with you we asked if anyone wanted to. Why did that upset me?

Jane: It didn't upset me because it was your particular problem.

Diana: You just used me for an example!

Jane: It just happened that it was you. It could have been Sally. It could have been Carol. But the thing that was making me feel. . . . I was starting to feel that I was some kind of oddity, as if I felt that every time I tried to say something. . . . I was conscious of the fact that I was sixty-nine years old. And at sixty-nine I didn't have. . . . I wasn't to have any opinions. And everything I said could be misinterpreted, and I thought, "Maybe sixty-nine years old is when you ought to die."

Amanda: Jane, you know something? You are far more conscious of your age than anybody else is. Much more conscious of it.

Sally: What does age have to do with . . . ?

Amanda: It just never crosses my mind how old you are . . . How young you are. I really don't think about it. Because, for one thing, the first half of my life I was always the youngest one in the group. For awhile I was the oldest in the group. And then. . . . I'm going back to my childhood . . . I have a lot of sweet friends who are anywhere from ten to fifteen years older than I am. I never think about it.

Jane: You know why I thought about it, Amanda? Because every time I said something I felt as if I was regarded as a grandmother. I was a mother. . . .

Amanda: . . . I'm as much a grandmother as you are!

Jane: . . . that I wasn't regarded as a human being with certain ideas that I wanted to express. You know, you

don't always express it the right way. And, unfortunately, I wasn't expressing it the right way. And many
times some people here. . . . I don't know who they
were . . . would say, "Well, you don't realize that
you have lived so much longer." You see. And when
they would say you've lived so much longer, I started
to get a complex about it.

Amanda: Well, I think the feeling was very real to you. I don't
question that. But I must say I honestly don't think
you are justified in feeling that way. I don't think that
was in the back of anyone's head to say you are
about to die with old age; so don't talk to me. After
all I'm but eight years younger than you are. I'm sixty-
one; I'll be sixty-two in September.

Sally: Well, I'm in between both of you!

Jane: And you know, I never. . . . Really! Until I came into
this group. I didn't feel my age . . . wasn't even aware
of it. I never even talked about it. In fact, I lied about it
all the time.

Amanda: Well, you told us that. I really do think twenty years
younger was a little excessive that time.

Jane: Yeah, I know it was. But, as I said, I don't like to do
things in half measures.

Steve: Can I share a feeling that I've had . . . and I feel
you've [to Jane] been under a heck of a lot of pressure here today. I feel the climate's good for me to
say this. I don't know if it's anger or not. But sometimes when I hear you talk in the group . . . and this
has happened in a number of situations. . . . The
group's focus turns from whoever was dealing with
their concern back to Jane. And I've had the feeling
too . . . and you've told me a number of times how
good I was doing in the group and all that. . . . When
I was saying to you privately that I didn't need to hear
that . . . that I felt confident about who I am and
about what I was doing. . . . And sometimes I had the
feeling that it was either in your awareness or possibly that you are unaware that it was a manipulation
of the group to get back to you and John . . . or you

and your age . . . or you and your relationship with the disease. And I'm not saying that it was intentional; but I'm saying that's a feeling that I had.

Jane: Well, let me assure you it was not that at all, because if I wanted to talk about it, I would not have beaten about the bush. I would have come out and talked about it!

Steve: What did. . . ?

Jane: . . . talked about my disease or whatever it was that I wanted to talk about. I would not have beaten around the bush!

Steve: I guess you are not hearing what I'm saying. I felt that you did that; that you talked about your relationship to the disease, your feelings of yourself at your present age, and your relationship to your son, John; and that unconsciously or out of your awareness, whenever we started to deal with, say Carol, or Diana, or with Sally, particularly the people in the group who had something to share with the group. . . . When you had a chance to give feedback to them, you brought the subject back to you and your disease, or you and John, or you and your age. And I felt like it was an unconscious attempt on your part to manipulate the group back helping you.

Jane: I'm not worried about my disease! That's the funny part. And you keep telling me that I talked about it so much that I don't think about it. I have so much confidence in the oncology department that I never even worry about it.

Steve: I guess now I feel like I've hurt you again. I feel like you've taken what I've said as an accusation instead of concern.

Jane: No, I don't feel it's an accusation!

Steve: It's just an expression of how I feel.

Jane: I can just tell! And this is an expression of how I feel! I'm not worried about it because every time they've changed my medication, I've felt better; so I'm not worried about it. I know that Doctor Norris. . . . As he says . . . always has some trick up his sleeve. So I don't worry about it. I have all this confidence.

Steve: I guess I wasn't saying that you were worried about it. I don't remember using the word worry.

Jane: No, you didn't *I* was using it!

Steve: I think sharing about how you feel about your disease and how you feel about your relationship with your son and how you feel about your age would be more accurate than worried. At least the feeling . . . and again I'm not saying this as an accusation. . . .

Jane: You know how I feel right now? I feel so saturated with all of these three subjects that I never. . . . I'm never going to talk about my age unless I lie! And I'm never. . . . I don't want to talk about my son! I want to resolve that because that was one of the most constructive things that happened here. So that is a thing that I like talking about. Really! Until at lunch when I mentioned something there. But I would not have said anything. . . .

Steve: I'm not asking you to do that.

Jane: . . . And as far as my condition is concerned, I don't want to talk about that *either*! It's not the most pleasant subject. But nevertheless, it isn't anything that frightens me. But it doesn't make good conversation; so I'm not going to talk about it.

Carol: Well, it makes good conversation if you are speaking to someone who has the same problem. But if someone doesn't have that problem, they can't. . . .

Jane: But in this group even, *it* became excessive! See, even if a thing is valid, if you talk about it too much, it can become annoying; so evidently that's what I was doing.

Steve: I guess, Jane. . . . I guess what my feeling is that what you just said is pretty accurate because I think that's part of Diana's confusion and its been part of my confusion. . . . On the one hand you say you haven't been talking about a lot in the group, and on the other hand my feeling and my experience is that you have talked a lot about these things in the group. And I think that's where the discrepancy and the confusion is coming into being.

Jane: See, this could be. . . . See, a group like this is emotionally charged, and many times you say a lot of things that you don't even remember saying and that you don't say intentionally. And then when you hear it. . . . If I probably heard that played back, I might be horrified.

The ability to examine anger as a feeling was a real testimony to the beneficial aspects of this type of group. In the following excerpt one can see illustrated the fruition of efforts of the therapist through techniques of counseling and through an understanding of group process, particularly with regard to problems with cancer patients.

Jane: Hey! You know, I'll tell you one thing I can honestly say. This is a step ahead for me, and this is really constructive for me because in the past I would not have had the nerve to be honest with the group and to say exactly how I feel. I would have kept quiet. And this, I think, is a step ahead because I have been able to feel. And I really feel this is a loving group. I don't take offense. Actually . . . honestly . . . at what is being said. I think that we express what sounds like that may be sort of superficial and something that I can accept because I know how it's offered. I know that people here aren't malicious with their words. I think they are kind. But sometimes just as I don't say, "Well I feel and mean any words that should convey my emotion and my interest" . . . other people have the same right. I think basically there should be no malice. And for me, I've already forgotten about it.

Amanda: Now! You see, you have worked through it! You've come full circle!

Jane: But I felt that I wanted to show you all I wasn't sissy. And, as some of you said, tell the group. I was going to tell the group. I couldn't have in the past. Do you know what I would have done?

Amanda: Just not come back?

Jane: I would not have appeared!

Amanda:	Well, that's good!
Steve:	It must have taken a lot of courage for you to come here today.
Jane:	. . . I'll tell you it put steel rods in my back.
Steve:	A *lot* of pressure.
Jane:	It put steel in my back!
Amanda:	Jane, your backbone's going to be so strong by the time you get out of here.
Jane:	Yeah! I'll be an acrobat! An emotional acrobat!
Steve:	I hope we can help that a little bit . . . putting a little stability into that.
Jane:	I hope so. I know my frailties, my emotional frailties. I know them. But as I say, this is a step ahead for me because I never would have said it. And I did say it! I hope. . . . I tried to say it in the best way. But I know that I was a little abrasive in certain areas, and I apologize. But I've said my piece.

After becoming somewhat defensive, Jane recognized what she had been doing in the group. Thus, from a therapeutic standpoint, the techniques used facilitated Jane's awareness of not only how she came across in the group, but how she was interacting with people in the real world. Significantly, within several weeks after the group ended, Jane died. During the process of her death, she confided to another counselor that the group experience had been one of the most meaningful experiences during the course of her thirteen-year battle with cancer. It helped her put her relationships in perspective and gave her a new understanding of the possibility of human relationships. She was able to experience a sense of growth through the group process. Much of the confrontation that took place during this session was necessary to that growth.

Sociometry

Figure 9-3 illustrates the seating arrangement for session 9. Figure 9-4 illustrates the primary patterns of communication for session 9. During the main portion of this session, Amanda took upon herself the role of facilitator. It was her presence that affected good communication. Carol and Sally interacted minimally. The two-way

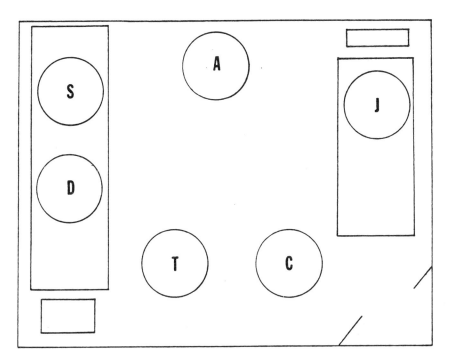

Figure 9-3. Session 9: Seating

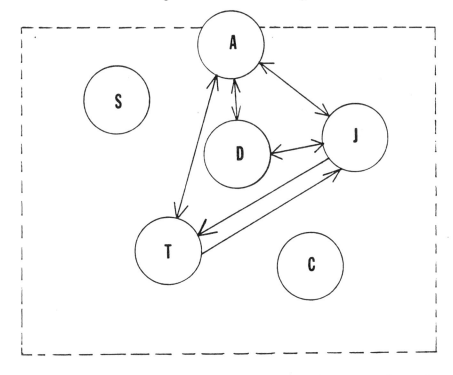

Figure 9-4. Session 9: Primary patterns of communication between members and members and therapist

arrows between the therapist and Jane signify one member confronting the other with the therapist in a member role during a particularly intense period of communication.

Journal

Our ninth session was a very confrontive one. Jane was upset with me and Diana. Jane, after session 8, was crying. As I comforted her, she said how good I was, how good the group was, etc. I told her that while I appreciated her good feedback (she does this often after each session), I didn't need such effusive praise. I felt good about myself and my skills. She was angry at me for this, and in the group she confronted me. She was angry at the group (particularly Diana) for not wanting to keep hearing about her problems with her son. I confronted her by saying that I, and perhaps the group, felt like she was manipulating the group's attention back to her. At any rate, we spent most of the session on that theme. I'm shaky about Jane. With only one session to go, I'm beginning to see the need to have more like twenty sessions versus ten. We are just now really getting into deeper action.

SESSION 10: TERMINATION PHASE

Termination was the main theme of the session. The beginning of the session involved discussion of medications and chemotherapy. This was the first session in some time during which the group members had focused on this theme. It represented an avoidance of termination. Attention was given to housekeeping chores such as completion of forms and tests for the research being conducted.

The object of this session was to give each of the members an opportunity to offer feedback to the group and to the leader. This was done in a structured fashion. Each person was offered the opportunity to speak if they so desired. There were several interesting aspects of the feedback. One aspect is exemplified in the following excerpt. It seemed that Jane had developed an awareness of her attempts to try to monopolize the group sessions. She had seen herself as the victim and was dissatisfied with being in that role. She thanked the group for helping her realize and internalize her new awareness.

Jane: I'm always the victim. You know what I was thinking as I imagined what would be a constructive remark? That when people have a tendency, as I have, to talk indeterminately, if there would be a period at which the leader could say or could introduce. . . . As a matter of fact, originally . . . "Now since our time is limited and since we have a certain number of people here and there may be some people who would like to ventilate their feelings as well, we must of necessity limit the time." . . . So that when I say to you, "Now . . . I'm talking to the person who is talking. . . . We have three minutes left, or five minutes left," that person can then wind up what they are saying.

Amanda: That's not a bad idea. In fact it's contrary to the whole premise of. . . .

Steve: I think what she's saying is. . . . She is saying, instead of confronting the person all of a sudden with awareness of domination in the group, that the leader should put a little more structure in and say, "OK. It is your turn to talk, and here's your limitation."

Jane: . . . And so I don't monopolize the whole session.

In addition to dealing with the spillover from session 9, Jane also gave some feedback regarding the entire group experience.

Jane: I got two very significant advantages. The first advantage I got was the feedback I got when I talked about my son so much. And the second thing that I really got . . . and after thinking about it . . . that I had a tendency to voice my opinion about how another person should feel. And I think that another person has the right to express anger . . . to express anything they want to express. If they want to tear the walls down, I think that that should be their prerogative. And I didn't recognize it until I gave a great deal of thought to it. And I thought particularly of Diana and how she must have felt when I said that, and I felt that she had a perfect right to be angry.

Steve: What I'm hearing you say is that in this group you felt

	OK about anger being expressed in the group . . . that you learned that it's possible to do that and still maintain relationships.
Jane:	Yes! Yes!

Diana shared some feedback about the group in the following excerpt. In the process of sharing, she expressed her anxieties about continuing in such a group for fear of having to confront others. Interestingly, Diana never was able to internalize the dissonance between her nonverbal expression of anger as being rage versus her verbal expression of anger, which was one of avoidance.

Diana:	But I don't think, since we all have something very vital in common, our very life. . . . I don't care what happens between any of us. I still feel like we've got a sisterhood, and we care about each other. I may never talk to Amanda or Sally and Jane again after today, but I'm going to think about them. And I'm going to. . . . I'm sure going to talk to Cindy and see how they are. You can't meet like we've met for ten sessions without caring about the other person. . . . Of course, I'm not right interested in going ahead with the group. But I had reservations, because maybe the way I've been brought up. . . . The atmosphere I'm accustomed to. I don't want to start sitting on Sally and tearing down what's inside . . . and somehow last week if you think that was good, *I* don't! I didn't enjoy it the day Jane was the focus of attention. I really had much regret about that. Maybe that's the way I was brought up; that you don't attack. In a sense you are attacking each other. I could never be comfortable in that situation.
Amanda:	I agree with you Diana. I was *extremely* uncomfortable!
Steve:	Maybe good or bad isn't a choice of words . . . a good choice of words. Maybe in the group process this is often *necessary*.

Notice Diana's verbalization of sisterhood. There was a feeling of closeness that could only be described as sister-like.

Interestingly, there was still spillover from session 9: the confrontation between Jane, Diana, and myself. Before offering her feedback to the group, Sally shared her reaction to the intensity. In response to Sally's remarks, during the same session, Amanda recalled feelings, which she had earlier described as uncomfortable. Again, one can see the manifestations of difficulties with confrontation and anger that seems to be a common thread in many adult cancer victims.

Sally: That upset me so last week that I lost my lunch.

Steve: Really?

Sally: When I got home, it was just churning on the inside. That's just the only way I know how to express it. It was so unpleasant to me. *You could cut that tension with a knife!* It was just like that.

Steve: That tense . . . ?

Sally: Oh, yes! It just tore at me so much. I don't know. I just feel like I have a problem with those things. Well, that's the way I react! But I did! *I lost my lunch,* and I could not eat my dinner that night because I still hadn't gotten over it. And it took me a long time to have a conversation with myself to try to get myself straightened out the best way I know how.

Amanda: Well, I didn't react quite that way; but I did find it very uncomfortable. I think it's good for people to open up to each other as far as they want to. I could not be as generous as you [to Jane]. I would resent it to the core of my being, and I would let you know about it. I mean, if we had had the same interaction as you and Diana had had, I couldn't. . . . I don't believe I could say, "Well, you were right, and I shouldn't have done that." I think you have a remarkable facility for that, Jane, and not many people have it. . . . To be very objective about your own attitude. . . .

Jane: I was able to divorce myself from the situation and say, "What was I doing? What precipitated this?" And I was very fair about it, I felt. I was doing something to her [Diana] which I don't really feel I had a right to do.

Diana: But I care about you, and I care about your feelings. And even though maybe I put words on them you didn't agree with, I felt the motherly instinct from you. I would not do anything to hurt you. And if that means I've got to suppress something in me, I'd rather suppress it in me than there to be a problem between you and I because I care about your feelings. I care about how you feel and how you feel when you leave this place. And I certainly don't want to be responsible for any problems you or Sally or anybody else might have.

Jane: Yeah! But I felt responsible for your feelings!

Amanda: You are responsible for each other!

Jane: I felt that!

Diana began to feel guilty about confronting Jane so vigorously at the previous session. In an effort to understand what had happened, she almost apologized for expressing her anger. Jane defended the group as being a special kind of group, one in which members could look at and examine in-depth their frailties, fears, and other personal difficulties in a safe setting.

Diana: I feel that we got in a position last week that was not natural . . . that we wouldn't have. . . . That wouldn't have happened under normal situations.

Amanda: No! I think Diana's right, and it may reflect the differences in priorities between a therapist and people who just live ordinary lives. To Steve the main thing is truth as he sees it. And to us . . . truth up to a point but not at the sacrifice of everything. And I agree with Diana. It may be the way we were brought up. And you [Steve] tease me a lot about being a tension breaker, but I cannot help it. I simply cannot help it. I think it is your duty to make people feel as comfortable as possible.

Jane: You see, but we are a special kind of group. . . .

Amanda: You see, I don't want to be in that kind of group.

Jane: . . . The purpose being that we can look at ourselves . . . look at our frailties, and so forth. And I feel that I have many that I want to make an effort to correct.

And I think if I correct them, my relationship with others improves . . . many things. . . . For everything you have to pay a price. All right! So it was said to me not in a vicious way. It wasn't said in a vicious way. I think the people here cared about me, and I think when I glean from it, it was very helpful because I was listening to what you were saying. And only if I listen to what you say can I correct what appears to be offensive. That's why I wasn't hurt. As a matter of fact, I was very grateful because then I could hear what I'm actually saying and doing. And if I want people to like me as much as I do, because I want very much for people to like me . . . I told you that . . . then I have to do certain things which are not irritating.

Several excerpts are noteworthy in and of themselves. Those regarding the purpose of the group itself and treatment are two subjects addressed in these excerpts. The first excerpt finds Amanda agreeing with Diana's contention that no one can solve all of her problems. In effect, what Diana said was that the group is only a faint spark of hope in the darkness of reality.

Diana: But I kind of look at our group as like a pie, and our whole life is a pie. And a little bitty one-sixteenth of an inch . . . here's the group and there's the whole rest of this big pie that. . . . No one in this group, you [Steve] included, are even remotely aware of my life. . . . So there's no way that you can take one-sixteenth of my life and try to solve all my problems.

Amanda: That assesses the whole situation!

Sally agreed with Diana's assertion about the pie. Her consent was followed by Amanda's succinct cynicism.

Sally: Feelings and all, you just can't put us in a bunch and say you belong in this bunch over here or in this category over there, because then when you get down to it, it's just like Diana says about the pie. It takes all of us to make the whole.

Amanda: We are part of all that's been before! That's the way it is!

As the group returned to task, Amanda shared one of the aware-
nesses that she had learned as a result of our group.

Amanda: Well, it seems to me that one of the good things that
all of us have gained, and it's true in my own
case. . . . You just don't talk about your aches. It just
bores the heck out of people or else it scares them to
death. And if it's your own family, they get all anxious and unhappy and worried. So it's kind of nice to
be able to talk to people very openly and matter of
fact. . . .

After some discussion initiated by Sally with regard to persons
wallowing in self-pity and after being encouraged by Diana to get
back to task, Sally offered her feedback.

Sally: Well, I just don't have too much to say. I mean I've
never been in a group like this. And I think the fact
that I've been in this one. . . . And I don't have too
much to say . . . is the fact that I'm sort of like
Amanda. I keep a lot inside of me. But I have enjoyed the group. And in another way. . . . I'll be
perfectly honest . . . I have not. Because many times
I felt real depressed when I left here. And last week,
as I've already said, I was real upset because it was
just a situation. . . . And I guess the best way to say it
is what I was sensing, and I didn't like it. And I
thought, "Well, you have to accept each individual
for what they are." They express themselves, and I
express myself. But if we express ourselves and if you
don't agree with our expression, that's fine. It's all
right with me. But don't get all in a tizzy over it and
get all angry and show that sort of feeling. Give the
other fellow the right to the way he thinks and the
way he believes because, as I've already said, there
are not two of us alike. But it did upset me, and that's
just the way it affected me. Then there have been
times when I've gone away and I have been depressed because I have a feeling for people, and you
feel helpless. I have at times when I left here. And I
thought, "Gee, I wish I had some facility or some

way to help somebody feel a little bit better," . . . say particularly when I think about Diana and how young she is and what she's facing. I think, "Well how would I feel in her situation?" I don't know because I'm not in it. But I would like very much to do something to help.

Notice that Sally also had ambivalence about the relative merits of the group. On the one hand she seemed to enjoy the sharing aspect of the group; on the other hand she seemed to have a very difficult time with the affect. Perhaps one of the implications here is that a supportive group may be much less threatening to larger numbers of cancer patients than a group directed at behavioral change and growth through overt therapeutic interaction.

Amanda tried to give Sally support, stating that she was a very important member of the group even though at times she had been quiet. During the process of support, Diana verbalized the anticipation of the loss of some meaningful experiences that occurred outside of the group in the form of informal discussions at lunches we would often enjoy preceding the group meetings.

Diana: But still, Steve . . . and I looked at you for lunch to-day . . . and last week you all met and ended up here. . . . I feel like we've gotten more feedback, more communications between each other when we sat and had lunch. You know . . . just sat and talked . . . you know, we opened up . . . you know, you talked about your feelings that maybe you didn't talk about in here, and I enjoyed that. I miss that even today.

The implication here is that if one is going to conduct a supportive or therapeutic group with cancer patients, some opportunity should be allowed for socialization in the form of a *coffee klatch* atmosphere. Much meaningful communication and group building seem to occur during such opportunities for interaction.

Finally, Amanda shared her feedback with the group. In spite of her resistance and ambivalence, Amanda felt that the group was a worthwhile experience. Diana, Sally, and Jane echoed similar feelings.

Amanda: My feedback is really what I said before . . . that the opportunity to talk about the fact that you have cancer and that sort of thing in a group that doesn't say, "Oh! Do you really feel all right?" and "Don't you think you ought to lie down?" . . . That kind of thing . . . It's very very helpful because I cannot do it any place else simply because it is socially unacceptable.

Diana: The way we were brought up!

Amanda: Right!

Sally: A lot of people are not interested!

Amanda: It's nice to get to know people. Although as Diana said, we may never see each other again.

Jane: When I first met Steve and we talked, that was precisely what I talked about: the power of the mind. I said I thought the mind was the focal point of the body and could control so much. And do you remember my telling you that? And I really felt that. And I felt that I had survived many situations only because I didn't become alarmed about it. I felt that my mind could discipline the situation.

Amanda: I don't want to rely on that entirely. I need a little spiritual help every so often . . . don't you say?

Sally: I do too!

Amanda: I don't know if the rest of you agree with Sally and me, but I think we are kind of in accord on that.

Just prior to the end of this feedback and the dissolution of the group session toward chitchat regarding research, housekeeping, and so on, Jane offered a remark that was both moving and telling in terms of the group experience.

Jane: But probably, you see, each person decides for himself what technique he wants to employ in a situation, and to me that was always the way I felt about it. I felt that with the strength of our minds . . . the determination . . . that I would not disturb many functions in my body, that what I would do would actually contribute to the healing process.

Technique

The basic technique applied during the termination phase of the

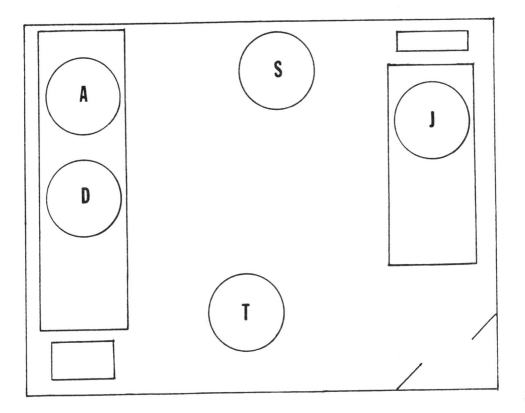

Figure 9-5. Session 10: Seating

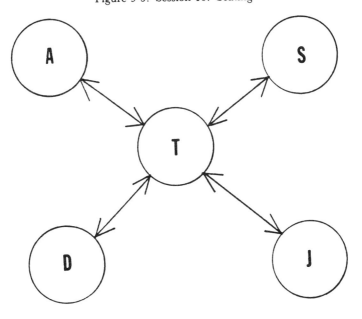

Figure 9-6. Session 10: Primary patterns of communication between members and therapist

group involved facilitation. Facilitation coupled with clarification enabled the group to deal with the emotions and thoughts relating to ending the group without encouraging the development of new subject material.

Sociometry

Because of her illness, Carol was not present during this session. Figure 9-5 illustrates the seating arrangement during session 10. It is noteworthy that Amanda chose to sit on the couch next to Diana. This symbolism suggests that Amanda had really felt a part of the group and felt supportive of Diana at its termination.

Figure 9-6 illustrates the primary patterns of communication during session 10. It was a pattern in which two-way communication between therapist and group members was pronounced, with little direct communication between each respective member. The session was somewhat structured and directive.

Journal

We had our tenth session yesterday. Carol could not attend because she wasn't feeling well. The other week the doctors found that she was a diabetic. Who would think that we would be happy that someone would have diabetes? We thought she was dying. Diabetes was after all treatable.

Jane wrote a letter to her son, finally. She looked pretty good. Amanda is feeling the effects of chemotherapy and showed us a more mellow, vulnerable side.

Diana has a "clean bill of health;" she's in remission. Sally threw up after last week's session and couldn't eat dinner for the same reason. She could not handle the pressure and the tension of the confrontation between Jane, Diana, and myself. I think that Sally, Jane, and Carol will be back for follow-up beginning March 16. Diana may attend occasionally if the group continues.

All in all, the group was successful and very meaningful to me. Diana, Amanda, and Sally expressed their wish that people should suppress their feelings and honesty in deference to others. Feelings should be controlled etc. Jane disagreed. The literature points to a cancer-prone personality as one in which feelings are suppressed and maintaining meaningful relationships is difficult.

So teach us to number our days
That we may get us a heart of wisdom.
Psalm 90:12

SUGGESTED READINGS

SECTION I

Chapter 1

Feifel, Herman: Death-relevant variable in psychology. In May, Rollo (Ed.): *Existential Psychology*, 2nd ed. New York, Random House, 1969.

Gengerelli, J., and Kirkner, F. (Eds.): *Psychological Variables in Human Cancer.* Berkeley, University of California Press, 1954.

Holland, James: Psychological aspects of cancer. In Holland, James, and Frei, Emil (Eds.): *Cancer Medicine.* Philadelphia, Lea and Febiger, 1973, pp. 991-1021.

Kastenbaum, Robert, and Aisenberg, Ruth: *The Psychology of Death.* New York, Springer Publishing Co., Inc., 1976.

Kubler-Ross, Elisabeth: Dying as a human psychological event. *Concilium: Theology in the Age of Renewal, 4,* 1974.

McCoy, John Warton: *Psychological Variables and Onset of Cancer.* Unpublished doctoral dissertation, Oklahoma State University, 1976.

Richmond, Julius B., and Weisman, Harry A.: Psychological aspects of management of children with malignant diseases. *Am J Dis Child, 89*: 42-47, 1955.

Rothenberg, Albert: Psychological problems in terminal cancer management. *Cancer, 14*:1063-1073, 1961.

Ryan, Eleanore A.: *The Psychological Aspects of Breast Cancer and Mastectomy.* Unpublished doctoral dissertation, Northwestern University, 1978.

Schuly, Richard: *The Psychology of Death, Dying, and Bereavement.* Reading, MA, Addison-Wesley, 1978.

Shands, Harley C.: Psychological mechanisms in cancer patients. *Cancer, 4*: 1159-1170, 1951.

Stehlin, John S., and Beach, Kenneth H.: Psychological aspects of cancer therapy: A surgeon's viewpoint. *JAMA, 197*:100-104, 1966.

Sutherland, Arthur M.: Psychological impact of cancer and its therapy. *Med Clin North Am, 40*:705, 1956.

Chapter 2

Feifel, Herman: Attitudes toward death in some normal and mentally ill populations. In Feifel, Herman (Ed.): *The Meaning of Death.* New York, McGraw-Hill, 1959.

Feifel, Herman: The taboo of death. *Am Behav Sci, 6*:66, 1963.

Garfield, Charles: *Psychosocial Care of the Dying Patient.* New York, McGraw-Hill, 1978.

Glaser, Barney G., and Strauss, Auselm L.: The social loss of dying patients. *Am*

*J Nurs, 64:*119-121, 1964.

Gordon, W., Freidenberg, I., Diller, L., Rothman, L., Wolf, C., Ruckdeschel-Hibbard, M., Ezrachi, O., and Gerstman, L.: *The Psychosocial Problems of Cancer Patients: A Retrospective Study.* Paper presented at American Psychological Association meeting, San Francisco, September 1977.

Jamison, Kay, Wellisch, David K., and Pasnau, Robert O.: Psychosocial aspects of mastectomy: The women's perspective. *Am J Psychiatry, 135:*432-436, 1978.

Lewis, Franses M., and Bloom, Joan R.: Psychosocial adjustment to breast cancer. A review of selected literature. *Int J Psychiatry Med, 9:*1-17, 1978-79.

Schoenberg, Bernard, Carr, Arthur C., Peretz, David, and Kutscher, Austin H.: *Psychosocial Aspects of Terminal Care.* New York, Columbia University Press, 1972.

Silberfarb, Peter M., Haurer, L. Herbert, and Crouthamel, Carol S.: Psychosocial aspects of neoplastic disease: functional status of breast cancer patients during different treatment regimens. *Am J Psychol, 137:*450-455, 1980.

Sudnow, David: *Passing On: The Social Organization of Dying.* Englewood Cliffs, NJ, Prentice-Hall, 1967.

Weisman, Avery D.: Psychosocial death. *Psychol Today, 6:*77-78, 1972.

Wortman, Camille B., and Dunkel-Schetter, Christine: Interpersonal relationships and cancer: A theoretical analysis. *J Soc Issues, 35,* 1979.

Chapter 3

Borstein, Irving J., and Klein, Annette: Parents of fatally ill children in a parents group. In Schoenberg, Bernard, et al.: *Anticipatory Grief.* New York, Columbia University Press, 1974, pp. 164-170.

Desmond, Helen Anne: *The Psychological Impact of Childhood Cancer on the Family.* Unpublished doctoral dissertation, California School of Professional Psychology, 1977.

Doyle, Nancy: *The Dying Person and the Family.* New York, Public Affairs Committee, 1972.

Evans, Jocelyn: *Living with a Man Who Is Dying.* New York, Taplinger, 1971.

Friedman, S. B. et al.: Behavioral observations on parents anticipating the death of a child. *Pediatrics, 32:*610-625, 1963.

Gyulay, Jo-Eileen, and Miles, Margaret S.: The family with the terminally ill child. In Hymovich, Debra, and Bernard, Martha U.: *Family Health Care.* New York, McGraw-Hill, 1973, pp. 438-457.

Krant, Melvin J., Doster, Nancy J., and Ploof, Susan: Meeting the needs of the late-stage elderly cancer patient and family: A clinical model. *J Geriatr Psychiatry, 13:*53-61, 1980.

Krieger, George W., and Bascue, Laurence O.: Terminal illness: Counseling with a family perspective. *Fam Coord, 24:*351, 1975.

Kubler-Ross, Elisabeth: Crisis management of dying persons and their families. In Resnick, H.L.P., and Ruben, H.L. (Eds.): *Emergency Psychiatric Care: The Management of Mental Health Crises.* New York, Charles Press, 1974, pp. 143-156.

McNutt: An experience of a therapeutic family reunion. *Transnational Ment Health Res Letter, 20*:1-8, 1978.

Pincus, Lily. *Death and the Family: The Importance of Mourning.* New York, Vintage Books, 1976.

Prichard, Elizabeth R., and Collard, Jean: *Social Work With the Dying Patient and the Family.* New York, Columbia University Press, 1977.

Schnaper, Nathan, et al.: *Management of the Dying Patient and His Family.* New York, Mss Information Corp., 1974.

Schoenberg, Bernard, et al: *Anticipatory Grief.* New York, Columbia University Press, 1974.

Verwoerdt, Adriaan: Death and the family. *Med Opinion Rev, 1*:38-43, 1966.

Walker, Cynthia: *Effects of Group Psychotherapy on Bereavement with Spouses of Dying Cancer Patients.* Unpublished doctoral dissertation, California School of Professional Psychology, 1977.

Wiener, Jerry M.: Reaction of the family to the fatal illness of a child. In Schoenberg, Bernard, et al.: *Loss and Grief: Psychological Management in Medical Practice.* New York, Columbia University Press, 1970, pp. 87-100.

Witkin, Mildred H., and Whitney, Payne: Helping husbands adjust to their wives mastectomies. *Med Aspects Hum Sex* pp. 93-94, October 1978.

Chapter 4

Becker, Ernest: *The Denial of Death.* New York, Free Press, 1973.

Feifel, Herman (Ed.): *New Meanings for Death.* New York, McGraw-Hill, 1977.

Feifel, Herman (Ed.): *The Meaning of Death.* New York, McGraw-Hill, 1959.

Feinberg, M., Feinberg, G., and Tarrant, J.: *Leavetaking.* New York, Simon and Schuster, 1978.

Henderson, Stephen R.: *Facing Life Through Death.* Staunton, VA, Counseling Services Associates, 1976.

Kavanaugh, Robert E.: *Facing Death.* Baltimore, Penguin, 1972.

Keleman, Stanley: *Living Your Dying.* New York, Random House, 1974.

Krant, Melvin J.: *Dying and Dignity: The Meaning and Control of a Personal Death.* Springfield, Thomas, 1974.

Kubler-Ross, Elisabeth: *Death, the Final Stage of Growth.* Englewood Cliffs, NJ, Prentice-Hall, 1975.

Kubler-Ross, Elisabeth: *On Death and Dying.* New York, Macmillan, 1969.

Kubler-Ross, Elisabeth: *Questions and Answers on Death and Dying.* New York, Macmillan, 1974.

Schneidman, Edwin S.: Aspects of the dying process. *Psychiatr Ann, 7*:391-397, 1977.

Weisman, Avery D.: *On Dying and Denying: A Psychiatric Study of Terminality.* New York, Behavioral Pubn's Inc., 1972.

Death and Dying: Attitudes of Patient and Doctor. New York, Group for the Advancement of Psychiatry, 1965 (no author).

Chapter 5

Achterberg, J., Matthews, S., and Simonton, O.C.: Psychology of the exceptional cancer patient: A description of patients who outlive predicted life expectancies. *Psychother: Theor, Res, Practice, 14*, 1978.

Greenberg, M.S.: *Patient Reported Disturbances in Hospital Treatment of Cancer Patients as Elicited by the Critical Incident Technique.* Unpublished master thesis, University of Houston, 1961.

Hotchkiss, S.: After mastectomy. *Hum Behav, 5*:40-41, 1976.

Jones, William H.: Loss in a hospital setting: Implications for counseling. *Pers Guid J, 59*:359-362, 1981..

Katz, Ernest R., Kellerman, Jonathan, and Siegel, Stuart E.: Behavioral distress in children with cancer undergoing medical procedures: developmental considerations. *J Consult Clin Psychol, 48*:356-365, 1980.

Kerr, M.: Emotional factors in the onset and course of cancer. In Sagar, R.R. (Ed.): *Georgetown Family Symposia, 4*, 1979.

Neff, Essie: *Children with Leukemia: A Study of Certain Emotional Responses Related to Their Treatment.* Unpublished doctoral dissertation, California School of Professional Psychology, 1978.

Nerenz, David Ross: *Control of Emotional Distress in Cancer Chemotherapy.* Unpublished doctoral dissertation, University of Wisconsin, Madison, 1979.

Peterson, Linda G., and Popkin, Michael K.: Neuropsychiatric effects of chemotherapeutic agents in cancer. *Psychosom, 21*:141-153, 1980.

Rosenbaum, Ernest H.: *Living with Cancer.* New York, Praeger, 1975.

Silberfarb, Peter M., et al.: Psychosocial aspects of neoplastic disease: affective and cognitive effects of chemotherapy in cancer patients. *Am J Psychol, 137*:597-601, 1980.

SECTION II

Chapters 6, 7, 8, and 9

Abraham, Ada: Death and Psychodrama. *Group Psychotherapy and Psychodrama, 25*: 84-92, 1972.

Bascue, Laurence, and Krieger, George: Death as a counseling concern. *Pers Guid J, 52*:587, 1974.

Bascue, Laurence, and Krieger, George: Existential counseling for the dying. *J Rehab, 38*:18, 1972.

Blake, Susan, and Paulsen, Karen: Therapeutic intervention with terminally ill children: A review. *Professional Psychol, 12*:655-663, 1981.

Franzic, M.A., Geren, J.J., and Meiman, G.L.: Group discussion among the terminally ill. *Int J Group Psychother, 26*:43-48, 1976.

Hora, Thomas: Existential psychiatry and group psychotherapy. In Gazda, George M. (Ed.): *Basic Approaches to Group Psychotherapy and Group Counseling*, 2nd ed.

Springfield, Thomas, 1975.

Kaufmann, W.: Existentialism and death. In Feifel, Herman (Ed.): *The Meaning of Death*. New York, McGraw-Hill, 1959.

Keeling, Wayne: Live the pain, learn the hope: A beginner's guide to cancer counseling. *Pers Guid J, 54*:502, 1976.

Koestenbaum, Peter: *The Vitality of Death; Essays in Existential Psychology and Philosophy*. Westport, Greenwood, 1971.

LeShan, Laurence, and LeShan, Eda: Psychotherapy and the patient with a limited life span. *Psychiatry, 24*:318, 1961.

Lindenberg, Steven P.: *The Effects of an Existential-Type of Group Psychotherapy on a Time-Limited Group of Members for Whom the Imminence of Death Is a Pressing Reality*. Unpublished doctoral dissertation, University of Georgia, 1977

May, Rollo (Ed.): *Existential Psychology*, 2nd ed. New York, Random House, 1960.

Pervin, Lawrence A.: Existentialism, psychology and psychotherapy. *Am Psychol, 15*:305-309, 1960..

Spiegel, David: Psychological support for women with metastatic carcinoma. *Psychosomatics, 20*:780-787, 1979.

Spiegel, David, and Yalom, Irvin D.: A support group for dying patients. *Int J Group Psychother, 28*:233-245, 1978.

Spiegel, David, Bloom, Joan R., and Yalom, Irvin: Group support for patients with metastic cancer: A randomized prospective outcome study. *Arch Gen Psychiatry, 38*:527-533, 1981.

Squire, Morris: Death, dying and hard-time therapy. *Int J Soc Psychiatry, 23*:5-7, 1977.

Yalom, Irvin D., and Greaves, Carlos: Group therapy with the terminally ill. *Am J Psychiatry, 134*:396-400, 1977.

Zuehlke, Terry E., and Watkins, John T.: Use of psychotherapy with dying patients — an exploratory study. *J Clin Psychol, 31*:729-732, 1975.